Contexts of
NURSING
An introduction

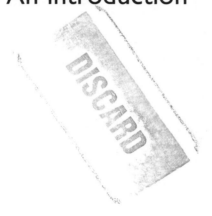

Contexts of
NURSING
An introduction

Edited by
John Daly
Sandra Speedy
Debra Jackson

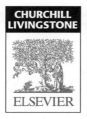

Sydney Edinburgh London New York Philadelphia St Louis Toronto

Churchill Livingstone
is an imprint of Elsevier

Elsevier Australia. ACN 001 002 357
(a division of Reed International Books Australia Pty Ltd)
Tower 1, 475 Victoria Avenue, Chatswood, NSW 2067

This edition © 2014 Elsevier Australia. Reprinted 2014.

3rd edition 2010; 2nd edition 2006; 1st edition 2000

eISNB: 9780729581523

National Library of Australia Cataloguing-in-Publication Data

Contexts of nursing / edited by John Daly, Sandra Speedy, Debra Jackson.

4th edition.
9780729541527 (paperback)
Includes bibliographical references and index.

Nursing—Australia.
Nursing—Social aspects—Australia.
Nursing—Study and teaching—Australia.
Nursing ethics.
Medical care—Australia.

Daly, John, 1958.
Speedy, Sandra.
Jackson, Debra, 1959.

610.730994

Senior Content Strategist: Libby Houston
Content Development Specialists: Liz Coady and Vicky Spichopoulos
Project Managers: Martina Vascotto and Rochelle Deighton
Edited by Jo Crichton
Proofread by Tim Learner
Picture research by Sarah Thomas
Cover design by Trina McDonald and Lisa Petroff
Internal design by Lisa Petroff
Index by Robert Swanson
Typeset by Midlands Typesetters
Printed in China

CONTENTS

CONTRIBUTORS

Alan Barnard RN, PhD
Senior Lecturer, School of Nursing, Queensland University of Technology, Queensland

Jen Bichel-Findlay HScD, MN, MPH, FACN, FACHI, AFCHSM
Director of Studies, Health Services Management, Faculty of Health, University of Technology Sydney, NSW

Sally Borbasi PhD, RN
Associate Dean Teaching & Learning, Professor of Nursing, Faculty of Health Sciences, Australian Catholic University, Queensland

Esther Chang RN, CM, DNE, BAppSc (Adv Nur), MEdAdmin, PhD
Professor of Nursing, School of Nursing and Midwifery, University of Western Sydney, NSW

Jane Conway RN, BHlthSc, BNurs (Hons 1), Grad Cert HRM, DEd
Conjoint Associate Professor, School of Nursing and Midwifery, Faculty of Health and Medicine, The University of Newcastle, NSW

Greta G Cummings RN, PhD, FCAHS
Centennial Professor, Faculty of Nursing, University of Alberta, Edmonton, Canada

John Daly RN, PhD, FACN, FAAN
Dean and Professor of Nursing, Faculty of Health, University of Technology, Sydney, NSW

Philip Darbyshire RNMH, RSCN, DipN (Lond), RNT, MN, PhD
Professor of Nursing, Monash University, Victoria and Flinders University, South Australia

Christine Davey RN, RM, Grad Cert RHP, Grad Cert PSM, MNP
Clinical Manager, Midwifery Services, West Coast Health Board, New Zealand

Patricia M Davidson RN, BA, MEd, PhD, FACN, FAHA, FPCNA, FAAN
Dean and Professor of Nursing, School of Nursing, John Hopkins University, Baltimore, MD, USA

Cathy Doran MHSc (Health Informatics), MSc (Health Policy and Management), RN, FACHI, AFCHSM
Senior Business Analyst, Justice Health and Forensic Health Network, NSW

Leah East RN, BN (Hons), PhD
Senior Lecturer, Southern Cross University, School of Health & Human Sciences, NSW

Doug Elliott RN, PhD
Professor of Nursing, Faculty of Health University of Technology, Sydney, NSW

Jean Gilmour RN, PhD
Senior Lecturer, School of Nursing, Massey University, New Zealand

Madonna Grehan RN, RM, Gr Dip Hlth Eth, PhD
Honorary Fellow, Nursing, School of Health Sciences, The University of Melbourne, Victoria

Amanda Henderson RN, RM, BSc, GradDipNurs (Ed), MScSoc, PhD
Nursing Director (Education), Princess Alexandra Hospital, Woolloongabba, Professor, School of Nursing and Midwifery, Griffith Health, Griffith University, Queensland

Anne Hofmeyer RN, PhD, MACN
Senior Lecturer, School of Nursing and Midwifery, University of South Australia, South Australia

Vicki Holliday RN, GradDip Indigenous Health Studies, MA (Indigenous Health Studies), GradCert in Educational Studies (Higher Education)
Lecturer, School of Medicine and Public Health, Discipline of Indigenous Health, University of Newcastle, NSW

Colin A Holmes PhD, MPhil, BA (Hons), TCert, Adjunct Professor
School of Nursing, Midwifery & Nutrition, James Cook University, Queensland

Annette Huntington BN, PhD, FCNA (NZ)
Associate Professor & Head of School, School of Nursing, Massey University, New Zealand

Marie Hutchinson RN, PhD
Associate Professor, School of Health and Human Sciences, Southern Cross University, Lismore, NSW, Australia

Debra Jackson RN, PhD
Professor of Nursing, Faculty of Health, University of Technology, Sydney (UTS), NSW

Megan-Jane Johnstone PhD, BA, RN, FACN
Professor of Nursing/Director, Centre for Quality and Patient Safety Research, Deakin University, Victoria

Margaret McMillan RN, BA, DNE, PhD, Grad Cert Management
Conjoint Professor, School of Nursing and Midwifery, University of Newcastle, NSW

Anne McMurray AM, RN, PhD, FACN
Emeritus Professor, School of Nursing & Midwifery, Adjunct Professor, Research Centre for Health Practice Innovation, Griffith University, Queensland
Emeritus Professor, School of Nursing and Midwifery, Murdoch University, Western Australia

Judith Mair PhD, LLB, DNE (NSW Coll Nsg)
Formerly Senior Lecturer, The University of Sydney

Jane Mills PhD, RN, BN, MN, MEd, GradCertEd, FACN
Associate Professor, Faculty of Health Science, School of Nursing, Midwifery and Nutrition, James Cook University, Queensland

Judith Parker AM, RN, BA Hons, PhD, MD (Hon Causa)
Emeritus Professor, The University of Melbourne, Victoria

Steve Parker RN, DipT (Nurse Ed), BEd, PhD
Associate Dean (Teaching & Learning), School of Nursing & Midwifery, Flinders University, South Australia

Siriorn Sindhu DNSc, MS, BEd, RN
Department of Surgical Nursing, Faculty of Nursing, Mahidol University,
Thailand
Isabelle Skinner RN, RM, MPH&TM, MBA, PhD
Professor of Nursing: Rural and Regional Practice Development, University
of Tasmania/Department of Health and Human Services, Tasmania
Sandra Speedy RN, BA (Hons), DipEd, MURP, EdD
Emeritus Professor, Southern Cross University, Lismore, NSW
Kim Usher PhD, DipNEd, BA, MNSt, FACN, FACMHN
Head School of Health, University of New England, NSW
Roianne West PhD, MMHN, RN, BN
Expert Advisor and Professor for Indigenous Health
Townsville Hospital and Health Service and Griffith University, Queensland
Sarah Winch RN, BA (Hons 1), PhD (Q), Centaur Fellow
Senior Lecturer Health Care Ethics, School of Medicine, The University of
Queensland, Queensland

REVIEWERS

Anita Bamford-Wade DNurs, MA, Dip Bus, RN
Senior Lecturer, Faculty of Health and Environmental Sciences, Auckland University of Technology, Auckland
Simulation Australia: Deputy Chair Learning and Development and Human Factors Committee
Australian Society for Simulation in Healthcare
New Zealand Association for Simulation in Healthcare
Nurses for a Smoke free Aotearoa New Zealand, Steering Committee

Murray Bardwell DipAppSc, BN, MnSt (Flinders)
Mental Health Clinician
Perinatal Mental Health Services St John of God Healthcare
Credentialed Mental Health Nurse

Sue Floyd RN, BN, MN, MCNA(NZ)
Nursing Practicum Manager Eastern Institute of Technology, Taradale, New Zealand

Karen Jackson MSc, PGDip Adult Ed, RN, CN
Lecturer, Deakin University, Geelong

Helen Kelly BN (Hon), Grad Cert Cardiac Nursing, Grad Cert University Teaching, MACN
Lecturer, School of Nursing, The University of Notre Dame, Sydney, Australia

Annabel Matheson RN, BNurs (Hon 1), PhD (in progress)
Lecturer, School of Nursing, Midwifery & Indigenous Health, Charles Sturt University, Bathurst, NSW

Md Nadim Rahman MBBS, AMC (Primary Assessment), PGT (General Practice), RN, BN, GCHPE
Lecturer, Faculty of Medicine, Nursing and Health Sciences, Monash University, Melbourne, VIC, Australia

Marilyn Richardson PhD, MEdStud, BAppSc (AdvNsg), CertClinTech (UK), CertAnaesth(UK), CertOR Tech&Man, RN, RCNT (UK)
Senior Lecturer, College of Health and Biomedicine, Victoria University

Natashia Scully BA, BN, PGDipNSc, MPH, PhD (candidate), MACN
Lecturer in Nursing, University of New England, Armidale, NSW, Australia

Lynn Thompson RN (Div 1), RM, MEdLead, DipTeach (Nursing), ChildFamilyHealthCert
Lecturer, School of Nursing, University Notre Dame, Sydney, Australia

Bev Turnbull RN, RM, PhD, FACON
Senior Lecturer, Charles Darwin University, NT, Australia

Lisa Wirihana BN, RM, MN
Lecturer, School of Nursing, Queensland University of Technology, Brisbane, QLD, Australia

PREFACE

Welcome to the fourth edition of *Contexts of Nursing*! As with the previous editions, this volume introduces students to the theory, language and scholarship of nursing and healthcare. Since we prepared the first edition, our major objective has been (and remains) to provide a comprehensive coverage of key ideas underpinning the practice of contemporary nursing. This book is a collection of views and voices; consequently, the chapters are not all identical in nature. This reflects our position that it is important that students/readers engage with various (and sometimes conflicting) views to challenge and extend them. This will hold them in good stead for the future, as the discipline and profession of nursing continues to evolve, mature and develop within Australia and New Zealand and globally.

We have specifically sought out a range of contributors who not only reflect the dynamic nature of nursing scholarship in Australia and New Zealand, but who are helping to shape contemporary nursing in this part of the world. These scholars have been chosen not only because of their expert knowledge, but also because of their professional standing, leadership and the sometimes controversial stances they take on various contemporary issues. We have not sought to silence the controversies or quieten the debates; rather, we present them to you, the reader, as a stimulus for reflection, discussion and debate and as a catalyst to further develop your own positions on various issues.

We have explained previously why the notion of 'contexts' has appeal for us in conceptualising nursing knowledge as a fabric composed of theoretical threads. This 'knowledge-as-fabric' metaphor provides access to a number of other related ideas, such as weaving and tapestry. Some new threads have been woven into the fabric of nursing knowledge presented in this work. Selection of these topics was based on extensive consultation with nurses who found previous editions useful in undergraduate and graduate courses and in their educational development and practice. Of course student evaluations of the previous issues were also considered. In addition, a number of experienced nurse authors and editors provided useful critique and feedback, which has helped us in shaping this new volume. We hope that the new contexts and topics we have included in this edition will make the book truly comprehensive and contemporary.

Though we have updated and added new content to this edition of *Contexts of Nursing*, it is based on the same aims and objectives that underpinned the design and development of the first edition of the work. Nursing knowledge and its foundational elements are explored and considered in relation to professional nursing practice and the context of healthcare. Our emphasis on pedagogic strength and accessibility, and the use of reflective questions and exercises to stimulate critical thinking and learning, has been maintained.

The editors acknowledge Elizabeth Coady, Libby Houston, Martina Vascotto, Jo Crichton, and the entire team at Elsevier, for their ongoing enthusiasm, encouragement, support and assistance in the preparation and production of this new edition.

Most of all, we thank our contributors, who have risen again to the challenge of developing engaging, scholarly and learning- and teaching-oriented work to stimulate reflection, discussion and debate.

John Daly
Sandra Speedy
Debra Jackson

Sydney, July 2013

CHAPTER 1

Presenting nursing ...
a career for life

John Daly, Debra Jackson and Sandra Speedy

LEARNING OBJECTIVES

By reading and reflecting on this chapter, readers will be able to:

- list some of the myths, legends and stereotypes that surround nursing
- arrive at a personal beginning definition of nursing
- establish their passion for nursing
- discuss some of the choices that a nursing degree offers for graduates
- describe the meaning of the term 'professional conduct'.

KEY WORDS

Nursing, stereotypes, critical perspective, career codes of conduct, lifelong learning

WHY NURSING?

Nursing is a unique and wonderful career choice. It is a curious mix of technology and myth, of science and art, of reality and romance. It blends the concrete and the abstract. It combines thinking and doing, 'being with' and 'doing for'. Nurses have privileged access to people's homes and share some of the most precious and highly intimate moments in people's lives—moments that remain hidden from most other people and professions. Nurses witness birth and death, and just about everything in between. Nurses share in people's most difficult moments of suffering and pain, and also bear witness to times of great joy and happiness. Because of the special place in society that nurses hold, nurses enjoy a high level of community trust. Indeed, in Australia and New Zealand, nurses continually rank very highly in surveys of public confidence.

Nursing can be a career for life. A degree in nursing provides a foundation for lifelong learning. It is the entry requirement to a fulfilling career, to a range of post-graduate courses in areas as diverse as paediatrics, midwifery, cancer care, community nursing, women's health, nurse education and nursing research. Age and experience are valued in nursing. Unlike many other professions and career choices in which people experience increasing difficulty in obtaining work as they get older, nurses can remain productively employed until retirement, and even post-retirement. Career interruption because of family responsibilities (or other reasons) can be extremely disadvantaging in some professions, but many nurses have effectively blended very successful careers with raising families. Nursing opens many doors. Internationally, Australian and New Zealand registered nurses are well respected and are able to gain registration in many other countries.

In this opening chapter, we aim to share what captured us and created our passion and enthusiasm for the wonderful career that is nursing—the passion and enthusiasm that has sustained and carried us successfully through our nursing careers. We also describe the different types and levels of nurse in Australia and New Zealand, and aim to introduce you to some of the ideas of interest to nurses and nursing, many of which are discussed in more detail in subsequent chapters of this book.

REFLECTION

What are the main reasons you have chosen a career in nursing?

NURSING: MYTHS, LEGENDS AND STEREOTYPES

Perhaps more than any other professional group, nursing and nurses are the subject of myth and popular belief; there are also many romantic connotations. Certain of these myths and beliefs are almost folkloric, yet they strongly influence the ways in which nurses are perceived by the general public, and also in the ways that nurses see themselves. Through the media, nursing is often portrayed as a dramatic, exciting, glamorous and romantic activity, with nurses frequently represented in the role of handmaiden/helper to medical doctors.

Several of the almost legendary attributes that surround nursing are derived from myths about Florence Nightingale and her work in the Crimean War. For example, the romantic notion of the 'angel of mercy', the quiet, modest and self-effacing woman who, with a religious-like fervour, would tirelessly and uncomplainingly nurse the ill and injured back to full strength, and the image of the 'lady with the lamp' fearlessly working at the frontline of a war zone, and instilling calm, peace and tranquillity where only chaos and suffering had reigned, have become enduring and mythologised popular images of the nurse (Bostridge 2008).

Because of her continued allure, much of Nightingale's life has been reconstructed and, in the process, subject to various forms of poetic licence. An excellent example of this poetic licence is explored by Jones (1988) in her critical examination of *The White Angel*, a motion picture released in 1936, which purported to be a biographical representation of the life of Florence Nightingale. On its release, this film was widely acclaimed, both within and outside the nursing profession, with influential professional nursing journals promoting the movie as 'a good educational picture', and commending it to the nursing profession, 'especially those concerned with information and education' (Jones 1988:222). However, although the movie was widely accepted as factual, even by the nursing community, Jones (1988) proposes that the screenplay contained a series of key errors, which served to trivialise major events in the life of Nightingale, and reinforced the myth that her decision to become a nurse was made in the manner of a religious calling.

> [S]he is dressed in white, thus fulfilling the image of the title [*The White Angel*], but the image does more than just show Nightingale in white. Her dress and veil are like a bridal gown and veil in style as well as color. The association of white with virginity and purity is important, as is the bridal association. At the same time she announces her decision to be a nurse, Nightingale announces to her parents that she will never marry. Because she is visually presented as a bride at the same time that she rejects marriage, the subliminal message is that her marriage is to her profession, just as a nun's marriage is to Christ.
> (Jones 1988:225–226)

However, notwithstanding the influence of myth and legend, nursing does have a noble history, and there are many stories of the fortitude, bravery and courage shown by Australian nurses in wartime and other times of community hardship (e.g. Biedermann 2004, Hallett 2007, Scannell-Desch 2005). In Chapter 2 of this book, you will find an in-depth discussion of the history of modern nursing and, after reading it, you will have greater insights and understandings of the origins of some of the myths that surround nursing.

Nursing is endlessly fascinating to many people and this is reflected in the number of television shows, novels and movies that feature nursing and nurses as a major component. There is not the same level of interest in bank workers or bus drivers or beauty therapists, for example. Nursing is ripe with imagery. Many of the images associated with nursing are seemingly at odds with one another, yet all may be conjured up by the word 'nurse'. Images of selflessness (Fealy 2004), kindness, compassion and dedication, hard work, long hours, submission and low pay are among the things that come to mind for some people when they think of nursing (Maher & Lindsay 2008). But though nursing has current or historical elements of all these things, there is so much more to nursing than these portray.

Nursing and nurses are subject to various entrenched stereotypes (Fletcher 2007), and some of these are at least partly derived from the myth that surrounds nursing. In the early 1980s, Kalisch et al (1983) identified some major ways that nursing and nurses were stereotyped, and though this work was undertaken in the United States more than two decades ago, it remains relevant to nurses in Australia today, as well as nurses in other parts of the world (see also Muff 1988). The media and popular literature also tend to present nurses as having stereotyped personal characteristics such as youthfulness, femaleness, purity and naivety, altruism and idealism, compliance, and diminutive stature and 'good character' (Fealy 2004, Fletcher 2007).

Nurses are also credited with having certain qualities and virtues that are grounded in romanticism. De Vries et al (1995), in their study of images of nurses as portrayed in popular medical romances, found that nurses are almost always represented as youthful, pure, virginal, kind, petite, beautiful, subservient, sensitive, considerate, competent and able females. In addition to these personal characteristics, the heroines of these stories are typically presented as Caucasian, with blonde hair and green or blue eyes. They are also portrayed and represented as being emotional and hence not to be taken seriously (Ceci 2004).

Darbyshire (1995), in his exploration of the depiction of Nurse Ratched in the popular film *One Flew Over the Cuckoo's Nest*, discusses a counter image of nursing— the battleaxe/torturer. Unlike the nurses found in the medical romance genre, Nurse Ratched is not petite or subservient, nor is she acquiescent or particularly beautiful. Hunter (1988), in her discussion of the book upon which the film is based, proposes that the Nurse Ratched character is but one example of misogynistic literary tendencies which, she argues, frequently satirically portray the battleaxe/torturer/oppressor nurse as female, and the tender, gentle carer nurse figure as male. Hunter (1988) supports this notion by exploring the images evoked in Tolstoy's description of the gentle hero Gerasim (*The Death of Ivan Ilyich*, 1886) and Whitman's poem 'The wound dresser' (*Leaves of Grass*, 1891), and comparing them with those evoked by Kesey's Nurse Ratched (*One Flew Over the Cuckoo's Nest*, 1962). In Chapter 4 of this book, Philip Darbyshire scrutinises some current and past nursing stereotypes in more detail.

REFLECTION

Consider the popular stereotypes of nurses. How many can you identify? Did any of these stereotypes influence your decision to become a nurse?

Though we still see nurses portrayed in various stereotypical and sometimes highly sexualised ways, which is exemplified in the myth of 'nurse as whore', these stereotypes coexist with some of the noble and romantic images of nursing. Failure to challenge these stereotypes is dangerous for nurses and nursing (Fletcher 2007): various stereotypes give the nurse the status of a worker–handmaiden rather than a health professional (Fealy 2004). Stereotypes of this nature also help to perpetuate an anti-intellectual bias against nursing, which is manifest in the view that good nurses are primarily practical people, rather than highly educated health professionals.

Coexisting with the romantic myths and stereotypes surrounding nursing is the reality of nursing. This reality is that nurses become acquainted with the visceral and raw aspects of humanity that are usually hidden from the world, because of the illness, the incapacity, the frailty, the disability or other needs of those who are the recipients of nursing care. Nursing provides opportunities for human connectedness and growth that few other careers can offer.

But why is this significant? It is clear, as Fealy states, that it is:

> ... naive to assume that ideology will not continue to influence the development of nursing, and that factors such as class and gender relationships, power brokerage and economics, will not continue to reside at the heart of commentary on the nurse.
> (Fealy 2004:655)

It is for this reason that nurses need to be aware of the danger lurking in latent meaning and rhetoric, and recognise that a reality is being created on behalf of nursing—a reality that is not necessarily theirs. It is important to recognise that the concept of 'nurse' is socially constructed, and that nurses may want to believe in their power and control, but the broader societal context situates nurses in a much more fragile position. Nursing exists within a male-dominated healthcare system, bound by authority and power of that class. The sense of 'self as nurse' is thus subject to what David (2000) refers to as 'received behaviours', which can result in 'horizontal violence' or bullying—behaviours of aggression towards other nurses—in order to maintain fragile perceptions of self. These behaviours are self-defeating, as they destroy collegial relationships, and 'limit freedom of thought and action, and preserves nurses' borderline status' (David 2000:84). More recently, disruptive behaviour is the term that has been used to include both bullying and lateral violence (the latter defined as 'nurse to nurse aggression' (Center for American Nurses 2008)). Furthermore, there are turnover costs as nurses on the receiving end of lateral violence may tend to leave nursing. New graduate turnover has been reported to be as high as 60% within six months, with intent to leave associated with workplace bullying (Stanley 2010).

HOW TO DEFINE NURSING?

The urge to define nursing has attracted the attention of nurse scholars for a number of years. While defining a nurse is relatively simple, as you will see as you read further in this chapter, nursing itself has proved somewhat more challenging to define. Though you can probably describe what you think nursing is, the nature and breadth of activities that comprise nursing have contributed to the difficulties associated with defining nursing. Some definitions centre on the functions of a nurse, rather than offering an intrinsic definition of nursing. In a now historical piece of writing which has endured, Henderson produced such a definition of nursing:

> The unique function of the nurse is to assist the individual, sick or well, in the performance of those activities contributing to health or its recovery (or to a peaceful death) that he [sic] would perform unaided if he [sic] had the necessary strength, will or knowledge. And to do this in such a way as to help him [sic] gain independence as rapidly as possible.
> (Henderson, cited in Tomey & Alligood 1998:102)

What needs to be noted in passing is the sexist language that continues to be used when referring to nursing. Language is 'not a neutral information-carrying vehicle', but creates meaning; this meaning changes over time, which makes language very powerful (Fealy 2004:650); its importance cannot be underestimated. David (2000) provides a useful analysis of how nurses collude with oppressors by uncritically accepting outsiders' social construction of nurses and nursing, suggesting that nurses need to socially construct themselves and their context in order to regain their identity and power. Stanley (2010) notes that a contributing factor to lateral violence is gender: that the socialisation of girls and gendered health organisations in which the minority gender has the power help to create an environment that tolerates lateral violence. Added to this, a recent EOWA (Equal Opportunity for Women in the Workplace Agency) report, 'Gender Pay Gap Statistics', found that the gender pay gap in the healthcare and social assistance sector increased by 4% between 2011 and 2012, due to the stereotype that these professions are viewed as women's work, underpaid and undervalued (Australian Ageing Agenda 2012).

The complexities and difficulties associated with defining nursing means that some definitions may seem cumbersome and quite ambiguous. But remember that this is more a reflection of the complex nature of nursing than any lack of clarity on behalf of those who have proffered a definition. The International Council of Nurses (ICN), a coalition of nurses' associations that represents nurses in more than 120 countries, has captured some of the complexities in its definition:

> Nursing encompasses autonomous and collaborative care of individuals of all ages, families, groups and communities, sick or well and in all settings. Nursing includes the promotion of health, prevention of illness, and the care of ill, disabled and dying people. Advocacy, promotion of a safe environment, research, participation in shaping health policy and in patient and health systems management, and education are also key nursing roles.
> (The International Council of Nurses (ICN), www.icn.ch/about-icn/icn-definition-of-nursing/)

In 2003, the Royal College of Nursing (RCN) published a definition of nursing that was the culmination of 18 months' research, and included extensive consultation. The RCN proffered a definition and six key characteristics that capture the essence and varied activities of nursing. The six characteristics are quite detailed and cover issues such as values, relationships and interventions. The full statements can be seen online at www.rcn.org.uk/downloads/definingnursing/definingnursing-a5.pdf. The RCN definition reads as follows:

> Nursing is the use of clinical judgement in the provision of care to enable people to improve, maintain or recover health to cope with health problems and to achieve the best possible quality of life whatever their disease or disability, until death.
> (Royal College of Nursing)

REFLECTION

- Why do you think nursing has proved difficult to define?
- So what is it that excited us about becoming nurses? And, more importantly, what has sustained us on our journeys?

CHOOSING NURSING

Nursing was a gender choice given the societal and historical context of the time (early 1960s and 1970s). It was certainly viewed as an appropriate career choice for females, but also offered potential for achievement, growth and development. It was also a profession that attracted people motivated by altruism and the desire to make a difference to people suffering because of illness and disadvantage. Indeed, this is still a significant motivator of people who choose nursing today. Since the 1970s nursing has made stronger claims to a focus on health promotion, and this now has greater emphasis in construction of nursing knowledge and in conceptualisation of practice. But further to that, there was an overriding quest for understanding and caring for people. This was demonstrated in an egalitarian approach that proved to be unacceptable in nursing at the time (1963–77), when spending time with and caring about patients was viewed as naive and misguided. Such a view denied empathy and concern, and existed through the 1980s and 1990s (McVicar 2003). The concept of nurses distancing themselves from their patients has long been superseded by recognition of the importance of the nurse–patient relationship or the 'therapeutic alliance' (Speedy 1999). The therapeutic relationships that occur between nurses and patients, clients and families mean that nurses have to care for their emotional wellbeing. The 'emotional labour' (McQueen 2004) that is expended on these relationships can result in compassion fatigue if self-protective measures are not in place (Yoder 2010).

NURSING: WHAT SUSTAINS US

One of the most sustaining things about nursing and being a nurse is the opportunity to contribute a perspective that is informed by feminism. A feminist perspective is 'concerned with gender, power relations, patriarchy and hegemony in society, emphasising gender as a key factor in determining the experiences of women in … nursing' (Fealy 2004:650). Feminist theory can be used to examine power relationships in nursing and healthcare, resulting in the exposure of the 'doctor–nurse game', and more recently in the 'health administrator–nurse game' (Dendaas 2004), which elaborates on how nurses can be losers in the power stakes.

The issue of gender is important for nurses, and is an issue that continues to generate critical discussion in nursing (see, for example, Anthony 2004, Center for American Nurses 2008, Tracey & Nicholl 2007). Gender is critical to the maintenance of power relations, and the formation of an identity in nursing. This issue is discussed further in detail in Chapter 12. Nurses are socialised early in their development to adopt 'appropriate' behaviours and beliefs about how to behave as professionals, and how to, as women (predominantly), 'look, talk and feel' (Peter 2004). Their age, gender, family and life experiences all contribute to and influence the way they perceive the power structures and dynamics of the world that is nursing work (Roberts 2000). To be unaware of the impact of power relations and the oppression arising from these is to be locked in a cycle of relationships that serve to severely disadvantage nurses and nursing, perpetuating disunity and disempowerment (Wynter 2006).

Recognising the importance of the perceptions and experiences of nursing students with regard to nursing work, Curtis et al (2007) conducted research that concluded more than half of the surveyed second- and third-year students identified experiencing or witnessing horizontal violence and indicated that this would impact on their future career and/or employment choices. This may have negative implications for the future of nursing (Norris 2010).

It should be noted in passing that many young women of today appear to have an uneasy relationship with feminism, and some have totally rejected its meaning for them. However, the real problem can be identified as: 'can I be who I think I am and be feminist?' (Baumgardner & Richards 2003:448). This confusion is understandable, since young women are unclear about what feminism requires of them (and does not require of them). For example, can they still like fashion, have boyfriends, be forthright and self-determining and be who they want to be? They 'often think of feminism as telling them what they can't do, rather than as a philosophy that *shows them the potential for what they can do*' (Baumgardner & Richards 2003:448, emphasis added), and hence what they can contribute. This suggests that young women may be developing greater clarity about this situation (see Chapter 12). For example, Wynter (2006) suggests that the emphasis on feminism has shifted to a more global activity and social perspective. Thus, issues of 'discrimination, sexuality and gender' have given way to 'corporate governance, poverty, foreign affairs and globalism'.

A natural consequence of a feminist perspective was an interest in the theory and practice of feminist research, which demanded refocusing on the experiences of women. This required some fortitude and commitment, because at that time there was scepticism and ridicule directed towards those who advocated its usage, particularly from researchers who promoted a 'hard science' perspective as the only valid and reliable form of research. However, research that is informed by feminist (and other postmodern) perspectives is now more readily accepted as an appropriate methodology in many (but not all) research camps.

A sustaining factor within a nursing career is the opportunity to provide leadership in as many ways as possible, be it research, management or practice. Effective leadership requires particular attributes, such as high-level communication skills, awareness of one's beliefs, values, attitudes and emotions, respect for others, commitment, passion, flexibility and adaptability (Jackson 2008).

Transformational leadership is dominant in the nursing literature and though quite uncritically embraced by nursing (Hutchinson & Jackson 2012), it is said that such leaders are able to create shared visions, act as role models, inspire, motivate, intellectually stimulate and mentor others (Reinhardt 2004). In many ways, 'leadership is a process of drawing out rather than putting in' (Kitson 2004:211). This implicitly suggests that everyone has a responsibility to exercise leadership qualities. Acknowledging that nursing has many talented participants, Kitson implores us to desist from 'eating our young', or cutting our leaders down ('tall poppy syndrome'), and suggests that, as we work with patients, families, colleagues and managers, we:

> … draw out our vision, our values and beliefs about nursing; our notion of service; our understanding of our own humanity and our ability to face pain, suffering, anxiety, anger and all the other human emotions that nurses face on a daily basis.
> (Kitson 2004:211)

By developing these understandings, we can understand and accept ourselves, and see beyond to the dysfunctionality of organisations and workplaces in order to reform them. This requires nurse leaders to be political, astute (Antrobus 2004, Dendaas 2004, Donnelly 2003) and acquainted with the current literature, which stresses the issues of trust and employee engagement for optimum leader performance (Clarke 2011).

Women have specific leadership skills that can be harnessed. The research literature suggests that, in general, successful women leaders value interconnectedness, inclusivity and relationships, whereas male leaders value competition, dominance, ambition, aggression and decisiveness (Robinson-Walker 1999). Rudan (2003), in focusing on leadership in nursing, identified a warm demeanour, personal and professional interest in followers, nurturing behaviour, promotion of growth in others and the use of humour and interpersonal talk as some of the characteristics that make for successful nurse leadership. Clarke (2011) highlights that 'trust based on the motives and integrity of others, and trust based on their perceived competence and ability' are also essential characteristics (p. 1). These are all the skills that nurses at every level of the profession have, to a greater or lesser degree, which provides them with opportunities to assume leadership roles whatever the level and location of their work.

Over the years of our own nursing careers we have witnessed many changes— from changes in how students are prepared for registration as nurses, through to changes to the environment in which nurses work. Nurses work in climates of continual change, and are challenged by the demands of ageing and increasingly complex clients, as well as themselves.

In addition to these challenges, nursing is currently making attempts to address an international widespread shortage of experienced nurses, particularly specialist nurses (American Association of Colleges of Nursing 2012). Recruitment and retention issues have contributed to an ageing nursing workforce, increasing casualisation of that workforce and increasing international recruitment (Center for American Nurses 2008, Norris 2010). Furthermore, issues including bullying, abuse and violence, professional autonomy, imposed organisational change, occupational health and safety issues and constant restructuring (Center for American Nurses 2008, Jackson et al 2001) have been associated with difficulties in retaining a viable nursing workforce in that they contribute to a working environment that can be experienced as hostile and difficult (Hutchinson et al 2008, Rodwell & Demir 2012). The Center for American Nurses supports the 'development of zero tolerance for abuse in the workplace' as a strategy to remove disruptive behaviour altogether (2008:4), since such behaviours are not conducive to a culture of safety (including medication errors) (Institute of Medicine of the National Academies 2006). If nursing is to continue to be an attractive profession on which satisfying and rewarding careers can be built, it must embrace cultural change to 'eliminate the effects of disruptive behaviour including lateral violence and bullying at the personal, organizational, national and international levels' (Center for American Nurses 2008:5).

REFLECTION

What has been your experience of nursing? What motivated you to become a nurse? What now sustains you?

TYPES OF NURSE IN AUSTRALIA AND NEW ZEALAND

There are a number of entry points into nursing. In Australia and New Zealand, the title 'nurse' refers to someone who is recognised as such by duly authorised national or state-registering authorities. Nurses belong to a regulated professional group that is responsible to the community it serves for supplying healthcare to a constantly high standard, through the maintenance of professional standards and personal integrity. In both New Zealand and Australia, nurses are required to meet certain standards in order to become registered. Currently, there are two types of nurse who practise in a wide range of health and community settings (see the box overleaf for some examples). These are the Division 2 or enrolled nurse and the Division 1 or registered nurse.

Division 2 or Enrolled nurse

The enrolled nurse (EN) is one who has completed an approved educational course leading to enrolment with nurse-registering authorities. The EN course is shorter than courses leading to registration as a nurse, usually being of 12–18 months' duration. There are a number of career development opportunities available to ENs and these can include access to professional development courses that permit an extended role, such as medication administration. Some ENs wish to study further to complete qualifications to become registered nurses. Many universities and colleges give some recognition of prior learning to ENs, meaning that they may be able to undertake a shortened version of the Bachelor of Nursing degree.

Division 1 or Registered nurse

The term *registered nurse* (RN) refers to one who has undertaken and completed an approved program leading to nurse registration as a nurse, holds an appropriate qualification, has met all the requirements of registering authorities and whose name appears on a register of nurses in accordance with the relevant national legislation. The RN is considered to be a first-level nurse and, as such, is permitted to practise without supervision and is accountable and responsible for actions taken and decisions made.

RNs have various career progression paths and various titles, depending on where they are located, so as you enter hospitals and community health settings you will encounter RNs with varying degrees of experience and status. These can include clinical nurse consultants (CNCs), clinical nurse specialists (CNSs), nurse managers, nurse educators, nurse researchers and other levels of nurse.

Clinical practice settings for nurses

Nurses practise in a wide range of health and community settings, including:
- acute hospital settings
- day surgery nursing
- daycare clinics
- residential care facilities (such as nursing homes)
- school nursing
- drug and alcohol nursing
- general community nursing
- specialist community nursing (such as mental health nursing)
- occupational health nursing
- general practice (or practice) nursing
- justice health (including remand centres, prisons and juvenile justice settings), and
- rural and remote area nursing.

Assistant in nursing or nurse's aide

The *assistant in nursing* (AIN) or *nurse's aide* is a person who carries out some nursing duties under the direct supervision of a registered nurse. Most often, the duties are associated with activities of daily living, such as hygiene, feeding and personal care. Many undergraduate students undertake employment as an AIN while they are studying their undergraduate degree at university.

There are various titles given to people fulfilling the AIN (or very similar) role, and these titles are applied in various locations. Some of the other titles are nurse's aide, care worker or personal care assistant. AINs (and similar workers) are known as unregulated health workers, and they do not come under the auspices of nurse-registering authorities. Rather, the registered nurse under whose supervision they are working is accountable in the event of an adverse situation occurring.

PROFESSIONAL REGULATION AND CONDUCT

Nurses are expected to be people of integrity who conduct themselves with a high level of personal honour and veracity. It is important that members of the public feel safe in hospitals, and believe themselves to be in trustworthy and competent hands. If people do not feel safe, they would not be able to feel secure in leaving their loved ones in the care of nurses and healthcare facilities. Nursing authorities act to ensure the safety of the public by holding nurses accountable for their actions and making nurses answerable for their behaviour and any complaints that are made against them. In order to gain initial registration, nursing applicants need to demonstrate they are of good character.

REFLECTION

What do you see as essential personal qualities for nurses?

Nurses are answerable to registering authorities that have the power to question nurses, and suspend or remove them from the register. These same authorities can also place conditions on registration, restricting practice or, in certain circum-stances, requiring a nurse to participate in educational programs. The conduct of nurses is also guided by various codes that inform professional conduct. Though these vary depending on country, they are remarkably similar in substance. This is because the values of nursing cross national and international boundaries. It is an interesting exercise to use the internet and search for the Code of Conduct that governs you in your location.

REFLECTION

What are some examples of good and poor professional conduct? Can you think of some from your own practice experience?

CONCLUSION

Nursing attracts people from all walks of life. Many readers of this text will be entering nursing as school leavers, but others will be mature-aged students who come to nursing with a variety of life experiences. Welcome to nursing, and congratulations on making a choice that will open many doors for you and provide you with a career for life. You may find it challenging and, possibly, not quite what you expected. But go with your passion, and believe in yourself—because you can create your life. The road you have chosen is not an easy one, but you need to believe in yourself, as we do, to succeed. We may have had a more facilitative environment, so for that we are grateful, and we need to be. What a blessed life we have had, on behalf of nursing.

RECOMMENDED READINGS

Fletcher K 2007 Image: changing how women nurses think about themselves. Literature review. Journal of Advanced Nursing 58(3):207–215

Hinson T, Spatz D 2011 Improving nurse retention in a large tertiary acute-care hospital. Journal of Nursing Administration 41(3):103–108

Jackson D, Daly J 2004 Current challenges and issues facing nursing in Australia. Nursing Science Quarterly 17(4):352–355

Jirwe M, Rudman A 2012 Why choose a career in nursing? Journal of Advanced Nursing, 68:1615–1623

Scannell-Desch E 2005 Lessons learned and advice from Vietnam War nurses: a qualitative study. Journal of Advanced Nursing 49(6):600–607

Tracey C, Nicholl H 2007 The multifaceted influence of gender in career progress in nursing. Journal of Nursing Management 15:677–682

REFERENCES

American Association of Colleges of Nursing. Web source: www.aacn.hche.edu

Anthony A S 2004 Gender bias and discrimination in nursing education: can we change it? Nurse Educator 29(3):121–125

Antrobus S 2004 Why does nursing need political leaders? Journal of Nursing Management 12(4):227–228

Australian Ageing Agenda 2012 Gender pay gap largest of all industries. Online. Available: http://www.australianageingagenda.com.au/2012/06/05/article/Gender-pay-gap-largest-of-all-industries/PVDYRFKLTV.html

Baumgardner J, Richards A 2003 The number one question about feminism. Feminist Studies 29(2):448–454

Biedermann N 2004 Tears on my pillow: Australian nurses in Vietnam. Random House, Sydney

Bostridge M 2008 Florence Nightingale: the making of an icon. New York Farrar, Straus and Giroux

Ceci C 2004 Gender, power, nursing: a case analysis. Nursing Inquiry 11(2):72–81

Center for American Nurses 2008 Lateral violence and bullying in the workplace. February 1–12

Clarke M 2011 Employee engagement: too much 'trust', not enough debate? Business Leadership Review VIII 11 April:1–4

Curtis J, Bowen I, Reid A 2007 You have no credibility: nursing students' experiences of horizontal violence. Nurse Education Practice May 7(3):156–163

David A 2000 Nursing's gender politics: reformulating the footnotes. Advances in Nursing Science 23(1):83–94

Darbyshire P 1995 Reclaiming 'Big Nurse': a feminist critique of Ken Kesey's portrayal of Nurse Ratched in *One Flew Over the Cuckoo's Nest*. Nursing Inquiry 2(4):198–202

Dendaas N 2004 The scholarship related to nursing work environments: where do we go from here? Advances in Nursing Science 27(1):12–21

De Vries S, Dunlop M, Goopy S, et al 1995 Discipline and passion: meaning, masochism and mythology in popular medical romances. Nursing Inquiry 2(4):203–210

Donnelly C 2003 Leadership: professional, inspirational or dysfunctional? Journal of Nursing Management 11(2):65–67

Fealy G M 2004 'The good nurse': visions and value in images of the nurse. Journal of Advanced Nursing 46(6):649–656

Fletcher K 2007 Image: changing how women nurses think about themselves. Literature review. Journal of Advanced Nursing 58(3):207–215

Hallett C 2007 The personal writings of First World War nurses: a study of the interplay of authorial intention and scholarly interpretation. Nursing Inquiry 14(4):320–329

Hunter K 1988 Nurses: the satiric image and the translocated ideal. In: Jones A (ed) Images of nurses: perspectives from history, art and literature. University of Pennsylvania Press, Philadelphia

Hutchinson M, Jackson D 2012 Transformational leadership in nursing: towards a more critical interpretation. Nursing Inquiry doi: 10.1111/nin.12006bib17

Hutchinson M, Jackson D, Wilkes L, Vickers M H 2008 A model of bullying in the nursing workplace: organizational characteristics as critical antecedents. Advances in Nursing Science 31(2):E60–E71

Institute of Medicine of the National Academies 2006 Preventing medication errors: quality chasm series. Online. Available: http://iom.edu/Reports/2006/Preventing-Medication-Errors-Quality-Chasm-Series.aspx

The International Council of Nurses (ICN). Available: www.icn.ch/about-icn/icn-definition-of-nursing/

Jackson D 2008 Servant leadership: a framework for developing sustainable research capacity in nursing. Collegian 15(1):27–33

Jackson D, Mannix J, Daly J 2001 Retaining a viable workforce: a critical challenge for nursing. Contemporary Nurse 11(2–3):163–172

Jones A 1988 The White Angel (1936): Hollywood's image of Florence Nightingale. In: Jones A (ed) Images of nurses: perspectives from history, art and literature. University of Pennsylvania Press, Philadelphia

Kalisch P, Kalisch B, Scobey M 1983 Images of nurses on television. Springer Publishing, New York

Kitson A 2004 Drawing out leadership. Journal of Advanced Nursing 48(3):211

Maher J M, Lindsay J 2008 Times for caring? Nurses from work to home. Australian Sociological Association, Re-imaging Sociology, University of Melbourne, December

McQueen A C H 2004 Emotional intelligence in nursing work. Journal of Advanced Nursing 47(1):101–108

McVicar A 2003 Workplace stress in nursing: a literature review. Journal of Advanced Nursing 44(6):633–642

Muff J 1988 Of images and ideals: a look at socialization and sexism in nursing. In: Jones A (ed) Images of nurses: perspectives from history, art and literature. University of Pennsylvania Press, Philadelphia

Norris T L 2010 Lateral violence: is nursing at risk? Tennessee Nurse 73(2)

Peter E 2004 Nursing resistance as ethical action: literature review. Journal of Advanced Nursing 46(4):403–416

Reinhardt A C 2004 Discourse on the transformational leader metanarrative or finding the right person for the job. Advances in Nursing Science 27(1):21–32

Roberts S J 2000 Development of a positive professional identity: liberating oneself from the oppressor within. Advances in Nursing Science 22(4):71–83

Robinson-Walker C 1999 Women in leadership and health care: the journey to authenticity and power. Jossey-Bass, San Francisco

Rodwell J, Demir D 2012 Oppression and exposure as differentiating predictors of types of workplace violence for nurses. Journal of Clinical Nursing 21:2296–2305

Royal College of Nursing. Available: www.rcn.org.uk/downloads/definingnursing/definingnursing-a5.pdf

Rudan V 2003 The best of both worlds: a consideration of gender in team building. Journal of Nursing Administration 33(3):179–186

Scannell-Desch E 2005 Lessons learned and advice from Vietnam War nurses: a qualitative study. Journal of Advanced Nursing 49(6):600–607

Speedy S 1999 The therapeutic alliance. In: Clinton M, Nelson S (eds) Advanced practice in mental health nursing. Blackwell Science, Oxford

Stanley K M 2010 The high cost of lateral violence in nursing. Presentation at Sigma Theta Tau International Leadership Summit, Atlanta, Georgia April 24

Tomey A M, Alligood M R 1998 Nursing theorists and their work. Mosby, St Louis

Tracey C, Nicholl H 2007 The multifaceted influence of gender in career progress in nursing. Journal of Nursing Management 15:677–682

Wynter V 2006 Feminism is passé because it worked. Online and available at www.onlineopinion.com.au/view.asp?article= 4781 6 August 2008

Yoder E A 2010 Compassion fatigue in nurses. Applied Nursing Research 23:191–197

CHAPTER 2

Visioning the future by knowing the past

Madonna Grehan

LEARNING OBJECTIVES

After reading this chapter, students should be able to:

- understand the benefits of having a knowledge of the history of nursing
- develop a critical understanding of received accounts of the history of nursing
- identify the lineage of nursing and its occupational relatives
- identify significant events that have influenced the evolution of nursing in Australia
- describe aspects in nursing and midwifery that warrant historical research.

KEY WORDS

History, nursing, midwifery, regulation, education, hospitals

---

Disclaimer:

Aboriginal and Torres Strait Islander people are warned that this publication may contain images of deceased people.

HISTORY AND ITS RELEVANCE TO NURSING

History, heritage, tradition and the past are concepts that may be familiar to most of us, but what is their relevance to nursing? This chapter explains why having an understanding of the history of nursing is useful for all nurses, whether working in practice, education, administration or the policy arena. For some, history consists merely of important dates, events and the contribution of celebrated individuals. These elements certainly have a place in history's narrative, but history has so much more to offer than just time lines and famous faces. History is often equated with heritage and tradition, but an Australian historian, Graeme Davison (2000), argues that these concepts are concerned with sentimentality, not the accuracy and objectivity of history that is critical and self-aware. Later in this chapter we will return to the notions of 'heritage' and 'tradition'.

So why is history important for nurses to know about? Davison writes that, among other things:

> History ... tells us who we are, gives us an imaginative and sympathetic insight into the lives of others, encourages a critical attitude to question social and political change, and equips us to participate in a political community.
> (Davison 2000:263)

An understanding of history can help us to understand how things have come to be, why some things change and others do not, or are difficult to change (Davison 2000). Scholars point out that history can illuminate the background to issues in contemporary healthcare, many of which are not new (Connolly 2004, Fairman & Lynaugh 1998, Lewensen 2004, Nelson 1997, 2004). For example, concerns about current shortages of nurses and midwives, educating nurses and regulating nursing practice have been perennial issues in Australian nursing (Grehan 2009a). History can also help us to understand the place of nursing within healthcare and society (Connolly 2004).

History can offer valuable insights into what the future might bring, although clearly it is impossible to be certain about the future. But if we understand what has influenced the development of nursing, by knowing about the perennial issues in the history of nursing, it may be possible to devise novel responses to these longstanding issues. How, then, can nurses learn about the history of nursing?

Traditional views of history

Most nurses are familiar with stories of famous nurses, such as Florence Nightingale, feted for her work in the Crimean War (1853–1856) and possibly the story of Sister Elizabeth Kenny, the nurse who pioneered controversial physical therapies for poliomyelitis. Up to the late twentieth century what was commonly accepted as the history of nursing derived from popular culture, especially cinema and television. In the early twentieth century histories of nursing by nurse luminaries in the United States of America (Nutting & Dock 1907) and Britain (Tooley 1906), recorded the triumphs of nursing.

The accepted view of the history of nursing went something like this: the care of the sick and of childbearing women was unskilled work of low status until Nightingale nurses worldwide transformed bedside attendance from an age of darkness into one of light, from ignorance into science. This triumphal tale was subsequently reiterated by nurses who authored histories of Australian nursing (Walsh 1955, Webster

1942) and New Zealand nursing (Maclean 1932). Commonly accepted histories along these lines are referred to as 'received' history. They offer a simplistic view of a much more complex history. In so doing, they tend to ignore the contribution of everyday nurses, and aspects of history that do not 'fit' the story of the progress of nursing. In recent decades, more enlightened views of the history of nursing have emerged.

An enlightened view of the history of nursing

Australian historians (Godden 2006, Nelson 2000, Strachan 2001) and others (Baly 1987, Connolly 2004, D'Antonio 1999, Helmstadter & Godden 2011, MacPherson 1996, Nelson & Rafferty 2010, Strachan 1997) have used the tools of critical history to reappraise these conventional narratives. Critical history rejects long-held assumptions, such as the idea that history is about progress or that complex events can be explained simply, and considers nursing as a fundamental part of the society it serves, within political and social contexts (Connolly 2004).

Critical history can address the contribution of those not included in received history, such as Aboriginal and Torres Strait Islander nurses. Indigenous women like Sadie Corner (pictured) and Lowitja (Lois) O'Donohue had to overcome considerable odds to train as nurses and work in Australia's white healthcare system. Examining the role of indigenous nurses in Australia and New Zealand will entail consideration of politics, race, social attitudes and geography. The contribution of indigenous nurses is just one of many fascinating and instructive episodes in Australian and New Zealand nursing history worthy of critical inquiry.

This chapter offers merely a snapshot of the history of nursing, looking past received historical accounts to other explanations of the evolution of nursing. It briefly considers the antecedents of contemporary nursing and examines the formations of care in Australia and New Zealand that established patterns of care provision. It considers some of the historical influences on nursing, mile-

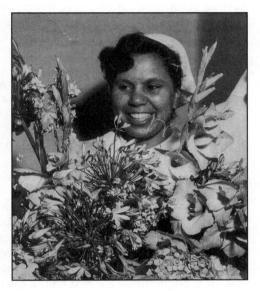

Figure 2.1
Sadie Corner.
Reproduced with the permission of the Salvation Army Australia, Southern Territory Archives and Museum, Melbourne and Sadie Canning, née Corner.

stones in the evolution of nursing, and discusses the relationship between history and professional identity. The chapter concludes with remarks on the future of nursing.

THE ROOTS OF MODERN NURSING

Given that the act of nursing is as old as the human race (Nelson 2000), it is difficult to identify nursing's so-called 'roots' as a starting point, so here we begin with the present. If we accept the premise that nursing in the twenty-first century is 'modern', from that standpoint we can draw out nursing's antecedents, which have evolved to produce the modern form.

In the twenty-first century, a large proportion of healthcare is provided in what historians call the 'modern' hospital. The concept of a 'modern' hospital emerged in the Western world in the late nineteenth century, a time when medicine was developing a sophisticated understanding of disease and illness, applying germ theory and experimenting with novel treatments such as vaccinations and surgery (Rosenberg 1987). Received medical history held that the modern hospital was an innovation for having replaced disorder with order and hierarchical systems of caregiving; the emergence of modern nursing, with its own hierarchical structures, was lauded as a parallel element in this medical innovation (Nelson 2000). However, scholars of nursing and health history, including the Australian nursing historian Sioban Nelson (2000), have challenged this view. Nelson argues that hospital, as a place for delivering systematised care, was not a 'new' concept. Rather, the modern hospital and modern nursing constituted new ways of doing 'old' things in which structure and standards were replicated but were evangelised as 'modern' and innovative. The antecedents of modern nursing can be found in these older ways of care provision.

Pre-modern nursing

The historical antecedents of modern nursing lie with the care of the sick poor as strangers, provided by religious orders as 'an integral part of Christian practice' (Nelson 2000:3). In the early Christian era and beyond, religious orders emulated the work of Jesus Christ in tending to his flock by providing care in hospices (early forms of hospitals), feeding the poor, tending the infirm and applying palliative treatments (Nelson 2000). One group of nurses who has sustained this philosophy of care for centuries is the Catholic religious order the Sisters of Charity of St Vincent de Paul, mentioned later in this chapter.

The care of the sick poor was also practised by Protestant organisations. Female followers of Christianity, among them Elizabeth Fry, Jane Shaw Stewart, Agnes Jones and Sister Dora [Pattison], in the nineteenth century formed nursing 'sisterhoods' through which nursing care was provided to the poor in a similar way (Summers 1989). Recent work by Carol Helmstadter and Judith Godden (2011) has demonstrated that, in London during the first half of the nineteenth century, some sisterhoods were contracted by the hospitals of that city to provide requisite nursing care to the inpatients. Gradually, the prominence of religious orders waned, and by the mid-nineteenth century philanthropically minded Christian people organised care provision to the poor as a charitable gesture (Grehan 2009a). The difference was that the latter organisations were underpinned by a strong moral compass. This had a foundational influence on the development of care provision in Australia and New Zealand.

HEALTHCARE IN EARLY AUSTRALIA AND NEW ZEALAND

When the British Empire expanded in the eighteenth and nineteenth centuries, its conventions of caregiving were replicated in the newly claimed colonies of Australia and New Zealand (Grehan 2004). Records, primarily coronial inquests that describe nursing and midwifery care in the early years of the colonies, reveal that it was often primitive, performed without modern-day technologies of sanitation, in circumstances where water was obtained from a nearby stream or a stagnant pond, where 'watching' the patient at night was done by candlelight and where help in the form of a doctor or nurse was several days' travel away by horse or on foot (Grehan 2009b).

Establishing institutions

Australia's colonial governments established general hospitals in the convict settlements of Sydney and Hobart Town, lunatics were housed in government asylums and midwives were appointed by the NSW government to specific geographic locations (Grehan 2009a). Institutional healthcare in the colonies emerged from the 1840s, developed by the charity sector and directed at the poor. Known as 'voluntary' hospitals or 'charitable institutions', these services were funded by subscription, so that, in return for their financial support, subscribers were able to recommend individuals for hospital treatment (McCalman 1998). Where colonists expanded the white frontier, hospitals were established in response to accidents in mines and other industrial catastrophes (Collins 1999). Lying-in institutions for poor pregnant women [maternity hospitals] were established for indigent women, mirroring similar institutions in England, Scotland and Ireland (McCalman 1998).

Hospitals, however, were thought to harbour miasmas, the noxious vapours said to emanate from filthy conditions, suppurating wounds, ill-ventilated rooms, cesspits and cemeteries; 'sanitary' science was the method employed to minimise miasmas (Nelson 1998). The practice of sanitary science meant that certain conditions were excluded from admission to hospital: smallpox, tuberculosis and forms of cancer. Pregnancy was considered a healthy state, to which miasmas posed a risk, meaning pregnant women also were excluded from hospital admission (Grehan 2009a).

Institutional nurses

Hospitals in the colonial world were hierarchical places, just as they were in England and Scotland. What a nurse was expected to do depended on the type of establishment where she was employed, and on what basis she was employed—that is, as a head nurse, assistant nurse or pupil nurse. Some hospitals were operated by a married couple who attended to the patients, cooked their food and did the laundry (Grehan 2011). Asylums (Monk 2008) and other establishments employed men and women as attendants (Collins & Kippen 2003).

The nurse's role was to maintain the cleanest environment possible, and the work of the nurse involved an extensive regimen of cleanliness and ventilation practices (Nelson 2000). With hospitals unsewered until the late nineteenth century, it was the nurses' job to dispose of bodily wastes such as blood, faeces and urine, emptying the excreta stored in buckets at the end of wards into cesspits within hospital grounds (Templeton 1969). Institutional nurses' work included scrubbing floors, brushing carpets, dusting, polishing brassware and furniture, washing the patients and providing nourishments for those who could not do it for themselves. Nurses had to clean and fumigate straw mattresses, known as palliasses, in special airing rooms, and carry soiled linen to the laundry for washing (McCalman 1998). Some institutions required the nurses to sleep at the end of wards so that they could attend the patients when necessary.

Mid-nineteenth-century nursing consisted of a mixture of bedside attendance and domestic work—extremely hard work for little reward. With newspaper reports of nurses being drunk on duty or cruel to patients, little wonder that few were attracted to the position of 'hospital nurse' (Grehan 2004). To weed out potential troublemakers, institutions such as The Women's Hospital in Melbourne required pupil nurse applicants to provide a testimonial from a minister of religion or medical practitioner, vouching for the nurse's character (McCalman 1998). However, such institutions were for the poverty-stricken. For most people who had a family, an individual's home or 'domicile' was the primary domain for receiving care (Grehan 2009a).

Care provided in the community

A variety of people were available to attend the sick and childbearing women in colonial Australia, among them: doctors, nurses, midwives, herbalists, oculists, druggists and dentists (Grehan 2009a). Similarly in New Zealand, a range of people practised (Bryder 1991). Who the patient chose depended on who was available, what the purchaser expected of his or her care and what the patient was willing to pay. In the cities and in rural areas, often local women attended births and cases of sickness as a neighbourly gesture (Grehan 2009a). Some women even combined their 'attending' work—tending the sick, preparing the dead for burial and acting as midwife—with running the local postal service (Forth et al 1998).

There is no doubt that employment for women in the colonial world was hard to find, making nursing and midwifery practice easy to adopt as paid work when family circumstances changed. A study by historian Glenda Strachan (2001), of all births registered in an isolated rural district of the Colony of New South Wales during the years 1856 to 1896, confirms this feature of maternity attendance. Australian nursing historian Joan Durdin cites the example of Mrs Elizabeth Knight, a well-respected midwife in the Mount Gambier region of South Australia who began her work at the age of 70, following the death of her husband (Durdin 1991).

Some women attending births had only their experience of childbearing and rearing, while others had none. Some women learnt their craft by apprenticeship, while others attended public lectures given by doctors. A proportion held qualifications obtained from formal training schemes, which included theoretical and practical elements. These schemes were available to women from the late eighteenth century, in centres such as Edinburgh (Grehan 2009a). Without any regulation of those practitioners, their practice or their prices, obtaining an attendant at birth or at times of sickness was like a lottery. It is unsurprising, too, given the plurality of attendants, that women who attended others for payment were referred to by the derogatory term 'handywomen', in the same category of the handyman who performs a multitude of tasks around a house (Grehan 2004). In this environment, a perception prevailed that the majority of nurses were unsuited to the important duty of caring for the sick and for childbearing women, and that perception mattered.

Worldwide calls to reform nursing

Criticism of domiciliary and institutional nurses was fuelled in part by the writings of author and social commentator Charles Dickens whose serialised novel *The Life and Adventures of Martin Chuzzlewit* (1843) opened a window on private nursing. *Martin Chuzzlewit* brought to the imagination of the reading public two fictitious but infamous London characters, Sarah Gamp and her friend Betsy Prig. Mrs Gamp, styling herself as a nurse and midwife, was available for all work: births, tending to the sick and laying out of the dead. Prig, a hospital nurse by day, moonlighted as a 'private' nurse in people's homes. Illustrated with graphic pen and ink sketches, Dickens' narrative depicted the two 'nurses' as ignorant, unrefined and untrustworthy reprobates. Sarah Gamp came to symbolise all that was perceived to be wrong with female nurses and nursing throughout the English-speaking world (Grehan 2004).

Within 15 years of the premiere of *Martin Chuzzlewit* and the story of Sarah Gamp, a charitable organisation in England, the 'Nightingale Fund for Nursing', was established. It followed a subscription campaign aimed at acknowledging Miss Nightingale's work with the war wounded in the Crimea. So much money was raised that the Fund's committee decided to direct it to the training of nurses. The Nightingale Fund's enduring message was that nursing needed educated 'ladies' of good character who could act as role models for the less educated nurses around them (Baly 1987). Australians donated to the Fund and the news that nurses would be trained 'properly' as a result was welcomed (*Argus*, 10 July 1856).

As Florence Nightingale and Sarah Gamp became household names throughout the English-speaking world, the Nightingale Fund established two training schools in London. At St Thomas's Hospital, nurses were to train for general work in public hospitals and infirmaries; at King's College Hospital nurses were to train in midwifery nursing to attend the poor, but this school was closed after only five years (Baly 1987). While Nightingale lent her name to the school at St Thomas's, in practical terms she had little to do with it. However, her published views on all things associated with nursing—on nurses, training, caregiving, hospital design and sanitary science—were lauded by most critics of colonial healthcare.

The context within which Miss Nightingale's ideas gained traction was relevant because calls for reform in nursing coincided with the emergence of the modern hospital. The introduction of new treatments and operations required a team of staff to guarantee success (Helmstadter & Godden 2011, Rosenberg 1987). The nurses providing pre-operative and post-operative care needed to be literate, cooperative and diligent; they needed to be able to observe changes in the patient's state, apply new technologies such as the thermometer, use a watch to count pulsations (Grehan 2004) and deliver complex regimens of nutrition and pharmacological agents via enemas. Nurses who would willingly work the long hours, and perform the new skills required of them, were not always easy to find. Thus, in the last quarter of the nineteenth century, hospitals introduced their own training schemes for pupil nurses (Grehan 2009a).

Institutional training schemes

Nurse 'training' in hospitals, it has to be said, was far less sophisticated than the term suggests. It involved on-the-job learning, combined with lectures by medical practitioners, which pupil nurses attended only if they could be freed from their ward work (Mitchell 1977). Up to the turn of the twentieth century at least, nurse training was organised around an institution's associated medical specialty, so that an eye and ear hospital's training scheme produced eye and ear nurses; children's hospitals produced children's nurses; lying-in hospitals produced nurses qualified for maternity and gynaecological care and so on. In fact nurse training in Australia was so specific to each hospital's needs that the nurse's skills were not always transferable to another hospital environment (Trembath & Hellier 1987).

Worse still was that hospitals, always starved of funds, sometimes hired out pupil nurses to private patients needing care at home, so that a pupil nurse could spend a substantial portion of her training time away from the hospital, without any supervision and learning very little (Templeton 1969). This variability meant that the concept

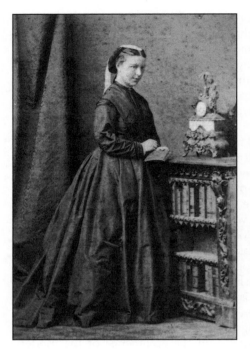

Figure 2.2
Lucy Osburn.
Reproduced with the permission of
South Eastern Sydney and Illawara Area
Health Service, NSW Government.

of a 'trained' nurse was fluid. Coupled with the plurality of attendants working outside institutions, it is little wonder that ideas of compulsory, uniform training, proof of claimed qualifications and superior senior nurses to implement these reforms were enthusiastically embraced in the colonies.

The first cohort of so-called Nightingale nurses arrived in Australia in 1868, superintended by Miss Lucy Osburn, to improve conditions at the Sydney Hospital. This transformative episode is much celebrated in the received history of Australian nursing, however it has emerged from Judith Godden's (2006) research that Sydney Hospital was not ill-managed and that this transformative episode is more myth than reality.

Nevertheless, the trend continued with the Australian colony of Tasmania welcoming three 'Nightingale' nurses in 1885, reportedly to institute necessary reforms at Hobart's General Hospital. Two of these nurses then worked in Victoria where, again, they are said to have instituted urgent and necessary reforms (Grehan 2004). New Zealand's nursing received history records analogous accounts of neglect and wretchedness in its hospitals that were subsequently transformed under the watch of reputable nurses. French (2001) notes Mary Lyons, Mrs Bernard Moore and Annie Crisp among them, the last-named credited with overhauling nursing at the Auckland Hospital and establishing its nurse training school. Crisp, awarded a Royal Red Cross in 1883, was a military nurse feted for her work in Africa (Masters 1993).

As the story goes, under the steady eye of these superior nurses, hospitals around Australia (Grehan 2004) and New Zealand (Hill 1982) adopted the so-called Nightingale scheme of nurse training, with its two categories of pupil. 'Lady' probationers paid for their training, were exempt from menial work and were expected to supervise their subordinates. 'Regular' probationers did not pay for pupillage but trained for longer; they did household work and scrubbing, and learned how to behave from the example set by their superiors. Received history tells us that the Nightingale model transformed the healthcare landscape (Grehan 2009a). The impression is that it was adopted successfully within all hospitals, in its entirety, and without a shred of resistance. Was this really what happened?

In fact, research by Godden (2006) and Grehan (2009a) shows that the evolution of nurse training in Australian institutions was far more complex than received history records. There is no doubt that some hospitals modernised training, but the process of doing so was difficult and expensive so change was achieved only incrementally. There was no miraculous shift from old to new models of training, and when changes were introduced no one individual, or group of individuals, was responsible for those developments, despite what received history would have us believe. Finally, reforms that were made in nursing and hospitals did not occur in isolation. As Nelson (2000) argues, they were just one element in a wave of lasting social change that swept throughout the English-speaking world in the late nineteenth century.

From the haphazard world of nineteenth century nursing and midwifery, our discussion now moves to the twentieth century, to consider some of the factors that have shaped nursing and midwifery practice as we know them today.

SOME HISTORICAL INFLUENCES ON NURSING

Nursing, just like other professions and occupations, is shaped by external factors because the profession exists as part of the society it aims to serve. In thinking about what has influenced nursing, we can point to obvious influences and constantly evolving technologies of care, such as the thermometer, fluid replacement: aseptic practices, infection control and myriad others. All of these developments have changed the way nursing is performed, and nursing today continues to respond to new technologies of care. New ideas about the concepts of health, wellbeing and illness have impacted on nursing practice too (Grehan 2009a). While these may seem obvious, there are those which are far less obvious; namely, the political, economic and social climate in which nursing is practised. Historically, one critical external influence on nursing in Australia has been the three tiers of government that hold differing responsibilities for aspects of healthcare provision. Other factors include financial conditions within which governments operate. Changes of government mean that the policy platform can change rapidly with effects on the clinical arena (Grehan 2008).

With a critical examination of the history of nursing, it is possible to reflect on the way that external factors and trends, momentous and less momentous events, have shaped nursing as we know it today. Two interconnected issues with a substantial influence on the development of nursing in Australia and New Zealand are: the consequences of a lack of government interest in healthcare in the nineteenth century; and the development of responsible government—in New Zealand as a national government, and in Australia initially as colonies and from 1901 as a federation of states and territories.

As we have discussed, in the last decade of the nineteenth century, pressure mounted to raise standards in nursing and midwifery attendance (Grehan 2009a). The New Zealand government's response was to adopt statutory regulation, a seamless process given that the population was small (Maclean 1932). In Australia most governments resisted that path, and disagreement persisted on how to run hospitals, how to teach nurses and what to teach nurses. Arguments also prevailed over the length of training and what it should consist of and even if it was beneficial (Grehan 2009a). In the absence of regulation by governments in Australia, sectors in the nursing fraternity opted for voluntary professional self-regulation.

Voluntary regulation

Efforts in Australia to introduce voluntary professional regulation for nurses and midwives mirrored those in Britain where a British Nurses Association was established in late 1887 (Grehan 2009a). Voluntary professional regulation was designed to do what legislation might have done: differentiate trained nurses from untrained people by setting standards in education and training, and by maintaining registers of trained nurses so that the public could choose trained nurses.

A Victoria Nurses Association formed in 1886 as a professional organisation of private nurses in Melbourne, but it endured for only two years. In 1891, Tasmanian nurses agitated to form a professional association in that colony, but subsequently looked to Victoria for a critical mass who could make this happen. A Nurses Association of Australasia then was founded in Melbourne in 1892; but it too failed to flourish (Grehan 2004). Two subsequent associations endured: the Australasian Trained Nurses Association (ATNA) based in New South Wales established in 1899; and the Victorian Trained Nurses Association established in 1901. After the VTNA was awarded Royal Charter in 1904, it became the Royal Victorian Trained Nurses Association (RVTNA) (Trembath & Hellier 1987).

Trembath and Hellier (1987) argue that the success of these organisations was marginal. There is no doubt that for nurses and midwives in many parts of Australia, especially those in private practice, voluntary regulation made little difference, while the ATNA's and RVTNA's different stances on registration precluded reciprocity between the states. But the long-term influence of these organisations deserves some credit. When legislation was eventually introduced for nursing and midwifery across Australia, the categories of nurse and curricula laid down by the ATNA and the RVTNA formed the basis of many initial statutes (Grehan 2009a). It is also worth pointing out that one of the likely reasons that these organisations did endure was that their membership base included doctors whose support was critical in securing the co-operation of the hospital sector so that uniformity in nurse training would be enforced (Grehan 2009a).

Voluntary regulation preceded statutory regulation in all states of Australia, but in New Zealand the reverse occurred. There a voluntary professional association for 'private' nurses, the New Zealand Trained Nurses Association, formed in 1909 as a response to developments in the international nursing arena (Maclean 1932). The International Council of Nurses (ICN), formed in 1899, was providing a voice for nurses worldwide but member countries needed to have a national nurses association that was governed by nurses (Grehan 2009a). Because the New Zealand Trained Nurses Association was a national organisation, governed by nurses and not doctors, that country became a member of the ICN much earlier than Australia. Only in 2011 did Australia's two colleges of nursing, the Royal College of Nursing Australia and The College of Nursing, the latter based in New South Wales, overcome long-held differences to unite as a national college, the Australian College of Nursing (Grehan 2012).

Statutory regulation

New Zealand's pathway to government regulation of nursing and midwifery was uncomplicated. New Zealand appointed a Scots-born, English-trained nurse, Mrs Grace Neill, to assist in developing its legislative framework. National regulation for nurses applied in New Zealand from 1901, and a Midwives Registration Act was passed in 1904 (French 2001). It was a rather different story in Australia where six independent colonies were established, each at a different time, and each with its own unique regulatory oversight for aspects of commerce, trade and legal matters (Macintyre 1986). Under the 1901 Australian Constitution, the states' capacity to make state laws was protected. Consequently, statutes and regulations pertaining to nursing and midwifery varied considerably across Australia, with reciprocity of registration between the states a major obstacle for nurses who sought employment opportunities across state borders. The first statutory regulation in Australia for nurses practising midwifery was passed in Tasmania in 1901. By the mid-1920s, legislation governing midwifery and nursing practice had been passed in the other states (Grehan 2009).

In recent years, development of trade agreements, the globalisation of workforces and worldwide shortages of nurses have forced change in the way that nurses and midwives in Australia are registered as healthcare practitioners. In 1992, the Australian and New Zealand national governments signed a Mutual Recognition Agreement, extending it in 1997 to include the Australian state governments under the Trans-Tasman Mutual Recognition Arrangement (Council of Australian Governments n.d.). Designed to 'promote economic integration and increased trade', these agreements have enabled the mutual recognition of most occupational qualifications in both jurisdictions. However, the problem of nurse and midwife shortages, rather than free trade requirements, has provided the impetus to ease regulatory restrictions on nurses and midwives. In July 2010 a national registration system for all nurses and midwives in Australia was introduced (Australian Nursing and Midwifery Council 2010), making qualifications within the nation portable.

The challenge of regulation in Australia's political landscape, developments in technology and shifts in understanding of health and illness are just some examples of the historical influences which deserve consideration when developing a vision of the history of nursing. Tumultuous events, also, have had a lasting influence on nursing as a profession. Some of these are considered next.

MILESTONES IN AUSTRALIAN AND NEW ZEALAND NURSING

Even in the relatively short history of nursing in New Zealand and Australia, there have been notable events and momentous occasions. Here we concentrate on two particular milestones in the history of nursing. The first is the role of war; the second is the development of nursing education and the eventual transfer to the tertiary setting. It is their context and their sequelae that are of interest in historical terms.

War

Conflicts have been a significant theme in nursing history in Australia and New Zealand, another consequence of being part of the British Empire. The work of Florence Nightingale with the war wounded of the Crimea and that of women in the American Civil War attracted the admiration of the public worldwide. As Sioban Nelson writes, 'the successes of the war nurses stimulated a shift in public perceptions of the role of the nurse' because, in the organised arena of tending the war wounded, 'nursing came to be seen as a useful profession' and a rather more lofty exercise than simply nursing the poor (Nelson 2000:148).

The Anglo-Boer War, World Wars I and II

There is little doubt that by the turn of the twentieth century, nurses believed their profession was useful indeed, as did many members of the public. During the Anglo-Boer War (1899–1902), nurses from the Australian colonies and from New Zealand volunteered (Speirs 2010). In late 1899 a group of NSW nurses formed the first Army Nursing Service Reserve in Australia, with 14 nurses despatched to South Africa and paid for by the NSW government. Others joined the Imperial service while yet others served as private citizens, with private subscriptions supporting them. In World War I (1914–1918), around 2500 nurses served with the Australian Army Nursing Service (AANS) in the Middle East, in the south of Europe, France, England and India on land and sea (Harris 2010). New Zealand nurses served in similar locations, on trains and hospital ships (Dahl 2009).

Australian nurses volunteered during World War II (1939–1945), serving in North Africa, the Middle East, the south of Europe and across the Pacific, as members of the three areas of the Australian military forces: the AANS, the Royal Australian Air Force Nursing Service and the Royal Australian Naval Nursing Service (Harris 2007). In 1943 nurses in the Australian forces were awarded military rankings, formally placing women in charge of men at a time when no comparable positions were open to women in civilian life (Milligan & Foley 1993). Similarly, New Zealand also recognised serving nurses as officers at that time (Clendon 1997).

Two particular events in World War II involving Australian nurses encapsulated the inhumanity of war and drew attention to the roles and sacrifices of ordinary women who risked their lives in their work as military nurses.

The sinking of the *Vyner Brooke* and the Bangka Island massacre

In February 1942, when the city of Singapore was invaded by Japanese forces, 65 AANS had been serving in a military general hospital there. The nurses were forced to evacuate with civilians, leaving Singapore harbour on a small coastal steamer, the *Vyner Brooke* (Shaw 2010). The *Vyner Brooke*, with more than 200 passengers aboard, made its way through the Malacca Straits. There, the vessel was one of several attacked by Japanese bombers from the air.

Some survivors of the *Vyner Brooke*'s bombardment and sinking managed to swim ashore to Radji Beach on Bangka Island, landing in two parties on different parts of the coast. One party was taken as prisoners of war; a second party of service personnel and civilians was discovered by Japanese soldiers two days after the landing on Bangka Island. Among that party were 22 nurses. The soldiers ordered the nurses to march into the sea, where they were shot. Vivian Bullwinkel, then aged 26, was the only survivor of this war crime. After hiding for 12 days in the jungle with a severely wounded British soldier, Bullwinkel surrendered to the Japanese army, and was reunited with the other party of 31 nurses. Until the end of the war, this group of women remained prisoners of war, and news of the Bangka Island massacre did not reach Australia until well after hostilities had ceased in 1945 (Jeffrey 1954).

The sinking of the Australian Hospital Ship *Centaur*

A second incident occurred in May 1943, just off the Queensland coast, north east of Brisbane. An Australian Hospital Ship, *Centaur*, was on its second journey from Sydney to Papua New Guinea to collect injured servicemen. *Centaur* carried 332 personnel: doctors, field ambulance officers, ship's crew and 12 AANS sisters (Milligan & Foley 1993). At 4.10 a.m. and without warning, *Centaur* was torpedoed by a Japanese submarine. Only one of the 12 nurses on board survived. During the 36 hours which passed until the *Centaur*'s survivors were rescued, this remarkable nurse, Ellen Savage, took charge of rationing food and attended to some of the 63 injured survivors. Her nursing work took place on a raft in the Pacific Ocean and despite her own severe injuries: a fractured palate, nose and ribs, as well as perforated ear drums and severe bruising (Milligan & Foley 1993).

The sinking of the *Centaur* was judged to be a war crime because its protection was supposed to have been assured by all parties engaged in hostilities, according to the Hague Convention (Milligan & Foley 1993). The loss of the 11 nurses was used in advertising by the Australian government, exhorting Australians to avenge the nurses' deaths by actively supporting the war effort. Subsequently, the Australian public gave generously to various war nurses memorials, including the Centaur Fund in Queensland and the War Nurses Memorial Centre in Melbourne, now called the Nurses Memorial Centre (Williams 1991).

On the home front

The duration of World Wars I and II had substantial impacts on nursing and midwifery, certainly in Australia. In World War I, deficits were created in every area of nursing across the nation when nurses joined up (Harris 2007). Some hospitals attempted to overcome this shortage by extending nursing training from three to four years, but this had an unintended effect of discouraging young women from applying for training places. 'War emergency nurses' were introduced in Australia in 1915 when there were no fully trained nurses to do

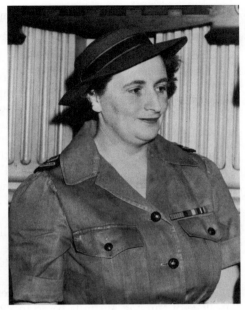

Figure 2.3
Ellen Savage.
Reproduced with the permission of
Australian War Memorial – Image 061952.

the work and after the war there were disputes about whether these nurses should be allowed to continue as nurses (Grehan 2009a). In the five years before World War I, a Bush Nursing scheme was formulated in Australia to provide healthcare, particularly maternity care, to Australians in rural and remote areas. Nurses who wanted to work as Bush Nurses had to hold qualifications in midwifery and general nursing. This strict policy had to be relaxed when the scheme could not attract nurses with a general nursing certificate (Grehan 2009a).

In World War II, out of an estimated workforce of 13,000, around 4000 nurses in Australia volunteered. Shortages of trained nurses were so dire that the Australian government recognised nursing's importance to national stability (Nelson & Rabach 2002). From 1942 until 1945, nursing was designated a protected industry and placed under the control of the Manpower Directorate, a federal authority. Any nurse who wished to either work or train interstate required the permission of the Directorate to leave the state in which she lived. Sometimes, canny nurses found someone who would exchange places before contacting the Directorate (Grehan 2009a).

Adjustment to civilian life after the war must have been difficult for these service nurses, but particularly so for those who had occupied positions of authority in the military. Colonel Annie Sage, Matron-in-Chief of the AANS from 1943 until 1947, in civilian roles was unable to reach the heights of leadership that were tacit in her military position. Sage's aspirations to lift Australian nursing out of the realm of women's work into an even more professional sphere were dashed at The Women's Hospital in Melbourne where her authority was challenged vigorously by civilian doctors (Nelson & Rabach 2002). But Sage and other nurses understood that advancing education was critical to the growth of nursing as a profession. Our discussion now turns to this aspect of the history of nursing.

Developing education

The apprenticeship mode of training nurses on the job in hospitals was the mainstay of institutional nursing education throughout the nineteenth and twentieth centuries. Education of nurses throughout the English-speaking world was in large part a service provision, with a smaller weighting on education (Trembath & Hellier 1987). But since the 1920s, Australian nurses had recognised that nursing lacked postgraduate education opportunities that were available to nurses in American universities, in England at the Royal College of Nursing and in New Zealand 'at the postgraduate school of nursing in Wellington' (Smith 1999:21). Aspirations to establish postgraduate education in Australia came to fruition after World War II, albeit in two different forms.

A national college of nursing in Australia was the goal of both NSW and Victoria but neither wished to be a state branch of the other, and the organisation had to be based in a large city. In the state of Victoria, postgraduate courses in teaching, administration and industrial (now occupational health) nursing were offered by the Royal Victorian College of Nursing (RVCN) which had metamorphosed from the RVTNA in the 1930s. A College of Nursing Australia based in Victoria was established formally in early 1949 and in May of the same year NSW established its own college, commencing postgraduate education programs with support from the New South Wales Nurses Association, the Australian Trained Nurses Association and the Institute of Hospital Matrons Nursing (Smith 1999).

Despite their differences, both entities cooperated on efforts to transfer nursing pre-registration education to the tertiary sector and, by the 1970s, momentum had gathered (Lusk et al 2001). In 1977, and after continued lobbying from the profession, the NSW state government transferred nursing education from the health portfolio to education, a move that enabled the state's Colleges of Advanced Education to assume responsibility for pre-registration nurse education. Other states followed. In 1984, under an Australian federal government plan, tertiary education for all nurses was formally approved (McCoppin & Gardner 1994). Midwifery education was transferred to the tertiary sector in the early 1990s. Also in the 1990s, alongside a program of closing psychiatric hospitals and moving the mentally ill into community care, hospital-based pre-registration psychiatric nursing ceased. Psychiatric nursing is now a postgraduate specialty. Collectively these shifts in Australia ended 140 years of nurses' learning by apprenticeship. Similarly in New Zealand, apprenticeship in hospitals was replaced gradually by diploma-based education in technical institutes, beginning in 1973 under pilot programs, and in the mid-1990s an undergraduate degree program was formally adopted as the only pre-registration pathway (Lusk et al 2001).

Streams of specialisation

Much of our discussion has focused on the 'general' nature of nursing, but an important element in the history of nursing has been the specialisms which have developed in clinical practice nursing. Some specialisms have emerged alongside the related medical specialty, such as eye and ear, orthopaedics and so on. Psychiatric nursing, formerly known as mental nursing, had its foundations in asylums which were geographically and philosophically far away from general hospitals and general nurse training schemes. Bush nursing was an early form of independent practice which developed for particular geographic populations with broad needs.

Some specialisms have presented in tandem with rapid developments in medicine in the treatment of disease conditions, and others as a result of new ways of understanding health and illness. Specialisms within nursing have emerged in association with a specific body of knowledge particular to an area of care, one being the intensive care nursing unit in the 1960s (Fairman & Lynaugh 1998). Maxine Dahl (2009), a historian of Australian military nursing, argues that Royal Australian Air Force air evacuation nurses were responsible for establishing the specialty of flight nursing and retrieval during military service in World War II and the Korean War (1950–1953).

Numerous specialties—community nursing, neonatal intensive care units, coronary care units, burns units, spinal units and myriad others—are now accepted as requisite by modern healthcare standards in the Western world, each of which infers a nursing specialty. Stomal therapy, diabetes education, mental health, infection control, occupational health, women's health, adolescent health, cancer nursing, tissue transplant nursing, paediatrics, health promotion and palliative care are just some examples of the specialty nursing practice areas to have emerged since the 1970s. The history of their individual development as specialisations in nursing will make for fascinating historical inquiry in the future. Another area of historical interest is the relationship between history and professional identity, to which our discussion now turns.

HISTORY AND IDENTITY

Earlier in this chapter, we noted that history can tell us about our identity as individuals and as members of a recognised profession. We have seen that nursing's identity in received histories is linked to a sense of the profession as a 'modern' entity with many branches. For the greater part of the twentieth century, midwifery was considered midwifery 'nursing'; that is, a branch of the practice of nursing. However, in recent years, midwifery's identity as a branch of nursing has been disputed, as part of a worldwide movement aimed at professionalising midwifery. This movement seeks to have midwifery in Australia recognised as it is in the Netherlands, New Zealand and other parts of the Western world: as a profession, separate and distinct from nursing (Australian College of Midwives Incorporated Victorian Branch 1999). To this end, a freestanding educational pathway leading to registration as a midwife, the Bachelor of Midwifery, has been underway since 2002 in Australia, emulating the direction taken by New Zealand in 1990 when midwifery and nursing were placed under separate legislation (Grehan 2009a). This brings us to the relationship between a profession, its identity and its history.

Midwifery's identity, not 'nursing'

As the argument goes, the main distinction between nursing and midwifery is that midwifery involves care in a natural healthy episode in the female life cycle, while nursing concerns the care of the sick (Fahy 1998). Midwifery is also said to have a history that is different from that of nursing (Australian College of Midwives Incorporated Victorian Branch 1999). So what is the relationship between profession, history and identity? 'Identity' histories, sometimes referred to under the banner of 'revisionist' histories, have been popular since the 1960s when second-wave feminism and the broader movement in social change at that time critiqued received historical narratives as a march of progress (Davison 2000). Revisionist history aimed to give 'voice' to groups whose contributions had been ignored in conventional interpretations of history: women, African Americans and other ethnic groups (Davison 2000).

Revisionist history that is focused on an identity in many ways is no less problematic than received history. Without doubt, it can acknowledge those whose voices have been ignored previously, but its very aim—that is, righting wrongs or locating origins that resonate with the present—raises concerns. When the aim of history becomes a search for roots, or righting history's wrongs, history can be crafted so that it 'fits' with the author's view of the world (Davison 2000, Ulrich 2002). In other words, this kind of history is not critical, does not question its assumptions, is not self-conscious and is not objective. The outcome can be that these interpretations are invested with nostalgia but masquerade as history (Ulrich 2002).

Two histories of midwifery, produced during the revival of midwifery in the 1990s, illustrate the effects of an uncritical approach to examining professional identity. The first is an oral history of midwifery in England; the second is a study of South Australian midwifery. Leap and Hunter, the authors of the English study, declare in their introduction that: 'We expected to uncover a treasure chest of forgotten skills: experience that would enhance midwifery practice and inspire the midwives of today' (Leap & Hunter 1993:xi). In the Australian text, Annette Summers examines the 'historical terrain which led to the demise of the community midwife, whose lost autonomy is lamented by the midwife of the 1990s' (Summers 1995:1).

Both texts are searching for forgotten skills and lost autonomy, concepts likely to resonate with contemporary midwifery's professional aspirations to regain what is believed to be its 'lost' independence and distinguish itself from nursing (Summers 1995). But searching for a preconceived kind of history is no less problematic than the received history of nursing's pursuit of Nightingale-style nurses and their transformation of healthcare. It is no surprise that Leap and Hunter, and Summers, for the most part find the history they were looking for, because neither applies the self-consciousness of critical history.

Leap and Hunter, for example, having interviewed handywomen who practised in the first half of the twentieth century, found no evidence to suggest that handywomen were in any way dealing out 'death and destruction' or any evidence that handywomen midwives were involved in performing abortions (Leap & Hunter 1993:22). This confident assessment is made despite ample documentary evidence in England confirming that some untrained women as well as trained midwives were ill-equipped (as were many doctors) for even the most common of complications in labour, such as haemorrhage, and evidence that female midwives facilitated the crimes of abortion and infanticide (Grehan 2009a). Likewise, Summers locates midwifery's 'lost' autonomy in South Australian midwifery at a time before the profession of nursing eclipsed this 'ancient' form of women's practice. Summers, too, ignores ample Australian documentary evidence that shows that some midwives played a role in abortion and infanticide, and that they lacked basic skills (Grehan 2009a).

Criticism of these revisionist histories is not to suggest that independent midwifery was not extinguished, nor is it to suggest that medicine and nursing did not wish to control midwifery that was practised by women. But when accounts of history inform the fundamentals of a professional identity and make special claims for status and privilege on that basis, it is critical for nurses and midwives to be conscious of how these histories have been constructed, and to understand the motivations of their authors because history written along these lines inevitably clouds the real picture. For those willing to investigate the history of nursing from the perspective of critical history, the rewards are great. In the next section, we raise some aspects of New Zealand's and Australia's nursing and healthcare history, which are worthy of critical inquiry.

Religious nurses

One can be forgiven for believing that no skilled nurses worked in Australia or New Zealand in the nineteenth century given the longstanding narrative that ignorant and incompetent nurses were those in practice until the arrival of 'Nightingale' nurses. Aside from midwives whose claimed training and qualifications have been confirmed (Grehan 2009a), the Catholic Sisters of Charity have a long history of care provision in Australia. As early as 1838, five religious sisters from Dublin were providing care in Sydney. Of these five Sisters of Charity, one had trained as a nurse while another had been sent to Paris to gain nursing experience (MacGinley 2002). The Sisters visited 'the sick poor in their own homes' as well as Parramatta's female factory or gaol where miscreants served their sentences (MacGinley 2002:72). In 1857, the Sisters of Charity opened the first St Vincent's Hospital in Australia, at Sydney's Pott's Point. Since that time, the St Vincent's network has expanded substantially, with their hospitals providing a considerable proportion of public health services.

The Catholic Sisters of St John of God cared for typhoid sufferers in isolated settlements in Western Australia and those affected by leprosy, while the Sisters of the People, associated with the Methodist Church, tended the indigent in cities (Grehan 2008). The role of religious or faith organisations in nursing and nurse training is one of the most interesting and challenging topics in Australian and New Zealand nursing history. Two Christian religious groups with enormous influence on Australian nursing are the Presbyterian Church and the Salvation Army for their pioneering of nursing provision to remote communities in Australia.

The Australian Inland Mission

The Australian Inland Mission (AIM), an offshoot of the Presbyterian Church, was another form of charitable assistance to rural and remote communities, devised in the early twentieth century by the Reverend John Flynn of Flying Doctor fame. Flynn established a network of health centres staffed by trained nurses in extremely isolated territory (Cockrill 1999). Nurses appointed in the AIM's early years were also deaconesses of the Presbyterian Church so in this sense they were evangelists for health and faith. They attended patients, conducted Sunday School and offered spiritual comfort to people in their communities (Cockrill 1999).

There is no doubt that AIM's nurses faced all kinds of challenges because of the isolation in which they worked, especially before the introduction of pedal radio. Not all were trained in midwifery nursing, but they were expected to attend births. In the early days of the service, the Women's Hospital in Melbourne agreed to prepare deaconess nurses by allowing them to undertake short terms of midwifery 'training'. Nurse Mary Ann Bett was a deaconess and nursing sister who completed a short stint of training prior to taking up her AIM position at Oodnadatta in South

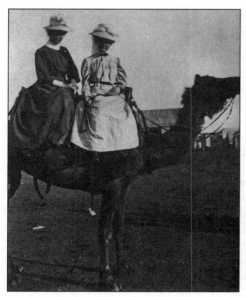

Figure 2.4
Jean Finlayson (right) and fellow
deaconess at Alice Springs c1915.
Reproduced with the permission of
Church Council, Adelaide House Museum.

Australia in 1909 (The Women's Hospital Board of Management Meeting Minutes 1909). Sister Jean Finlayson who worked at the AIM's Oodnadatta centre was then inaugural trained nurse at the Northern Territory's Alice Springs AIM Centre in 1915, later the Alice Springs Hospital (Cockrill 1999). In Figure 2.4, Jean is pictured on a mode of desert transport.

Aboriginal nurses

The Salvation Army (SA), another Christian organisation, had a pivotal role in the training of nurses that to date has not been investigated. As well as instituting district nursing services in cities, the SA ran a network of hospitals around Australia, some of which were big enough to become training schools for nurses. Bethesda, a SA hospital in the city of Melbourne, offered nurse training to Aboriginal women who came from mission stations, such as Mount Margaret in Western Australia and Colebrook in South Australia. While mainstream hospitals were reluctant to accept indigenous women as pupil nurses, the SA in contrast offered valuable educational opportunities for indigenous Australian women (Grehan 2008).

Miss Sadie Corner, pictured earlier in this chapter, moved from Mount Margaret to train as a nurse at Bethesda in the 1950s, beginning as a nurses' aide, then training as a general nurse, and then as a midwife. Subsequently, Miss Corner was the first Aboriginal woman to work as a trained nurse and hospital matron in Western Australia. As Mrs Canning, Sadie was later awarded an MBE and Queen's Jubilee Medal for her contribution to the health of the community of Leonora and surrounding district (Australian Legal Information Institute 2000). Another Aboriginal woman, Lowitja (Lois) O'Donohue CBE AM, from South Australia, was initially rejected for nurse training because she was of Aboriginal descent. Subsequently, Ms O'Donohue graduated from the Royal Adelaide Hospital in 1954 as a trained general nurse and later worked in Adelaide as a charge sister. She then spent time in India with a missionary society before taking up positions in national Aboriginal affairs (State Library of South Australia 2001).

In New Zealand, historian Pamela Wood reports there were organised efforts in the late nineteenth century to educate Māori women as nurses (Wood 1992). Recent research by Odette Best (2012), an indigenous nurse from Queensland, has revealed a similar program in that state, the Native Nurses Training Scheme, which existed in the 1940s on three mission stations. This emerging research demonstrates a nexus between faith organisations and their focus on training indigenous women as nurses. This aspect of the history of nursing is important and worthy of further research, as is faith organisations' pivotal role in buttressing the rural and remote nursing workforces in Australia and New Zealand.

THE FUTURE

At the beginning of this chapter, we proposed that sometimes history can offer insights that might be applied to the future. Of course, it is impossible to tell what the future will bring, but Graeme Davison, the Australian historian, emphasises that an understanding of history can tell us what is *unlikely* to happen, rather than what will happen, simply because history never repeats itself, although over a sweep of time it may show patterns. As this chapter has noted, the trends that have featured consistently in the history of nursing emphasise the perennial nature of some issues in nursing and healthcare. It is likely that arguments about professional identities are unlikely to dissipate and may even strengthen. Given the recent separation of midwifery from nursing, it is possible that in the future other branches of nursing might pursue a similar path. Psychiatric nursing had its foundations in asylums which were geographically and philosophically separate from general hospitals and general nurse training schemes, but educational reforms resulted in psychiatric nursing being positioned as a postgraduate specialty. Just as contemporary midwifery has argued its difference from nursing, so may psychiatric nursing reiterate its difference in foundations and history.

The role of nurses in war service has been a consistent element in nursing's narrative, indicating that this is likely to remain so. Nursing has been affected by chronic and acute shortages of personnel from time to time, necessitating novel ways of education and even government intervention in wartime to control the supply of nurses. There is no guarantee that government will not institute similar controls if it sees the need in the future to manage public health emergencies. Workforce shortages seem to be a perennial feature of nursing and midwifery, in Australia at least (Grehan 2009). Over the sweep of nursing's history since Europeans arrived in the colonies, the primary domain for care has shifted from the home, to the modern hospital, and recently returned to the home where patients can receive sophisticated treatments previously performed in hospitals. But a continuation of this cycle cannot be ruled out.

Technology has impacted greatly on the development of nursing. Technologies of care, coupled with sophisticated understandings of trauma and illness, have transformed the way in which care in hospitals and homes is provided and call for a style of education far different from that required in the 1960s. With technological advances part and parcel of modern nursing and healthcare, these are likely to remain so into the future.

CONCLUSION

In this brief survey of the history of nursing in Australia and New Zealand, there are many aspects of nursing history worthy of examination, using the tools of critical history. Some have been mentioned here: the contribution of women combining nursing with their evangelical missionary work, the role of Aboriginal women as nurses, migrant nurses and aspects of nursing practice—that is, doing, organising, planning and implementing the care of others. More historical inquiry will illuminate the background to contentious areas in the history of nursing, such as the relationship of nursing with midwifery and the care of women. Research on the impact of world events and globalisation on nursing may provide clues about how to deal with workforce shortages. What is important for nurses and nursing is to accept its past 'warts and all', celebrating ordinariness alongside triumphs (Nelson 1997:234).

The pursuit of critical history will provide a realistic vision of the history of nursing in the Australian and New Zealand context, one that factually illuminates the richness and complexity of that history.

REFLECTIVE QUESTIONS

1 How does knowing about nursing's past help nurses to understand the present and the future?

2 What have been some of the major historical influences on nursing and midwifery?

3 What new questions could be asked about aspects of nursing history?

RECOMMENDED READINGS

Bashford A 1998 Purity and pollution: gender, embodiment and Victorian medicine. St Martin's Press, New York

Fairman J, Lynaugh J E 1998 Critical care nursing: a history. University of Pennsylvania Press, Pennsylvania

Helmstadter C, Godden J 2001 Nursing before Nightingale 1815–1899. Ashgate, Farnham, England

Nelson S 2001 Say little, do much: nurses, nuns, and hospitals in the nineteenth century. University of Pennsylvania Press, Pennsylvania

Nelson S, Rafferty A M 2010 Notes on Nightingale: the legacy and influence of a nursing icon. Cornell University Press, Ithaca, New York

REFERENCES

Argus, 10 July 1856, Melbourne

Australian College of Midwives Incorporated (ACMI) Victorian Branch 1999 Reforming midwifery: a discussion paper on the introduction of Bachelor of Midwifery Programs into Victoria. ACMI Victorian Branch, Melbourne

Australian Legal Information Institute 2000 Council for Aboriginal Reconciliation archives, Members of Council 1991–2000. Online. Available: www.austlii.edu.au/au/other/IndigLRes/car/2000/16/appendices04.htm 20 Feb 2006

Australian Nursing and Midwifery Board 2010 Tenth meeting of the Nursing and Midwifery Board of Australia 29 July 2010. Online. Available: http://www.nursingmidwiferyboard.gov.au/News/Communiques-from-Board-meetings.aspx

Baly M 1987 The Nightingale nurses: the myth and reality. In: Maggs C (ed) Nursing history: the state-of-the-art. Croom Helm, New Hampshire, pp 33–59

Best O 2012 The native nurses of Queensland c.1940, Nursing History in a Global Perspective, International History of Nursing Conference, Kolding, Denmark 9–11 August 2012

Bryder L 1991 A healthy country: essays on the social history of medicine in New Zealand. Bridget Williams Books, Wellington

Clendon J 1997 New Zealand military nurses fight for recognition World War One–World War Two. Nursing Praxis in New Zealand–Journal of Professional Nursing 12(1):24–28

Cockrill P 1999 Healing the heart: 60 years of Alice Springs Hospital 1939–1999. Alice Springs Hospital's 60th anniversary reunion organising committee. Alice Springs

Collins Y 1999 The provision of hospital care in country Victoria 1840s to 1940s. Unpublished PhD thesis. Department of History of Philosophy and Science, University of Melbourne, Melbourne

Collins Y, Kippen S 2003 The 'Sairey Gamps' of Victorian nursing? Tales of drunk and disorderly wardsmen in Victorian hospitals between the 1850s and the 1880s. Health and History 5(1):42–64

Connolly C 2004 Beyond social history: new approaches to understanding the state of and the state in nursing history. Nursing History Review 12(3):5–24

Council of Australian Governments (n.d.) Trans-Tasman Mutual Recognition Arrangement. Online. Available: www.coag.gov.au/the_trans-tasman_mutual_ recognition_arrangement 20 Feb 2006

Dahl M 2009 Air evacuation in war: the role of RAAF nurses undertaking air evacuation of casualties between 1943–1953. Unpublished PhD thesis, Institute of Health and Biomedical Innovation, Queensland University of Technology, Brisbane

D'Antonio P 1999 Revisiting and rethinking the rewriting of nursing history. Bulletin of the History of Medicine 73(2):268–290

Davison G 2000 The use and abuse of Australian history. Allen & Unwin, Sydney

Dickens C 1843 The life and adventures of Martin Chuzzlewit. Chapman and Hall, London

Durdin J 1991 They became nurses: a history of nursing in South Australia 1836–1980. Allen & Unwin, Sydney

Fahy K 1998 Being a midwife or doing midwifery? Australian College of Midwives Incorporated Journal 11(2):11–16

Fairman J, Lynaugh J E 1998 Critical care nursing: a history. University of Pennsylvania Press, Pennsylvania

Forth G, Critchett J, Yule P (eds) 1998 The biographical dictionary of the Western District of Victoria. Hyland House, Melbourne

French P 2001 A study of the regulation of nursing in New Zealand. Victoria University of Wellington Graduate School of Nursing and Midwifery Monograph Series 2/2001, Wellington

Godden J 2006 Lucy Osburn, a lady displaced: Florence Nightingale's envoy to Australia. University of Sydney Press, Sydney

Grehan M 2004 From the sphere of Sarah Gampism: the professionalisation of nursing and midwifery in the colony of Victoria. Nursing Inquiry 11(3): 192–201

Grehan M 2008 A historical perspective of community nursing in Australia. In: Kralik D, Van Loon A (eds), Community health care nursing in Australia. Blackwells, Oxford, pp 1–16

Grehan M 2009a Professional aspirations and consumer expectations: nurses, midwives and women's health. Unpublished PhD thesis, School of Nursing and Social Work, The University of Melbourne, Melbourne

Grehan M 2009b A most difficult and protracted labour case: midwives, medical men and coronial investigations into maternal deaths in nineteenth century colonial Victoria. Provenance, Journal of Public Record Office Victoria 8:63–74

Grehan M 2011 Servants and serving at the Melbourne Lying-in Hospital and Infirmary for Diseases Peculiar to Women and Children, 1856–1900. Royal Women's Hospital History Website. Online. Available: at http://www. thewomenshistory.org.au/biogs/e0000102b.htm 29 Apr 2012

Grehan M 2012 Realising unity: the Australian College of Nursing's long gestation. Connections Royal College of Nursing, Australia 15(2):2–3

Harris K 2007 Not just 'routine nursing': the roles and skills of the Australian Army Nursing Service during World War I. Unpublished PhD thesis, History Department, University of Melbourne

Harris K 2010 More than bombs and bandages: Australian Army Nurses at work in World War I. Big Sky Publishing, Newport, New South Wales

Helmstadter C, Godden J 2011 Nursing before Nightingale 1815–1899. Ashgate, Farnham, England

Hill A 1982 The history of midwifery from 1840–1979: with specific reference to the training and education of student midwives. Unpublished MA thesis, Department of Education, University of Auckland

Jeffrey B 1954 White Coolies: a graphic record of survival in World War Two. Angus & Robertson, Sydney

Leap N, Hunter B 1993 The midwife's tale: an oral history from handywoman to professional midwife. Scarlett Press, London

Lewensen S 2004 Integrating nursing history into the curriculum. Journal of Professional Nursing 20(6):374–380

Lusk B, Russell R L, Rodgers J, Wilson-Barnett J 2001 Pre-registration nursing in Australia, New Zealand, the United Kingdom and the United States of America. Journal of Nursing Education 40(5):197–202

McCalman J 1998 Sex and suffering: women's health and a women's hospital. Melbourne University Press, Melbourne

McCoppin B, Gardner H 1994 Tradition and reality: nursing and politics in Australia. Churchill Livingstone, Melbourne

MacGinley M R 2002 A dynamic of hope: institutes of women religious in Australia, 2nd edn. Crossing Press for the Institute of Religious Studies, Sydney

Macintyre S 1986 A concise history of Australia: Vol. 4, 1901–41. The succeeding age. Cambridge University Press, Cambridge

Maclean H 1932 Nursing in New Zealand: history and reminiscences. Tolan Printing, Wellington

MacPherson K 1996 Bedside matters: the transformation of Canadian nursing 1900–1990. Oxford University Press Toronto

Masters D 1993 Annie Alice Crisp RRC Lady Superintendent of Auckland Hospital. Auckland Waikato Historical Journal April (62):36–37

Milligan C S, Foley J C H 1993 Australian hospital ship *Centaur*: the myth of immunity. Nairana Publications, Brisbane

Mitchell A 1977 The hospital south of the Yarra: a history of the Alfred Hospital Melbourne from foundation to the nineteen-forties. Alfred Hospital, Melbourne

Monk L 2008 Attending madness: at work in the Australian colonial asylum. Rodopi, Amsterdam

Nelson S 1997 Reading nursing history. Nursing Inquiry 4:229–236

Nelson S 1998 How do we write a nursing history of disease? Health and History 1(1):43–47

Nelson S 2000 A genealogy of the care of the sick: nursing, holism and pious practice. Nursing Praxis International, Hants, England

Nelson S 2004 History v youthful folly. Nursing Inquiry 11(3):129

Nelson S, Rabach J 2002 Military experience: the new age of Australian nursing and other failures. Health and History 4(1):79–87

Nelson S, Rafferty A M 2010 Notes on Nightingale: the legacy and influence of a nursing icon. Cornell University Press, Ithaca, New York

Nutting M A, Dock L L 1907 A history of nursing, Vol. 1. Putnam, New York

Rosenberg C E 1987 The care of strangers: the rise of America's hospital system. Johns Hopkins University Press, Baltimore

Shaw I 2010 On Radji Beach: the story of the Australian nurses after the fall of Singapore. Pan Macmillan, Sydney

Smith R 1999 In pursuit of excellence: a history of the Royal College of Nursing, Australia. Oxford University Press, Melbourne

Speirs K 2010 Nursing in the Boer War: the Nurses Database. Online. Available: http://www.boerwarnurses.com/joomla/index.php?option=com _ wrapper&view=wrapper&Itemid= 2 July 2011

State Library of South Australia 2001 Lowitja O'Donohue: Elder of our nation. In: Women and politics in South Australia: the Aboriginal voice. Online. Available: www.slsa.sa.gov.au/women_and_politics/abor1.htm 20 Feb 2006

Strachan G 1997 Employment conditions for nurses in Australia during World War II. In: Rafferty A M, Robinson J, Elkan R (eds) Nursing history and the politics of welfare. Routledge, London, pp 192–207

Strachan G 2001 Present at the birth: 'handywomen' and neighbours in rural New South Wales 1850–1900. Labour History 81:13–27

Summers A 1989 The mysterious demise of Sarah Gamp: the domiciliary nurse and her detractors c. 1830–1860. Victorian Studies 32(2):365–386

Summers A D 1995 For I have ever so much more faith in her ability as a nurse: the eclipse of the community midwife in South Australia, 1836–1942. Unpublished PhD thesis, History Department, Flinders University

Templeton J 1969 Prince Henry's: the evolution of a Melbourne hospital. Robertson & Mullens, Melbourne

Tooley S 1906 A history of nursing in the British Empire. SH Bousfield, London

Trembath R, Hellier D 1987 All care and responsibility: a history of nursing in Victoria 1850–1934. Florence Nightingale Committee, Australia, Victorian Branch, Melbourne

Ulrich L T 2002 The age of homespun: objects and stories in the creation of an American myth. Random House, New York

Walsh A 1955 Life in her hands: the Matron Walsh story told to Ruth Allen. Georgian House, Melbourne

Webster M E 1942 The history of trained nursing in Victoria. Typescript copy. Royal Women's Hospital Archives, Melbourne, unaccessioned

Williams J 1991 Victoria's living memorial: history of the Nurses Memorial Centre 1948–1990. Nurses Memorial Centre, Melbourne

Women's Hospital Board of Management Meeting Minutes 1909 Royal Women's Hospital Archives Melbourne, unpublished, Accession No. RWHA 1991/6/26

Wood P J 1992 Efficient preachers of the gospel of health: the 1898 scheme for educating Maori nurses. Nursing Praxis in New Zealand Journal of Professional Nursing 7(1):12–21

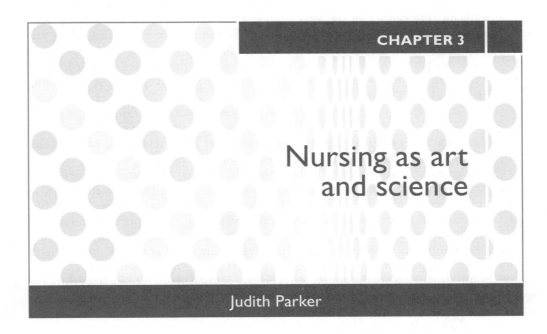

CHAPTER 3

Nursing as art and science

Judith Parker

LEARNING OBJECTIVES

Upon completion of this chapter, the reader should have gained:

- an understanding of the development of ideas about nursing as an art and a science within an historical context
- an appreciation of the meaning of the art of nursing within the Florence Nightingale school of thought
- an appreciation of debates about the art and science of nursing in the US context
- an appreciation of emerging ideas about art and science and the relationships between them in the current context of healthcare
- insight into the implications of these ideas for current nursing education, practice and research.

KEY WORDS

Art, science, nursing, gender, aesthetics, enlightenment, contemporary

NURSING: AN ART AND SCIENCE?

What is nursing? Is nursing an art? Is nursing a science? Is nursing both an art and a science? Is nursing neither an art nor a science? Over the years there has been extensive debate in the nursing literature about the art and science of nursing. Why are questions about the nature of nursing posed in these terms? What is it about how knowledge and practices are understood in our society that invites us to ask these questions about nursing? What are the implications of these perceptions for education, practice and research in nursing?

This chapter seeks to explore a number of these questions. It considers some of the history of the development of ideas about modern nursing as an art and a science. More specifically, it examines the division between art and science, and explores the impact that this separation has had upon ideas about nursing.

Two particular developments in the history of nursing ideas are discussed, one stemming from the United Kingdom and the other from the United States. One of these, often described as the Florence Nightingale school of thought, represents the first expression of nursing as an art in modern times. In this development, nursing as an art is conceived of in relation to the character of the nurse and the importance of character training in nursing education programs. The other concerns the development of nursing ideas within the university context of the United States. Of particular note in this discussion are the attempts to construct closed systems of thought through nursing theory development and the production of nursing science. It was in this context that contradictions between nursing as an art and as a science began to be recognised and attempts made to reconcile the two.

The chapter then examines some of the implications of these ideas for nursing in the contemporary context where many of the binary divisions that occurred historically, including those between art and science, are collapsing. It concludes with a discussion of the art and science of nursing within the emerging milieus of healthcare delivery.

WHAT IS AN ART? WHAT IS A SCIENCE?

Many modern ideas about art and science have their origins in the scientific revolution of the seventeenth century and the eighteenth century 'age of reason' that was generated by the philosophical movement known as the French Enlightenment.

The scientific revolution was a quest to understand, control and manipulate nature through rational, empirical means. As Capra pointed out in 1982:

> This development was brought about by revolutionary changes in physics and astronomy, culminating in the achievements of Copernicus, Galileo and Newton. The science of the seventeenth century was based on a new method of inquiry, advocated forcefully by Francis Bacon, which involved the mathematical description of nature and the analytical method of reasoning conceived by the genius of Descartes.
> (Capra 1982:54)

The Enlightenment project had the aim of civilising all—of implementing its ideal of social betterment through the power of reason. It was based on beliefs in the universal superiority of the knowledge and values produced by Western science and culture. Those who believed in the democratic ideals of the Enlightenment sought to perfect humankind through reason and create a better world—a civilised and cultured one aided by the new knowledge produced by science (Parker & Gibbs 1998). Two ways of thinking about art can be linked to the Enlightenment, one concerning the cultural production of knowledge and the other the art of living.

A separation between the arts and the sciences occurred in the educational structures and processes that emerged in the wake of the Enlightenment period and with the rise of modern professions. Knowledge came to be packaged into the two domains of sciences and arts within university faculties, and a division emerged between those who were educated in the sciences and those who were educated in the arts (humanities). Each of these produced different ways of thinking and acting, and different types of knowledge. According to CP Snow (1964), writing of the United Kingdom, scientific training produces 'doers' and training in the arts produces 'thinkers' (intellectuals). He argued that by the 1950s, the science/art professional rift was so deep that the two groups worked completely independently of each other, a trend he saw as potentially dangerous for society.

Another way of thinking about art that emerged out of the Enlightenment concerns the art of living. The search for human perfectibility, which was a major plank of the Enlightenment, became linked to a philosophy of humanism, which, as Nelson (1995:37) points out, 'stresses the centrality of the human subject and sets freedom as the subject's destiny'. The human subject, however, was male, and rationality was understood to be a masculine attribute. The art of living for men was linked to the pursuit of freedom through rationality, as 'doers' and 'thinkers'.

Women were seen as neither free nor rational. They were understood 'as an essential nature defined by purposeful organic functions' (Berriot-Salvadore 1993:387). Medical discourse defined the feminine ideal in terms of natural determinism as 'the mother, the guardian of virtues and eternal values' (Berriot-Salvadore 1993:388). Thus, while men, defined as human subjects, were separated and freed from the constraints of nature via reason and culture, women, defined in relation to nature and the feminine, were not. Nature and culture merged in this understanding of the feminine, and women were defined on natural and moral grounds. Good women exercised their womanly arts and civilised others through the practice of these arts. By and large, women were excluded from education into the professions.

ART, SCIENCE AND MODERN NURSING

The constitution of modern secular professional nursing as it has evolved since the days of Florence Nightingale has been influenced by some of these ideas. Of particular importance to this discussion is how the divisions that occurred between art and science were managed in nursing. These will be considered first in relation to the Florence Nightingale school of thought stemming from Britain and then in relation to university-based nursing in the United States.

The Florence Nightingale school of thought

The Florence Nightingale school of thought developed and was sustained within the nurse training schools that sprang up in hospitals, not only in Britain, but also in Australia, New Zealand and other countries. I argue that within nursing education and practice, nursing as an art was seen to involve the character of the nurse in the exercise of feminine virtues, and the importance of character training in the development of nursing as a female profession/occupation. In this context, science was out of place: the scientific enterprise was a male one and, in the hospital and medical context, belonged to the doctor.

Nursing in nineteenth-century industrial England was regarded as an inferior, undesirable occupation practised by morally suspect women. In *Martin Chuzzlewit*, Dickens epitomised the nineteenth-century English nurse in the character of Mrs Gamp, writing that 'it was difficult to enjoy her company without being conscious of a smell of spirits' (Dickens 1910:312–313). The contrast of Florence Nightingale's work in the Crimea, and the subsequent publicity, brought about her identification in the public mind as a 'ministering angel' (*The Times*, London, 20 November 1854). This image was instrumental in elevating secular nursing to a female vocation based on Enlightenment ideals of the womanly virtues and the exercise of the womanly arts through the care of the sick. Indeed, Florence Nightingale described nursing as 'the finest of the fine arts' (Donahue 1996).

Enormous effort went into the attempts to position nursing as epitomising feminine ideals of the good woman. Nursing transgressed many prevailing ideas about the role of women in society and it was extremely difficult for nursing to gain acceptance as a legitimate and respectable occupation. Mrs Gamp and the 'bad woman' were never far beneath the surface; it is therefore not surprising that Florence Nightingale and her followers placed so much emphasis on ensuring appropriate character formation among nurses in training (Parker 1990).

The first Florence Nightingale training school began at St Thomas's Hospital in London in 1860 and became the model for many training schools in Britain and its overseas territories in the latter half of the nineteenth century (Trembath & Hellier 1987). Student nurses were judged on their qualities of trustworthiness, neatness, quietness, sobriety, honesty and truthfulness (Smith 1982). Additionally, nurses were trained to ensure they did not wish to usurp any of the doctor's functions. Isabella Rathie, the first trained Matron of the Melbourne Hospital, noted, 'we are in a great measure the handmaid of the medical man and our function in this particular is to be obedient in every detail' (Rathie, cited in Trembath & Hellier 1987:19).

Thus, the division between art and science as it was manifest within modern secular professional nursing of the Nightingale school of thought can be described as a gendered division. Nursing as a feminine art was developed through character training that resulted in non-assertiveness, obedience and compliance with medical directives. Specific nursing arts comprised nursing procedures such as bathing, bed-making, positioning patients and comforting techniques. While some science content was included in nursing courses, '[t]here was minimal, if any, application of science content in nursing practice' (Peplau 1988:8). Nor were nurses educated in the arts subjects of the university, which produced the thinkers of society, for that was primarily the sphere of men. Rather, they were instilled with womanly virtues.

Nursing education was a process of systematically inculcating a task orientation and the moulding of a set of appropriate attitudes within hospital training schools to produce nurses who exemplified the feminine ideal. Science belonged to the rational and objective world of men, of which medicine was one domain. Men were subjects (minds), while women were objects (bodies); nurses were therefore not positioned as rational subjects shaping the Enlightenment project and their own destinies, but rather as passive and compliant objects, subservient to medicine.

Hospital-based nurse training lasted for more than 100 years in Australia and much longer in Britain. Many changes occurred over that time, including considerable strengthening of the science content, particularly from the 1950s onwards. However, the gendering of nursing as a feminine art, developed in the restrictive environment of the hospital, placed limitations upon the possibilities for nursing to develop as a modern profession. It also limited the possibilities for nurses to develop knowledge, skills and attitudes in ways that would enable them to act as autonomous subjects. Nevertheless, it equipped them powerfully to work as moral agents engaged in socially significant work and to develop in-depth knowledge of the human condition in sickness and in suffering, albeit in an unarticulated, scientifically untested form.

Nursing in the university

In the United States, a four-year entry-to-practice program had been established within a university by 1919. Within this system, it was possible to ensure the development of knowledge in a systematic and orderly way. By the late 1950s, programs for training nurse scientists had developed in a number of major universities, which stimulated interest in theoretical and scientific bases of practice. These were supported by a huge federal investment in nursing education during the 1960s and early 1970s (Gortner 1983). In the period from the late 1950s to the early 1980s, theories of nursing proliferated as nurse scholars sought to include in the concept of nursing an understanding of biological, behavioural, social and cultural factors in health and illness. Of particular note in this discussion were the attempts made to produce closed systems of thought through nursing theory development and the creation of nursing science.

This scientific orientation in nursing, however, came into conflict with ideas about the art of nursing. These stemmed not only from the Nightingale school of thought, but also from consideration of the art of nursing in relation to humanism and the nature of the human subject, by this time conceived of as including women. It is in this context that most of the debates about the art and science of nursing have occurred.

Nursing as a science

As has already been noted, a significant feature of the modern era has been the rise of professions, each clearly delineated by a separate body of knowledge. In the early modern era, nursing could not be regarded as a profession because it was seen to be subservient to and complicit in the medical tasks of diagnosis and treatment. With the location of nursing education within universities, and with the goal of securing professional status for nurses, a major task was to establish its own scientific base, separate from that of medicine.

One early nursing theorist, Johnson (1961), distinguished medicine from nursing by arguing that while the scientific basis of medical knowledge was biological systems, the scientific basis of nursing was behavioural systems. She proposed a behavioural subsystem model of the person 'with behaviour understood as the sum total of physical, biological and social factors/behaviours' (Parker 1995:334). These ideas were further developed by Roy (1980), who conceived of the person as an open, adaptive system, and nursing as the science and practice of promoting adaptation.

Other theorists, however, argued that these approaches did not sufficiently distinguish nursing from medicine. Like medical knowledge, the knowledge produced through study of systems was overly simplistic and mechanistic. Nursing, by contrast, needed to be conceptualised in broader, more encompassing, terms (e.g. Levine 1971). Ideas about nursing as a holistic science were developed by writers such as Rogers (1970) who conceived of the person as an energy field, coextensive with the environment, identified in terms of unified wholeness, openness, pattern, organisation and sentience.

Other writers further differentiated nursing science from medical science by emphasising the caring function of nursing in opposition to the curative function of medicine. Watson (1985), for example, pulled together two of the central ideas of the modern era by describing nursing as a humanistic science, with caring the central unifying dimension of nursing (Cohen 1991).

Thus, with the shift of nursing education to universities in the United States, strong schools of nursing thought emerged. Each was developed in opposition to medicine, and understood nursing as a behavioural science, a holistic science or a caring science. These conceptual models for nursing practice were the work of a number of nursing intellectuals who had undertaken higher degree work in a range of disciplines, particularly in social sciences and education. Each model was designed to capture the complex dimensions of nursing, although, naturally enough, each one tended to reflect the disciplinary base of its author.

Following the establishment of the basis for nursing science through these models, there were calls to test the models against practical experience and refine them. However, progress was slow, as Flaskerud and Halloran pointed out in 1980, and Fawcett in 1984. There was also concern that the proliferation of models would weaken the claims of nursing to be seen as a profession based in a single unique body of knowledge. Fawcett made the point that '[t]he discipline of nursing will advance only through continuous and systematic development and testing of nursing knowledge' (Fawcett 1984:84). Nursing authors sought to concentrate on the common ground in nursing conceptual models. Fawcett, for example, proposed a 'metaparadigm' (an explanatory framework) for nursing built on the central concepts of the discipline—person, environment, health and nursing—and attempts were made to further unify nursing knowledge around these concepts.

Many nurses, however, rejected nursing theories altogether as a means of establishing a science base for nursing. Nursing administrators and clinicians were particularly vocal in their rejection following frustrating experiences of trying to implement them in practice. Nursing theories were seen to reinforce the splits between the theory and practice of nursing, between the education students received and the realities of healthcare service provision, and between nursing thinkers (academics in universities) and nursing doers (nursing administrators and clinicians). In their attempts to develop nursing science through the advancement of nursing theory, nursing theorists, not surprisingly, replicated the binary modes of thought and the dividing practices of the general society.

While nursing theory was being developed, attempts were also being made to construct nursing science knowledge in ways that were linked more closely to practice. The nursing diagnosis movement attracted strong support following the first national conference on the classification of nursing diagnosis held in Missouri in 1973. Nursing diagnosis was developed to identify and classify the phenomena of nursing, to develop a common language for nursing and to facilitate the development and testing of nursing concepts and techniques. However, by 1983, the first broadscoped critical rejection of nursing diagnosis emerged (Kritek 1985).

This more practice-focused approach to developing nursing science suffered from the same fundamental problem as the theory-based approach. Once again, nursing was attempting to develop its science in opposition to medicine by identifying a discipline-specific scientific knowledge base that would legitimate nursing's claims as a separate profession. In doing this, nursing opened itself to some of the same type of critiques that were made of medicine. The creation of a dedicated nursing language separated nursing not only from medicine but also, more importantly, from patients. When viewed through the nursing diagnosis lens, the patients were reduced to objects of nursing diagnoses and treatments, a positioning that was in opposition to nursing's understanding of the patient as a holistic subject.

Two broad approaches to the development of nursing science have been identified: one that focused on defining the domain of nursing theoretically and then testing propositions empirically; and another that focused on the phenomena of nursing practice and on developing ways of defining and classifying them. Both approaches were consistent with prevailing philosophies of science. Neither appears to have been successful in providing a discipline-specific body of knowledge that would justify nursing's claims to professional autonomy and power.

Nursing as an art

Nursing's power seems to rest more in its moral claims than in its science base. Ideas that stem from the Nightingale school about the nature of nursing art as an expression of the essential goodness of feminine virtues persist in contemporary nursing practice. Peplau (1988), writing about the United States but presenting a view widely held internationally, points out that nursing has been called the conscience of the healthcare system, which 'suggests that nurses are major keepers of the morality, goodness, honesty, and ethics of client care' (Peplau 1988:9).

This positioning of nurses on the moral high ground in the battlefield of healthcare provision has been sustained by beliefs that nurses exemplify feminine ideals, and appears to have wide community support. It points to an ongoing belief in the Nightingale legacy that presents nurses as good women. It also suggests that nurses and nursing organisations recognise and exploit the ways in which this characterisation of nursing serves wider political agendas and social functions. Additionally, it supports the idea of nursing as a caring and holistic art that sets itself in opposition to the rationality and reductive practices of scientific medicine and healthcare organisation. As Tanya Buchanan (1999) noted, the 'Nightingale discourse generates myths about nursing that … appear to be eternal truths. We need to see past it' (Buchanan 1999:30).

And indeed, ideas that the art of nursing stems from essential female virtues have been challenged within the university setting. The essence of nursing has been claimed to lie in its humanistic philosophy and the artistic practice that flows from this philosophy. In a much-quoted paper, Munhall (1982) argued that nursing has identified itself as a humanistic discipline, adhering to a basic philosophy 'that focuses on individuality and the belief that the actions of men [sic] are in some sense free' (Munhall 1982:176).

Munhall focused attention on the extent to which university-based nursing education in the United States moved away from the Nightingale school of nursing thought based on female character training, and drew more upon a precisely set out philosophy of the discipline to provide the basis for artistic practice. However, this placed nursing philosophy in opposition to prevailing notions of nursing science. As Munhall pointed out, because nursing subscribed to a humanistic philosophy as well as a scientific research orientation, 'incongruities, paradoxes, and conflicting ideologies' (Munhall 1982:176) resulted between philosophy and research.

Munhall also drew attention to the attempts made within nursing education to accommodate both a scientific and a humanistic (arts) orientation. This suggests that professional university-based nursing education in the United States attempted to bridge the divide between the sciences and the arts that had been identified by CP Snow (1964) in the British higher education context. Nursing in the university aimed to produce practitioners who were both scientists in orientation and humanists in practice.

However, in educational preparation, the aims and scope of scientific and arts training differ significantly, and the transfer of both scientific and humanistic orientations to the realities of practice is a complex process.

Many writers have noted that the differing orientations of art and science have resulted in problems for nursing practice. Peplau (1988), for example, pointed out that science and art are both essential for excellence in the performance of nursing's mission, but indicates the difficulty for a discipline of accommodating these two forms of professional behaviour:

> Combining both the art and science of nursing, seeing and bringing to bear the distinctive characteristics of each form and of the relation between them, imposes a complexity in professional nursing that virtually defies description.
> (Peplau 1988:9)

Holden (1991), an Australian nurse, argued that the split between the arts and the sciences seriously complicates the notion of nursing. She pointed out that the caring role in nursing constrains nursing into the domain of the arts, while nursing that embraces high technology pushes into the domain of science. Jennings (1986) suggested that it is not a matter of choosing either art or science, but rather skilfully blending both for the betterment of nursing.

Peplau (1988) supported Jennings' view, pointing out that both science and art come together in practice, so that:

> There is surely a seamless quality, a graceful and delicately balanced movement, between art and science portrayed by experienced expert nurses that transcends as it uses the differences between these forms.
> (Peplau 1988:14)

She suggested further that this transcending of the differing forms of art and science enables nursing to be practised not only as a helping art, but also as 'an enabling, empowering or transforming art'. People, she noted, 'are touched (literally and figuratively) and sometimes changed at a very personal level by the art nurses practice' (Peplau 1988:9).

The aesthetic dimension—the creative expression—of nursing has received increasing attention over the last few decades. It has built particularly upon the work of Carper who noted in 1978 that the primary emphasis in the professional literature of the time was being placed on the development of the science of nursing. She pointed out:

> There is, nonetheless, what might be described as a tacit admission that nursing is, at least in part, an art. Not much effort is made to elaborate or to make explicit this aesthetic pattern of knowing in nursing—other than to vaguely associate the 'art' with the general category of manual and/or technical skills involved in nursing practice.
> (Carper 1978:16)

Chinn and Watson (1994) have been very influential in further developing ideas about aesthetics and nursing, drawing upon notions of nursing as a caring science.

Subsequently, Chinn et al (1997) described the development of aesthetic inquiry in nursing and the conceptualisation that has emerged is of nursing as an art form. Further work along these lines was undertaken by Johnson who conducted a philosophical analysis of conceptualisations of nursing art as a means of contributing to debate on the specific abilities required for artistic creation in nursing (Johnson 1993, 1994, 1996).

Despite these developments, other writers (e.g. Darbyshire 1994a, 1994b, Lafferty 1997) have suggested that science content is still emphasised in nursing curricula at the expense of humanities content, and, as a result, humanistic aspects of care believed to be essential to the artistic component of nursing are not being addressed sufficiently. Lafferty argued that nursing's dual identity as an art and a science requires a balance and calls for the promotion and acquisition of aesthetic knowledge by nursing students. She suggests that studying literature is a way of fostering this. Darbyshire makes a similar point, arguing that nursing as an art and a science is in danger of becoming a cliché unless attempts are made to reverse the marginalisation of arts and humanities within nursing curricula.

It can be seen that nursing as a contemporary secular profession has developed out of ideas about the essential nature of women, wherein nursing has been regarded as an art practised by virtuous women. This essentialist notion of nursing as a gender-based art may help account for the continuing failure to attract equal numbers of men into nursing. This view has also resulted in nurses sometimes regarding themselves, and being regarded by others, as the conscience of the healthcare system. Nursing as a gendered art is a continuing thread in professional nursing.

However, this notion was challenged significantly by the shift of nursing education into universities in the United States and by the attempts that have been made to discuss nursing as a science and a humanistic art. The literature explored indicates that nursing lies somewhat uneasily in the domains of both science and art, a division that stemmed from dividing practices in the cultural production of knowledge. Nursing developments, too, have replicated many of these dividing practices.

Nursing and contemporary healthcare

Many of the old divisions of the modern era are collapsing in both contemporary higher education and the health sector. This is certainly true in Australia, with implications for practices that sustained the conceptual, methodological and practical separations between art and science in nursing. The clear division between arts and sciences in higher education that reinforced the arts/sciences divide in knowledge development and the professions is clearly breaking down. It is becoming less possible for professions to define themselves in relation to discrete bodies of discipline-specific knowledge. The continuing knowledge explosion, together with the information technologies now available, are resulting in new fields of scientific enquiry and the proliferation of new professions that draw upon knowledge from a range of sources.

The nexus between professional knowledge and power is being subverted in a number of ways, not least through the processes of mass higher education and the access consumers now have to information that enables them to make their own decisions, independently of professional advice. These changes are taking place in a wider context in which global market influences are strengthening and humanist principles are weakening. This is an era of market contestability, privatisation, accountability and competition. It is an era in which performance is measured and evaluated on the basis of outcomes.

The 'reinvention' of nursing

The healthcare sector has been rapidly transforming in response to demands for identifiable, quantifiable indicators of cost-effective quality outcomes. Clinical areas have been responding to the changes wrought in diagnosis and treatment through the use of new investigative and surgical technologies. Nursing, like many other professions, has been seeking to 'reinvent' itself to meet emerging challenges (Parker & Rickard 1999).

The reinvention of nursing, I would suggest, has been occurring on several fronts, all of which have implications for the art and science of nursing. Measures undertaken in nursing education, research and practice are ensuring that nurses have the necessary repertoire of knowledge and skills to play a part in the transformations aimed at cost-effective quality outcomes of healthcare (Parker 2001). Efforts are being made to identify the nursing practices that positively influence health outcomes (Hinshaw 2000) and to develop, test and apply new practice interventions (Aranda 2008). Nurses are investigating traditional nursing practices to determine both their continuing appropriateness and the skill level necessary for their implementation.

Competencies for general, specialist and advanced practice are being refined to ensure greater accountability in relation to consumers, within the profession, in relation to other health professionals, and with regard to various contexts of practice (Australian Nursing and Midwifery Council 2010). Nurses, in collaboration with other health professionals, are also contributing to the development, testing, implementation and evaluation of standardised clinical pathways. They are developing evidence-based nursing practices and contributing to progress in evidence-based healthcare (Fineout-Overholt & Johnston 2007, Pape 2003, Parker 2002, Parker et al 2000). They are working with consumers of health services to satisfy their learning needs.

What is becoming clear in this aspect of its reinvention is that nursing is shifting away from attempts to define itself as an autonomous profession with its own discipline-specific body of nursing science knowledge. As it moves into an interdisciplinary, team-based and consumer-oriented approach to practice and research, it is drawing upon current science/technology and information systems, and focusing upon nursing contributions to health outcomes and accountability for practices.

Nurses today need to draw substantially upon scientific knowledge to inform their practice, and scientific training needs to be a significant component of nursing education programs. At the same time, nurses can contribute to the development of scientific knowledge in interdisciplinary and nursing-specific research projects. Questions for—and about—nursing emerge out of what nurses ask about their practices and the people and communities that they serve.

But how is the art of nursing manifest in this reinvention of the discipline? In a multitude of ways, I would suggest. We live today in an era of diversity, multiplicity and hybrid practices. Nursing can be practised as a gendered art; as a humanistic, aesthetic endeavour; and it can take fragments from both of these traditions and draw upon others as well. It can take up aspects of traditional art forms such as music, movement and touch, and incorporate them in diverse ways into repertoires of skilful practice.

In all of the multiplicity that is the art of nursing there is, however, a continuing thread, expressed as support of the sense of wholeness and integrity of individuals and communities rendered vulnerable through sickness and suffering.

CONCLUSION

In the current climate, many nurses are expressing reservations about the market-driven approach and the economic ethic that underlie contemporary health reforms. They are worried that standardised approaches to care will compromise their ability to meet the demands of particular and unique situations. They are troubled that the increasing rationalisation of health services is causing fragmentation of services, despite the rhetoric of continuity of care. They are concerned that greater reliance upon advanced technologies is resulting in delivery of dehumanised services.

It is important that compliance with current healthcare reforms and resistance to them are not seen to be mutually exclusive endeavours. We can no longer think about the art and science of nursing as mutually exclusive endeavours. We can no longer claim that nursing is a holistic and artistic enterprise with humanistic and expressive concerns developed in opposition to the scientific, technical and instrumental dimensions of care (Parker 1995). The therapeutic tools and technologies of care we use are not separate from us: they are part of us and we are part of them. As they change, so we change. As we change, they change too. They are integral to our self-expression as nurses. The art of nursing, then, involves the perception and understanding of the inseparability of expression and technology.

Working within the framework of a standardised pathway does not prevent a nurse from recognising the individual and unique needs of particular patients. An aesthetic sensibility recognises the extent to which there is congruence between the standard (form) and the individual (content). Aesthetic integrity is responsive nursing in which standard and individual, form and content, become shaped into wholeness. An aesthetic sensibility facilitates expression of the art of nursing as part of the complex, ambiguous and technologically expressive milieus in which nurses work. An aesthetic sensibility is responsive to unified experiences for both recipients and providers of healthcare. It resists fragmented experience and can also 'empower people who are … sick, weak, vulnerable or disturbed to demand that attention is given to the particularities, complexities and ambiguities of their individual situation' (Parker 1995:2).

Nursing as art and/or science has been addressed somewhat differently at different times and in different contexts. A continuing thread nonetheless exists, which demonstrates the significance that nursing has given as a discipline and a profession to both science and art, and the nature of their relationship in nursing. Modern secular professional nursing since its beginnings in the nineteenth century has been and continues to be a complex set of practices that contains many anomalies and contradictions. The art and science of nursing manifests itself within a broader and changing social, cultural and political agenda. Nursing's social mandate acknowledges the art and science of nursing. The challenge for nurses in the contemporary healthcare context is to exercise that mandate judiciously and creatively.

REFLECTIVE QUESTIONS

1　What do you think are the main reasons nursing has come to be viewed as an art?
2　Why has nursing made consistent attempts to align itself with science?
3　How do you think the art and science of nursing can interrelate in the current contexts of healthcare?

RECOMMENDED READINGS

Carper B 1978 Fundamental patterns of knowing in nursing. Advances in Nursing Science 1:13–23

Chinn P L, Maeve M K, Bostick C 1997 Aesthetic inquiry and the art of nursing. Scholarly Inquiry for Nursing Practice 11(2):83–100

Johnson J L 1996 The perceptual aspect of nursing art: sources of accord and discord. Scholarly Inquiry for Nursing Practice: An International Journal 10(4):307–327

Peplau H E 1988 The art and science of nursing: similarities, differences, and relations. Nursing Science Quarterly 1(1):8–15

REFERENCES

Aranda S 2008 Designing nursing interventions. Collegian 15:19–25

Australian Nursing and Midwifery Council (ANMC) 2010 National competency standards for the registered nurse. ANMC, Canberra

Berriot-Salvadore E 1993 The discourse of medicine and science. In: Davis N Z, Farge A (eds) A history of women in the West: Vol. 3. Renaissance and enlightenment paradoxes. Belknap Press, Cambridge, Massachusetts

Buchanan T 1999 Nightingalism: haunting nursing history. Collegian 6(1):28–33

Capra F 1982 The turning point: science, society and the rising culture. Simon & Schuster, New York

Carper B 1978 Fundamental patterns of knowing in nursing. Advances in Nursing Science 1:13–23

Chinn P L, Maeve M K, Bostick C 1997 Aesthetic inquiry and the art of nursing. Scholarly Inquiry for Nursing Practice 11(2):83–100

Chinn P L, Watson J (eds) 1994 Art and aesthetics in nursing. National League for Nursing, New York

Cohen J S 1991 Two portraits of caring: a comparison of the artists, Leininger and Watson. Journal of Advanced Nursing 16:899–909

Darbyshire P 1994a Understanding caring through arts and humanities: a medical/nursing humanities approach to promoting alternative experiences of thinking and learning. Journal of Advanced Nursing 19(5):856–863

Darbyshire P 1994b Understanding the life of illness: learning through the art of Frida Kahlo. Advances in Nursing Science 17(1):51–59

Dickens C 1910 Martin Chuzzlewit. Macmillan, New York

Donahue P 1996 Nursing: the finest art. Mosby, St Louis

Fawcett J 1984 The metaparadigm of nursing: present status and future refinements. Image: Journal of Nursing Scholarship XVI(3):84–89

Fineout-Overholt E, Johnston L 2007 Evaluation: an essential step to the EBP process. Worldviews on Evidence-Based Nursing First Quarter:54–59

Flaskerud J H, Halloran E J 1980 Areas of agreement in nursing theory development. Advances in Nursing Science 3(1):1–7

Gortner S R 1983 The history and philosophy of nursing science and research. Advances in Nursing Science January:1–8

Hinshaw A 2000 Nursing knowledge for the 21st century: opportunities and challenges. Journal of Nursing Scholarship 32:117–123

Holden R J 1991 In defence of Cartesian dualism and the hermeneutic horizon. Journal of Advanced Nursing 16(11):1375–1381

Jennings B M 1986 Nursing science: more promise than threat. Journal of Advanced Nursing 11(5):505–511

Johnson D E 1961 The behavioural system model for nursing. In: Riehl J P, Roy C (eds) Conceptual models for nursing practice, 2nd edn. Appleton Century Crofts, New York

Johnson J L 1993 Toward a clearer understanding of the art of nursing. Unpublished doctoral dissertation. University of Alberta, Edmonton

Johnson J L 1994 A dialectical examination of nursing art. Advances in Nursing Science 1(1):1–14

Johnson J L 1996 The perceptual aspect of nursing art: sources of accord and discord. Scholarly Inquiry for Nursing Practice: An International Journal 10(4):307–327

Kritek P B 1985 Nursing diagnosis in perspective: response to a critique. Image: Journal of Nursing Scholarship 17(1):3–8

Lafferty P M 1997 Balancing the curriculum: promoting aesthetic knowledge in nursing. Nurse Education Today 17:281–286

Levine M 1971 Holistic nursing. Nursing Clinics of North America 6(2):253–263

Munhall P L 1982 Nursing philosophy and nursing research: in apposition or opposition? Nursing Research 31:176–177, 181

Nelson S 1995 Humanism in nursing: the emergence of light. Nursing Inquiry 2(1):36–43

Pape T M 2003 Evidence based nursing practice: to infinity and beyond. Journal of Continuing Education in Nursing 34(4):154–161

Parker J 1990 Professional nursing education in the university context. Meredith Memorial Lecture, La Trobe University, Melbourne

Parker J 1995 Searching for the body in nursing. In: Gray G, Pratt R (eds) Scholarship in the discipline of nursing. Churchill Livingstone, Melbourne

Parker J 2001 The implications of international health policy trends on nursing education: an Australian perspective. Policy, Politics, and Nursing Practice 2(2):142–148

Parker J 2002 Evidence based nursing: a defence (editorial). Nursing Inquiry 9(3):139–140

Parker J, Gibbs M 1998 Truth, virtue and beauty: midwifery and philosophy. Nursing Inquiry 5(3):146–153

Parker J, Johnston L, Faulkner R 2000 Evidence-based nursing: integrating research into practice. In: Greenwood J (ed) Nursing theory in Australia: development and application, 2nd edn. Prentice Hall, Sydney, pp 396–412

Parker J, Rickard G 1999 Nursing town and nursing gown: time, space and the reinvention of nursing through collaboration. Clinical Excellence for Nurse Practitioners 3(1):36–42

Peplau H E 1988 The art and science of nursing: similarities, differences, and relations. Nursing Science Quarterly 1(1):8–15

Rogers M 1970 Theoretical basis of nursing. FA Davis, Philadelphia

Roy C 1980 The Roy adaptation model. In: Riehl J, Roy C (eds) Conceptual models for nursing practice. Appleton Century Crofts, New York

Smith F B 1982 Florence Nightingale, reputation and power. Croom Helm, London

Snow C P 1964 The two cultures: and a second look. New American Library, New York

Trembath R, Hellier D 1987 All care and responsibility: a history of nursing in Victoria 1850–1934. Florence Nightingale Committee, Australia, Melbourne

Watson J 1985 Nursing: human science and human care. Appleton Century Crofts, Norwalk, Connecticut

Heroines, hookers and harridans: exploring popular images and representations of nurses and nursing

Philip Darbyshire

LEARNING OBJECTIVES

After reading this chapter, students will be able to:

- explain the importance of nursing's image for contemporary nursing
- describe the various prevalent stereotypes of the nurse and nursing, and try to explain the persistence of these
- debate the issue of whether nurses should abandon the 'overworked angel' image and suggest what should take its place
- explain the difficulties involved in proposing a 'realistic' or 'truthful' portrayal of nurses and nursing
- explore the UK media coverage of 'bad nursing' and the 'crisis in nursing'; and discuss how nursing should respond to such criticisms
- propose a strategy or small-scale project that could help promote alternative media representations of nurses and nursing.

KEY WORDS

Images, iconography, media, stereotypes, portrayal, mythical, realism, 'crisis in nursing'

INTRODUCTION

Since the mid-1970s, there has been a burgeoning interest in the study of popular images of nurses and nursing; it seems that every conceivable aspect of the image of nurses has been scrutinised. Writers have focused on images of nurses and nursing on television (Anonymous 2003, Buresh & Gordon 1995, Holmes 1997, Kalisch et al 1983, Lenzer 2003), in cinema (Darbyshire 1995, Fiedler 1988, Jones 1988, Kalisch & Kalisch 1983c, Kalisch et al 1982), in novels and short stories (Hunter 1988, Jones 1988, Summers 1997), in news coverage (Berry 2004, Delacour 1991, Doolan 2000, Dunn 1985, Ferns & Chojnacka 2005, Kalisch & Kalisch 1984, Mason 2002, Takase et al 2002), in advertisements (Lusk 2000, Regan 2005), in greeting cards (Smith 2003), on the internet (Kalisch et al 2007) and even in YouTube (Kelly et al 2012). Why such fascination with the image of nurses? With the possible exception of doctors, why is there no comparable body of inquiry literature regarding the image of teachers, social workers, physiotherapists, accountants, occupational therapists or other professional groups?

In this chapter, I will explore some of the early history and iconography of nurses and nursing in order to clarify the origins of many of the issues and 'images of nursing' which are so hotly contested and debated today. The 'so what?' question is important here. Why, when there are so many other pressing issues and concerns facing nursing and healthcare, should we worry about nursing's image? At one fundamental level, this matters because how we see and understand ourselves as nurses impacts on how we think and work as nurses (Takase et al 2002, 2006) and sets up expectations among the public as to how nurses will treat them. Furthermore, understanding how and why nursing's image has been shaped and formed helps us understand vital lessons about how the world works. Delacour argues that:

> Certainly it is important that we analyse the process through which dysfunctional images and discourses are maintained. Moreover, it is useful to regard reading media as a politically situated and critical activity for the nursing profession.
> (*Delacour 1991:413*)

Developing a critical and questioning view of our historical and contemporary representations is thus important for every nurse's personal and professional development. What we should strive for is to move beyond a 'knee-jerk' response that this or that image is good or bad, and to develop the critical thinking and analytical qualities that help us understand the production, meaning(s) and possible effects of popular images of the nurse and nursing.

Perhaps of even greater concern is that in so many media 'medical shows' and stories, nurses and an informed, valuable nursing voice is airbrushed out. As the Kaiser Family Foundation report, 'As seen on TV: health policy issues in TV's medical dramas', from the United States showed:

> … the shows portrayed doctors as dominating discussions around health policy issues. Nurses, social workers, and other members of the health care team hardly existed in policy scenes.
> (*www.kff.org/entmedia/John_Q_Report.pdf, pp 27–28*)

NURSING'S EARLY ICONOGRAPHY

Representations and images of nursing are as old as nursing and healing themselves. By tracing the origins of modern nursing back to antiquity and to the earliest accounts of babies, pregnant women, family and other members of early communities being cared for, usually by women, we can see that 'the nurse as saintly domestic is no modern invention' (Kampen 1988). The earliest Greco–Roman depictions were almost entirely of 'baby nurses' and the image of the 'modern' nurse as tender of the sick or wounded was not to appear until the fourteenth century (Kampen 1988).

With the emergence of religious orders and associated charitable services came a new iconography of nursing which showed women extending their care practices from the immediate household and family arena to the care of strangers. This was not always welcomed, however, and the Middle Ages in Europe especially saw the slaughter of many 'wise women' who were burnt as witches (Darbyshire 1985). Commenting on fifteenth-century depictions of 'nurses' working with the sick, Kampen makes the significant observation that:

> Several features common to scenes of nursing sisters help to define the nature of their role: they nurse patients who are most often men lying in bed, they work in a distinctive location that does not look like a house, they wear distinctive costumes, their activities are domestic and religious rather than specifically medical, and most important, they are never subordinated to patients and doctors.
> (Kampen 1988:23)

It is salutary to think that, with the exception of the last phrase, this description would have fitted any typical Victorian infirmary almost 500 years later. So powerful is this depiction of nurses as tenders of the prostrate sick, reinforced no doubt by the iconographic imagery of Florence Nightingale wending her ethereal way through the wards of Scutari Hospital during the Crimean War, that nursing has often been seen in the public mind as being exclusively focused on this particular form of acute care nursing. McCoppin and Gardner (1994) noted how this one-dimensional view of nursing and nurses can occlude the view of all other forms and areas of nursing, which can somehow be deemed to be 'less than' or 'other than' 'real nursing', which of course was deemed to be practised exclusively at the bedsides of sick people:

> The stereotypical view of nurses as working only in acute care, high technology areas often portrayed in the media makes it very difficult to provide the alternative view of nurses working within the community which is more difficult to make 'attention grabbing'.
> (McCoppin & Gardner 1994:156)

It is not only the various forms of community nursing which may be seen as less than 'real nursing', but also the myriad other 'nursings', such as working in mental health, health promotion, school nursing, working with people with learning/intellectual disabilities and many others. This masking of what, even in 1985, was more than half of the whole nursing workforce (Dunn 1985) is significant as it can help narrow and restrict students' and other nurses' perceptions of what nursing fundamentally 'is'. For example, in Kiger's study of student nurses in Scotland, she found that: 'The picture of adult medical-surgical nursing as typical of real nursing persisted throughout [the students' concept of] working with people' (Kiger 1993).

The 'real nurse as general nurse' is, however, only one of many distortions and misrepresentations that have plagued nursing since its inception. Why nursing should be such a fertile ground for image construction and manipulation is a hugely complex issue and one that has been discussed and argued over many years. One way of beginning to understand the heady brew of images, social constructions, myths and contradictions and 'realities' which form the image(s) of nurses and nursing is to look more carefully at the persistence and power of the major stereotypes of nurses which still exist in either blatant or more subtle forms even today.

NURSING'S STEREOTYPES

Perhaps it could be considered something of a backhanded compliment that there are so many stereotypes associated with nursing. At least we are not seen as bland and instantly forgettable! Major stereotypes can, however, be so unrelentingly negative in their connotations and so wholly untenable in their relationship to any notion of a 'reality' of nursing. (This notion of a single nursing reality is itself contentious and I shall return to this later.) The problem with any stereotype is that it can become so pervasive that its effects become more than merely an annoyance. As Delacour observes:

> ... even stereotypes regarded as dubious may, after a measure of exposure, become internalized and naturalized, they are thereby metamorphosed into categories of the normal, the real, and the healthy and desirable.
> (Delacour 1991:413)

If the sole problem with nursing stereotypes was just that some get-well cards, tabloid newspaper stories or 'X-rated' films portrayed nurses as oversexualised bimbos, then perhaps we could laugh it off, but when the effects of stereotyping are more serious, then there is more at stake than nursing's collective need to 'lighten up'.

The images and perceptions of nursing, both within the profession and in society in general, are important for several reasons. We live in an era where image and the marketing of image has never been more important, and while we can certainly maintain that the 'core business' of nursing is caring for the health and wellbeing of people, we would be foolish to ignore the importance of nursing's image. If we are to attract creative, committed, intelligent and passionate people into nursing, then nursing needs to be seen as every bit as worthwhile and challenging a career as any other in the fields of healthcare or social service. The persistence of hackneyed old stereotypes does nothing to enhance the attractiveness of nursing as a career.

Muff (1982:211) has suggested six 'major nursing stereotypes': angel of mercy, hand-maiden to the physician, woman in white, sex symbol/idiot, battleaxe and torturer. Dunn (1985:2) credits the average tabloid newspaper with even less imagination, being interested in only three types of nurse: angel, battleaxe and nymphomaniac.

Angels with pretty faces

If nursing iconography has an enduring stereotypical image, it must surely be the nurse as 'angel' (Gordon & Nelson 2005). While much of the earliest artwork and imagery of nurses showed nurses ministering to the sick in various quasi-religious ways and settings, nurses in Australia, even in the late 1800s, were 'redefining the image of nurses as motivated primarily by self-sacrifice' (Bashford 1997). However, it was Florence Nightingale's story that captured the public imagination and stimu-lated a swathe of hagiographic accounts (which critic Leslie Fiedler called 'shameless schlock' (Fiedler 1988:103)) and movies such as *The White Angel* and *The Lady with the Lamp* (Jones 1988, Kalisch & Kalisch 1983b). So powerful were these images of the angelic presence which lit up the wards of Scutari with her lamp, that Florence Nightingale has become easily identified as the soul or spirit of nursing and as the embodiment of selfless, devoted, compassionate care that borders on the saintly. Despite some of the more critical and balanced scholarship concerning the life and work of Florence Nightingale (e.g. Hektor 1994), the stereotype of the nurse as selfless angel is still prevalent, especially in the public imagination.

There are several difficulties here. At first glance it may seem no bad thing to think that society views nurses as 'angels'. Who wouldn't like to be thought of in such a 'positive' light? Which nurse would not like to think that she was capable of such profound caring, which could earn such adoration? Is this not just being held in high regard by society? Don't we feel good when opinion polls put nurses near the top of the list for perceived honesty, trustworthiness and hard work? Salvage (1983) perceptively pointed out that nurses often collude in sustaining the 'selfless angel' stereotype while professing to scorn it. As she noted, 'The trouble is we are secretly flattered by the myths, especially those emphasising dedication and high-minded self-sacrifice' (Salvage 1983:14).

However, buying into the 'angels' stereotype may be a Faustian bargain, for there is a price to pay for this. 'Angels' may be saintly, but such perfection is impossible for mere mortal nurses to achieve or maintain; nurses are, after all, only human. Nor do angels seem to require any education or experience; their sanctity is more of a divine gift. For real nurses, however, becoming a skilled and competent nurse is hard work. We may be born with particular dispositions and talents (although some would dispute even this), but we cannot be 'born nurses'. That will take more than an accident of birth. Such shafts of grace as we achieve are often hard won through our sustained engagement in the lives of those people who place their trust in us.

Doctors' handmaidens

If the 'angel' myth is a remnant of nursing's religious order origins, then the unquestioning obedience of the doctor's handmaiden owes much to nursing's military origins. This stereotype touts the image of the nurse as a kind of 'lady in waiting', or the doctor's 'right-hand woman'. For decades this has been a hugely influential media view of nursing. Essentially, the nurse is there to provide faithful and obedient service to the doctor and, like the 'angel' myth, this view has often been sustained by nurses themselves, who were flattered by the idea that 'their' doctors or 'their' consultant says that he or she could not manage without them. In her analysis of the image of nurses in postwar Britain, Hallam (1998) noted also that: 'Within the broadcasting environment, nursing's professional discourse of "service" was interpreted as service to medicine, nurses themselves did little to challenge the picture' (Hallam 1998:37).

In this sense, the 'handmaiden' stereotype may be less mythical than nursing would like to acknowledge. While nationally and internationally particular nurses and nursing projects/initiatives have led healthcare advances (often in collaboration with medical colleagues), there are still many nurses who work with doctors who seem to not recognise nurses' ability and responsibility to make an equal contribution to care, and who assume that the nurse's role is to make coffee, not decisions. Despite claims of teamwork and 'multidisciplinary' cooperation, some nurses continue to work in 'teams' where teamwork is lots of people doing what one person says, and that one person is usually a doctor.

The battleaxe or monstrous figure

For images to be powerful and long lasting they must be capable of being both sustained and subverted. The battleaxe figure is in many ways a magnificent subversion of other stereotypes of the nurse. It is what Hunter (1988) calls, in a slightly different context, the translocated ideal. Where the 'angel' is often portrayed as pretty, feminine, Caucasian, slim, caring, white-clad for purity, fun, deferential and loved by patients, the battleaxe or matron figure was almost the exact opposite—tyrannical, fearsome, asexual, cruel, monstrously large, dark-clad and set on crushing all fun and individuality. On a BBC radio program that I compiled several years ago, I listened to a recording of a 1960s radio quiz show where one of the male panellists joked that the tragedy of nurses is that they were one day destined to become matrons. Matrons, like other nurses who refuse to fit the accepted stereotype of the pretty, kind, compliant nurse, are banished to the moral margins of societal acceptance where they become objects of fear or ridicule.

Think here of 'bad' nurses like Charles Dickens' Sairey Gamp (Summers 1997), Ken Kesey's 'Big Nurse/Nurse Ratched' from One Flew Over the Cuckoo's Nest (Darbyshire 1995), Annie Wilkes from Stephen King's Misery and the more comic figures of Hattie Jacques from the Carry On film series (Ferns & Chojnacka 2005) or Matron Dorothy from Australia's 1990 television series Let the Blood Run Free (Delacour 1991). The 'battleaxe' stereotype cries out for a feminist analysis that reveals the fate of any nurse who does not comply with the mythical norms of the ideal nurse and who challenges male power (usually patients and doctors). Worse than this, perhaps, is that the battleaxe figure is a powerful woman who is unattracted to them (Darbyshire 1995), thus proving that she cannot be a 'real' nurse, as one of the most prevalent and damaging stereotypes is the nurse as an easily available sex bomb.

Naughty nurses and nymphomaniacs

When I was lecturing in Scotland, I would discuss the question of nurses' image with the first-year students who had just begun their course. I asked them what a common reaction would be at a party if they happened to mention that they were nurses. After the laughter and ribaldry had settled, it was clear that a common, if not thankfully universal, reaction from some men was a 'knowing grin' and some suggestion that a night of unbridled sexual abandon might lie ahead. For this reason, many of the students said that they would make up an occupation rather than 'admit' to being a nurse. Why is the 'naughty nurse' stereotype so prevalent? Why are there no 'naughty lawyer' sexual stereotypes? Why are there no pornographic films made about the adventures of a group of occupational therapy students? Why don't sex shops sell physiotherapist uniforms? What is it about nurses that make them such a target?

This is a deep and complex issue, but consider the following points in relation to Hunter's (1988) notion of a 'translocated ideal'. Nursing is utterly implicated in social power relations, between nurses and doctors, nurses and other nurses, nurses and patients, nurses and relatives, and more. When patients enter hospital, the traditional power relations are reversed and they find themselves vulnerable and dependent, rather than strong and in control. At a societal level (for not every male patient will see his situation in this way), one way of redressing this balance is to metaphorically (or perhaps even practically) sexualise the encounters between nurses and patients.

We also know that nurses' practices in relation to patients' bodies are part of this process. Nurses are exceptionally privileged in that we are intimate body workers.

Nurses have access to people's most private body areas and bodily functions (Lawler 1991). One of the most important and demanding practices that a nurse develops is the ability to work with patients' intimate body parts without sexualising the encounter. To transgress this boundary would be both embarrassing and dangerous. In an almost-too-painful-to-watch scene in Dennis Potter's television play, *The Singing Detective*, a nurse has to anoint with cream the genital areas of the hero, 'Philip Marlowe', as he has extremely debilitating psoriasis and cannot do this for himself. As the nurse applies his cream he becomes sexually aroused and despite trying desperately to divert his thoughts, he develops an erection. The nurse, however, wants to get the procedure done and continues creaming, causing him to ejaculate and suffer an agony of humiliation.

Fagin and Diers (1983:117) are clear on the damaging implications of conflating sexualisation and intimate body work: 'Thanks to the worst of this kind of thinking, nursing is a metaphor for sex. Having seen and touched the bodies of strangers, nurses are perceived as willing and able sexual partners.' The 'naughty nurse' stereotype also encourages the subversion of another ideal—that of the saintly purity of the nurse as 'angel'. Beneath the pristine white uniform, tightly bunched and restrained hair and sheepish obedience to authority lies the pornographer's win–win scenario. Either the nurse is *really* a 'sex-bomb' being barely held in check by the rules and regulations of the institution and awaiting the slightest excuse to release all of this pent-up passion, or she *really* is completely subservient to (male) authority, in which case she will willingly agree to every sexual demand. If you think that these scenarios are far-fetched, consider a feature that ran many years ago in the United Kingdom tabloid newspaper, *The Sun*, which aroused furious opposition, and not only from nurses and their organisations. The feature had the headline 'Calling all you naughty nurses' and read:

> Yes, we know you're out there. Lots and lots of people tell stories about those saucy times when temperatures soared in the wards. Who hasn't heard about the time the young nurse turned a bed bath into a saucy romp? And delighted male patients are always revealing how they got some very special medicine from the attractive sister when the screens were drawn. So come on folks. Let's hear from the naughty night nurses—and their happy patients—about the fun times in Britain's hospitals. We're opening our own special phone line between 10 a.m. and 6 p.m. today. Ring the number below and tell us your stories.

Such was the wave of protest from nursing organisations and others that the feature was withdrawn within days. Sadly, such 'saucy nurse' stories remain a staple of tabloid journalism (Ferns & Chojnacka 2005).

NURSING'S IMAGE: BLAME THE MEDIA?

For any nurse who wants to place the blame for the worst excesses and misrepresentations of nursing's image, then the media in general offer a clear, if rather too easy, target. Too easy perhaps because we assume that the media is almost automatically the most pervasive form of image transmission. Yet a study of 1155 people in the United States found that less than 10% of the respondents felt that they obtained their information from the media. Most said that their opinions came from first-hand impressions gained during visits to a hospital (Begany 1994, Delacour 1991).

Delacour (1991:418) makes the important point that often it is not only the ways in which nursing is portrayed but also, more than that, it is that nursing is 'symbolically annihilated by the mass media' and virtually ignored. To test this claim, it would be interesting to keep a local and a national newspaper for a month or two with a view to checking how many health stories included authoritative comments from nurses compared with doctors. Many nurses would say that they could confidently predict the results of such a survey well in advance.

Considerable research has been undertaken into the role of the media in constructing and shaping the image of nursing. In the United States in particular, the team of Philip and Beatrice Kalisch in the 1980s produced numerous books and papers on many different aspects of this question (Kalisch & Kalisch 1983a, 1983c, 1984, 1987, Kalisch et al 1982). Latterly, such concerns about nursing's image has become truly international (Almalki et al 2011, Karanikola et al 2011, Varaei et al 2012, Wilson & Feringa 2011).

A blunderbuss criticism of 'tha meeja' as a 'root of all evil' continues unabated and in the wake of the UK News International 'phone-tapping' scandal that saw the closure of the *News of the World* newspaper, some governments have leapt at the opportunity to impose greater 'regulation' on the press. At a more personal level, Holmes (1997:137), for example, advises that we should (perhaps) give up watching medical 'soaps' on television as they are 'anodyne and legitimating rather than transformative and critical'.

While 'soaps' may well be 'anodyne', there are probably few viewers of *Grey's Anatomy*, *Getting On* or *Nurse Jackie* who bemoan that the show is no longer as 'transformative and critical' as it used to be. Blaming genres for not being what we would wish them to be is surely tilting at windmills. To simply stop watching 'soaps' because we disagree with aspects of their portrayal of nurses and nursing is scarcely a mode of engagement. Nor is it particularly astute to imagine that the media exist to 'accurately' (or should that be positively/flatteringly?) depict nurses and their work. Much as we may dislike the notion, the mass media exists primarily as a profit-making entertainment business. It is not nursing's tame public relations machine, nor do journalists or reporters have an obligation to be nursing's unpaid cheerleaders.

Critics of media portrayals of nurses often seem to misunderstand the different genres of representation. For example, criticising a film like *Carry On Nurse*, or a television series like *Scrubs*, for giving a false image of nurses and nursing makes little sense. These are not documentaries and their purpose was never to represent someone's preferred 'reality of nursing'. They are comedies, and comedy usually has a target. Comedy works by upsetting or translocating our understandings and expectations, in this case of medicine or nursing. Condemning a *Carry On* film for not being a true-to-life account of nursing is like criticising the family car for not being a beautiful mountain.

Stanley's detailed and carefully nuanced analyses of nurses in feature films avoids the simplistic characterisation of portrayals of nurses as being 'good/bad'–'angel/devil' (Stanley 2008, 2012). While a 'blame the media' approach has a seductive simplicity, it is unlikely to achieve any significant results. However, working with the media in order to help create more 'realistic' portrayals of nursing's work has been reported to help (Buresh & Gordon 1995). In the early days of the filming of the medical soap ER, there was virtually no consultation with nurses or ER departments. Emergency room nurses in the United States, however, did more than complain or stop watching—they became proactive and contacted the producers regularly with comments and criticisms, and also with offers of help, storyline ideas and the names of subspecialty ER nurses who were willing to help the show 'get it right'.

NURSING'S IMAGE: DEPICTING 'REALITY'?

In a news report, the warning of Joanne Rule, former head of the RCN (UK) public relations office, was repeated: 'if nursing were to succeed finally in shaking off the "angel" image it so professes to hate, it might be replaced by an image that it hated even more' (Rule 1995). One of the significant difficulties in challenging potentially damaging images of nursing is that it is very difficult to give an agreed account of what a 'good portrayal' should look like. As Bashford noted in her study of how early Australian nurses challenged their systems:

> ... resistance was never straightforward. Often, rather than new discourses offering empowering new subject positions, they produced confusion, contradiction and insecurity. Women were asked to think about their work in religious terms in one moment and in one context, in scientific terms in another, and as a type of professionalism in another.
> (Bashford 1997:74)

This historical dilemma will seem blindingly contemporary to today's nurses who are struggling with very similar issues around nurses' 'expanded role' and what this means for nursing's identity/identities. The other difficulty in looking for a 'realistic' image of nurses is that it would be precious and narcissistic for nursing to adopt a stance that stated that the only acceptable portrayals of nurses and nursing were those that were 'positive'. (And for 'acceptable', ask: Acceptable to whom? To me personally? To nurses at my hospital? To nursing in general?) It would be reassuring to think that nursing was a little more secure in its role and purpose than to require constant flattery from an unrelenting diet of uncritical media comments and compliments. This quest for the 'positive' portrayal of nursing has been questioned by Hallam who argued that:

> This search for a positive image of nursing identity poses two crucial problems. On the one hand, it tends to presume a professional consensus in terms of what this image is or could be ... the positive image approach can also be critiqued from the viewpoint of media reception, it conceptualises readers and viewers as uncritical receivers of messages who unquestioningly digest the authority of the image.
> (Hallam 1998:33)

Similarly, Cheek has observed that 'the task is not to look for real and authentic representations of nursing, but rather to look for the speaking and representation that is done about nursing' (Cheek 1995:239). This is not to say, however, that no 'positive' images and accounts of nurses and nursing can be found. For example, in his account of his serious injury and recovery, surgeon and rehabilitation specialist Tony Moore describes the artistic and technical expertise of the intensive care nurses who gave him a blanket bath:

> They worked like a ballet corps in slow motion, softly moving me forwards, to the side, sponging, touching, towelling with clean tenderness, and when one gently washed my genitals I felt nothing but the compassion of her care.
> (Moore 1991:11)

Richard Selzer was another surgeon who found himself a patient in intensive care following legionnaires' disease. He is hugely embarrassed by his dependency and incontinence, but again, his nurses are memorably skilled in what he calls 'the forgiveness of the flesh' (Selzer 1993). Unlike the unfortunate 'Philip Marlowe' in *The Singing Detective*, Selzer's nurses spare him the embarrassment and pain that could so easily become part of his intimate body care. One nurse who makes such a profound difference to Selzer's care and recovery is Patrick, whom Selzer describes as being 'the sort of nurse who can draw the pus out of a carbuncle with his gaze alone, and turn it into a jewel' (Selzer 1993:56). Selzer is emphatic that the power of skilled nurse caring is not merely 'nice to get', but that it is actually transformative. He describes his being carried back to bed by Patrick following a tub bath as the moment when his 'molecules rearranged themselves'. He says: 'It is the true moment of cure' (Selzer 1993:93). Note, that is cure, not care.

Read these authors' accounts of their care and then consider that bathing patients is deemed by some to be 'basic' nursing care—where for 'basic' read 'unimportant and thus able to be undertaken by virtually anyone'. There are many other 'positive' accounts in literature and popular culture of nurses and nursing which are valued, appreciated and have a markedly beneficial effect on the recipient. However, care is needed not to fall into the trap of 'collecting' these accounts as a kind of trophy for nursing. If we are to cultivate and develop our questioning and critical powers, then the positive accounts also need to be questioned and discussed.

Caring as foundational to nursing can easily be trivialised as being little more than sickly sentimentality with all the substance of a tacky greeting card. Nursing undervalues caring at its peril and society devalues caring every time that it is set up as an *alternative* to attributes such as knowledge, skill, intelligence, creativity, determination, passion and mindfulness. As Rhodes et al (2011) discovered, even relatively inexperienced student nurses seem to almost instinctively value nursing's caring ethos and orientation. Combine this ethos with a recognition of the wide range of additional knowledge, skills, experience and connoisseurship that successful nursing will require and it becomes clear why caring and 'smarts' are never mutually exclusive.

Great nursing is not easy and not everyone who merely 'wants to be a nurse' will be able to achieve this. What can happen when nursing and broader health services collectively 'take their eye off the ball' regarding what is truly vital is that standards of nursing care will suffer. When this happens, no amount of media management or spin will restore a tarnished image. Before considering the profusion of 'bad nursing' and 'nursing crisis' stories that have emerged in the UK media, please listen to the radio broadcast called 'Care to be a nurse?' by Christina Patterson (2012), a journalist and a young woman who has experienced six hospitalisations for surgery related to breast cancer. She has an 'insider view' of current nursing that needs to be listened to, regardless of how uncomfortable it may be to hear of nurses who 'aren't kind' and how:

> I tried to explain what it feels like to be lying in a hospital bed in so much pain you can't even reach out for water, and feel that if you press your buzzer, you're going to make someone cross. I tried to explain what it feels like to hear the groans of people around you whose calls for help aren't being answered. And what it feels like to hear nurses who aren't even trying to whisper complaining about the other patients, and you. I had, I said, and was embarrassed to say this in front of an audience, and embarrassed to talk about losing a breast, never felt so abandoned, or alone. And I said that I thought it was time for nurses to start recognising that they have a choice about whether to do their job badly, or well.
> (*Patterson 2012*)

The 'Crisis in Nursing' in the UK: Exposure or creation of 'bad nursing'?

In the UK in recent years, nursing has experienced an unprecedented level of media attention as part of what has been called by some the 'Crisis in Nursing'. Rule's 'be careful what you wish for' caution mentioned earlier (Rule 1995) may well be nursing's chickens coming home to roost. This media scrutiny has not been the fawning adulation of the 'aren't nurses wonderful' school of sycophancy but rather an unprecedented level and intensity of criticism, not of 'the system', but of individual 'bad nurse' and poor or non-existent nursing care that is being attributed to nurses themselves who 'couldn't care less'. From a time when criticising nurses was akin to kicking Bambi, it now seems to be open season on nurses and nursing.

Newspaper headlines such as 'Nurses denounced as dirty, lazy drunks', 'Many NHS nurses are still the finest in the world. But they let my poor father die like a dog' and 'Nasty nurses? Tell me something new' make for painful reading. As did the 2009 report from the UK Patients Association, detailing families' accounts of wretched care of elderly people in hospital, that began with:

> For far too long now, the Patients Association has been receiving calls on our Helpline from people wanting to talk about the dreadful, neglectful, demeaning, painful and sometimes downright cruel treatment their elderly relatives had experienced at the hands of NHS nurses.
> (*Patients Association* 2009:3)

Public and media reactions to such reports and news stories provided nursing with little comfort. Rather than massive public outrage that nurses and nursing could be described in such terms, it was as if the lid of Pandora's Box had been lifted and everyone who had an experience of poor care or a nursing 'horror story' now had 'permission' to take to the internet or to the newspapers to say what even five years ago would have been unspeakable. However uncomfortable or indeed angry such reports make us feel (and they certainly should), the substantive issues and care concerns that underlie them cannot be brushed aside as media sensationalism or as some kind of conspiracy against nursing. Official nursing organisations were quick to point out that such appalling care or lack of care was not 'the nursing norm'. Absolutely, but this does not obviate the need to understand and rectify such poor nursing. If nursing wants accountability, autonomy and responsibility then we cannot simply blame 'the system' and absolve ourselves of personal and professional responsibility the moment that something goes badly wrong. When I wrote about this issue for an Australian nursing magazine (Darbyshire 2011) in response to the *British Medical Journal*'s editorial, pointedly entitled, 'We need to talk about Nursing' (Delamothe 2011), I received the most feedback and positive commentary I have known in 30 years of writing about nursing. This is an issue that nursing cannot wish away.

NURSING'S IMAGE: FROM AFFRONT TO ACTION

During the past few decades, there has been a plethora of research and discussion regarding nursing's image and portrayals of nursing. We are now much more aware of the forces that shape and maintain many of popular culture's images of nurses and nursing. Perhaps the next few decades will see nurses moving from this position of greater awareness to one of more positive action. By this I mean that it is no longer enough to be outraged at the 'negative images' and stereotypes that we will continue to encounter. Indignation or 'refusing to watch' are not strategies for change. Nor will it be enough to merely call for negative images of nurses to be withdrawn or 'banned'.

The most pressing tasks ahead for nurses and nursing are to use the media in a much more 'streetwise' way than we have in the past (Buresh & Gordon 2006) and to 'raise the bar' for nurses' performance to the point where mediocrity or overt poor care are unacceptable and have definite consequences. As Morris (2010:19) notes in relation to one UK nursing image initiative, there is a clear need to 'manage poorly performing nurses robustly, and to support them constructively either to improve or to leave the profession'. Nursing cannot become a 'job for life' regardless of how it is performed. If we do not like the images that are being presented, then we have a responsibility to provide alternatives. If we think that media reports and stories about nursing are inaccurate or inadequate, then we need to interest the media in alternatives. If we feel that the media completely ignores a particularly important program, service or aspect of nursing, then why not alert them to this and highlight the importance of what it is that they are missing. No media like to feel that they are missing something interesting or important, especially in their local area.

We need to ask tough questions such as: What images would we want to see in the media? How do we base our appeal and image on the power and benefits of skilled, engaged nursing, rather than on a sense of entitlement that the media somehow has an obligation to run 'positive nursing stories'. How can we show the positive power of nursing to local and national media? Why would/should the media be interested in this program/innovation/nursing development? How can we 'sell' this idea or story to them in such a way that they can't ignore it? Whose expertise and support could we call upon to help us do this? (Belcher 2003, Buresh & Gordon 2006, Clark 1989, Monahan 1996, National Nursing and Nursing Education Taskforce 2006, Strasen 1992, Waters 2003).

CONCLUSION

We now know a great deal about representations of nurses and nursing in the various media and popular culture. Lack of knowledge or information is not our big issue. As nurses, our task now is not simply to 'adapt' to, or merely observe and comment on future changes, but also to get out there and make the changes happen.

REFLECTIVE QUESTIONS

1 Discuss with a group of your peers the reactions that you have encountered, both favourable and unfavourable, when you have told people that you are a nurse/student nurse and how you feel about such reactions.

2 Talk with your colleagues about their experiences if they, a friend or a family member has recently been hospitalised or otherwise receiving care from nurses. How do they describe these experiences and this care? What does this say about nursing's image and how we may be perceived by the public?

3 Visit the web's best site for 'Nursing's Image' resources, discussions and campaigns: http://www.truthaboutnursing.org/ and think about how you, your class or your ward/unit could make a contribution.

4 Plan how you would go about creating your own media story about nurses or nursing. What would you choose as the issue? Would it be a nurse-led clinical initiative, an ethical dilemma, a particularly successful patient outcome, an exciting new approach in nursing education or a particular nurse who is doing something really special in an area? How would you go about interesting the media in the story and how would you present it?

5 Read Christina Patterson's various articles on UK Nursing and consider whether these issues 'only affect UK nursing' or whether they may be more universal. (Can be accessed via links at www.independent.co.uk and from this article: http://www.independent.co.uk/life-style/health-and-families/health-news/how-can-a-profession-whose-raison-dtre-is-caring-attract-so-much-criticism-for-its-perceived-callousness-does-nursing-need-to-be-managed-differently-or-is-the-answer-to-develop-a-new-culture-of-compassion-7637490.html)

6 Discuss with peers how nursing should respond to stories and media coverage of 'bad nursing'. Can we defend nursing without being 'defensive'?

7 Visit www.philipdarbyshire.com.au and listen to 'The Professionals', a feature program on nursing's image as portrayed in the BBC Radio archives. Discuss if and how you think nursing would be portrayed differently in the current decade.

RECOMMENDED READINGS

Buresh B, Gordon S 2006 From silence to voice: what nurses know and must communicate to the public. Cornell University Press, New York

Darbyshire P 'The professionals'; nursing as portrayed in the archives of BBC Radio. Online. Available: www.philipdarbyshire.com.au

Davis C, Schaefer J 1995 Between the heartbeats: poetry and prose by nurses. University of Iowa Press, Iowa City

Donahue M P, Donahue P M 1996 Nursing: the finest art. Mosby-Year Book, St Louis

Friedman L 2004 Cultural sutures: medicine and media. Duke University Press, Durham

Gordon S 2005 Nursing against the odds: how health care cost-cutting, media stereotypes, and medical hubris undermine nursing and patient care. Cornell University Press, New York

Gordon S (ed) 2010 When chicken soup isn't enough: stories of nurses standing up for themselves, their patients, and their profession. Cornell University Press, Ithaca, NY

Hallett C, Lynaught J 2010 Celebrating nurses: a visual history. Barron's Educational Series, Hauppauge, NY

Jones A 1988 Images of nurses: perspectives from history, art, and literature. University of Pennsylvania Press, Pennsylvania

Jones C 2012 The American Nurse Project. Online. Available: http://www.welcomebooks.com/americannurse/ and http://americannurseproject.com/

REFERENCES

Almalki M, FitzGerald G, Clark M 2011 The nursing profession in Saudi Arabia: an overview. International Nursing Review 58(3):304–311

Anonymous 2003 American nurses speak out over portrayal in ER. Nursing Standard 18(14–16):5

Bashford A 1997 Starch on the collar and sweat on the brow: self sacrifice and the status of work for nurses. Journal of Australian Studies 52:67–80

Begany T 1994 Your image is brighter than ever. RN 57(10):28–34

Belcher D 2003 Nurses making a difference. Bridging the gap between nurses and the media: the grassroots. Center for Nursing Advocacy. American Journal of Nursing 103(5):130

Berry L 2004 Is image important? Nursing Standard 18(23):14–16

Buresh B, Gordon S 1995 Taking on the TV shows. American Journal of Nursing 95(11):18–20

Buresh B, Gordon S 2006 From silence to voice: what nurses know and must communicate to the public. Cornell University Press, New York

Cheek J 1995 Nurses nursing and representations: an exploration of the effect of viewing positions on the textual portrayal of nursing. Nursing Inquiry 2(4) 235–240

Clark G 1989 To be or not to be: it's time to market nursing's image. In: Gray G, Pratt R (eds) Issues in Australian nursing 2. Churchill Livingstone, Melbourne, pp 175–192

Darbyshire P 1985 Bedpans or broomsticks? Nursing Times 81(Nov 6–12):44–45

Darbyshire P 1995 Reclaiming 'Big Nurse': a feminist critique of Ken Kesey's portrayal of Nurse Ratched in One Flew Over the Cuckoo's Nest. Nursing Inquiry 2(4):198–202

Darbyshire, P 2011 We do, indeed, need to talk about Nursing. Nursing Review 3 August http://www.nursingreview.com.au/pages/section/article.php?s=Features&idArticle=21714 (Available at: http://e2.ma/webview/4qo/81b4efdfa78b70bba3a7106e836cc0aa)

Delacour S 1991 The construction of nursing: ideology discourse and representation. In: Gray G, Pratt R (eds) Towards a discipline of nursing. Churchill Livingstone, Melbourne, pp 413–433

Delamothe, T 2011 We need to talk about nursing. British Medical Journal 342:d3416

Doolan E 2000 Nursing: image politics and the media. British Journal of Perioperative Nursing 10(9):474

Dunn A 1985 Images of nursing in the nursing and popular press. Bulletin of the Royal College of Nursing (UK) History of Nursing Group 6:2–8

Fagin C, Diers D 1983 Nursing as a metaphor. The New England Journal of Medicine 309(2):116–117

Ferns T, Chojnacka I 2005 Angels and swingers, matrons and sinners: nursing stereotypes. British Journal of Nursing 14(19):1028–1032

Fiedler L 1988 Images of the nurse in fiction and popular cultures. In: Jones A (ed) Images of nurses: perspectives from history art and literature. University of Pennsylvania Press, Pennsylvania, pp 100–112

Gordon S, Nelson S 2005 An end to angels. American Journal of Nursing 105(5):62–69

Hallam J 1998 From angels to handmaidens: changing constructions of nursing's public image in post-war Britain. Nursing Inquiry 5(1):32–42

Hektor L 1994 Florence Nightingale and the women's movement: friend or foe? Nursing Inquiry 1:38–45

Holmes C 1997 Why we should wash our hands of medical soaps. Nursing Inquiry 4(2):135–137

Hunter K 1988 Nurses: the satiric image and the translocated ideal. In: Jones A (ed) Images of nurses: perspectives from history, art, and literature. University of Pennsylvania Press, Pennsylvania, pp 113–127

Jones A 1988 Images of nurses: perspectives from history, art, and literature. University of Pennsylvania Press, Pennsylvania

Kalisch B, Kalisch P 1983a An analysis of the impact of authorship on the image of the nurse presented in novels. Research in Nursing and Health 6(1):17–24

Kalisch B, Kalisch P 1983b Anatomy of the image of the nurse: dissonant and ideal models. American Nurses Association Publications G-161 3-23. Online. Available: www.nursingadvocacy.org/images/kalisch/anatomy_of_the_image_of_the_nurse_ocr.pdf 20 Sept 2008

Kalisch B, Kalisch P 1983c Heroine out of focus: media images of Florence Nightingale. Part 1: popular biographies and stage productions. Nursing and Health Care 4(4):181–187

Kalisch B, Kalisch P 1984 An analysis of news coverage of maternal-child nurses. Maternal-Child Nursing Journal 13:77–90

Kalisch B, Kalisch P, McHugh M 1982 The nurse as a sex object in motion pictures. Research in Nursing and Health 5(3):147–154

Kalisch B J, Begeny S, Neumann S 2007 The image of the nurse on the internet. Nursing Outlook 55(4):182–188

Kalisch P, Kalisch B 1987 The changing image of the nurse. Addison Wesley, Menlo Park, California

Kalisch P, Kalisch B, Scobey M 1983 Images of nurses on television. Springer, New York

Kampen N 1988 Florence Nightingale: a prehistory of nursing in painting and sculpture. In: Jones A (ed) Images of nurses: perspectives from history, art, and literature. University of Pennsylvania Press, Pennsylvania, pp 6–39

Karanikola M, Papathanassoglou E, Nicolaou C et al 2011 Greek intensive and emergency care nurses' perception of their public image: a phenomenological approach. Dimensions of Critical Care Nursing, 30(2):108–116.

Kiger A 1993 Accord and discord in students' images of nursing. Journal of Nursing Education 32(7):309–317

Kelly J, Fealy G M, Watson R 2012 The image of you: constructing nursing identities in YouTube. Journal of Advanced Nursing 68(8):1804–1813

Lawler J 1991 Behind the screens: nursing somology and the problem of the body. Churchill Livingstone, Melbourne

Lenzer J 2003 ER blamed for nursing shortage. British Medical Journal 327:1294

Lusk B 2000 Pretty and powerless: nurses in advertisements 1930–1950. Research in Nursing and Health 23(3):229–236

McCoppin B, Gardner H 1994 Tradition and reality: nursing and politics in Australia. Churchill Livingstone, Melbourne

Mason D J 2002 Invisible nurses: media neglect is one cause of the nursing shortage. American Journal of Nursing 102(8):7

Monahan B B 1996 The nurses' media handbook: a reference for nurses planning to meet the media. Massachusetts Nurse 66(5):2,6,12

Moore T 1991 Cry of the damaged man. Picador, Sydney

Morris V 2010 Nursing and nurses: the image and the reality. Nursing Management 17(1):16–19

Muff J 1982 Handmaiden, battle-axe, whore: an exploration of the fantasies, myths and stereotypes about nurses. In: Muff J (ed) Socialization, sexism and stereotyping: women's issues in nursing. Wareland Press, Illinois, pp 113–152

National Nursing and Nursing Education Taskforce 2006 Media and communication principles for nursing and midwifery. Online. Available: www.nnnet.gov.au/downloads/rec9_commprinciples.pdf 10 Sept 2008

Patients Association UK 2009 Patients ... not numbers, People ... not statistics. Online. Available: http://www.patients-association.com/

Patterson C 2011 Care to be a nurse? BBC Radio 4 'Fourthought' Broadcast, April 2011. Online. Available: http://www.bbc.co.uk/iplayer/episode/b010mrzt/Four_Thought_Series_2_Care_to_be_a_nurse/

Patterson C 2012 A crisis in nursing: six operations, six stays in hospital – and six first-hand experiences of the care that doesn't care enough. The Independent, 10 April 2012. Online. Available: http://www.independent.co.uk/voices/commentators/christina-patterson/a-crisis-in-nursing-six-operations-six-stays-in-hospital--and-six-firsthand-experiences-of-the-care-that-doesnt-care-enough-7-628092.html

Regan M 2005 Virgin's nurses and the public image of nursing. Nursing Philosophy 6(3):110–121

Rhodes M K, Morris A H, Lazenby R B 2011 Nursing at its best: competent and caring. OJIN: Online Journal of Issues in Nursing 16(2). Online. Available: http://www.nursingworld.org/MainMenuCategories/ANAMarketplace/ANAPeriodicals/OJIN/TableofContents/Vol-16-2011/No2-May-2011/Articles-Previous-Topics/Nursing-at-its-Best.aspx

Rule J 1995 Nurses may live to regret the 'angel' image era has ended (news item). Nursing Management 2(6):5

Salvage J 1983 Are you in the PINC? Distorted images. Nursing Times 79(1):13–15

Selzer R 1993 Raising the dead: a doctor's encounter with his own mortality. Penguin, Harmondsworth

Smith L 2003 Image counts: greeting cards mail it in when it comes to accurately portraying nurses. Online. Available: http://include.nurse.com/apps/pbcs.dll/article?AID=2003310010351 25 Sept 2008

Stanley D 2008 Celluloid angels: a research study of nurses in feature films. Journal of Advanced Nursing 64(1):84–95

Stanley D 2012 Celluloid devils: a research study of male nurses in feature films. Journal of Advanced Nursing, (E-pub ahead of print) DOI:10.1111/j.1365-2648.2012.05952.x

Strasen L 1992 The image of professional nursing: strategies for action. Lippincott, Philadelphia

Summers A 1997 Sairey Gamp: generating fact from fiction. Nursing Inquiry 4(1):14–18

Takase M, Kershaw E, Burt L 2002 Does public image of nurses matter? Journal of Professional Nursing 18(4):196–205

Takase M, Maude P, Manias E 2006 Impact of the perceived public image of nursing on nurses' work behaviour. Journal of Advanced Nursing 53(3):333–343

Varaei S, Vaismoradi M, Jasper M, Faghihzadeh S 2012 Iranian nurses self-perception – factors influencing nursing image. Journal of Nursing Management 20(4):551–560

Waters A 2003 Image makeover brings in recruits for US nursing. Nursing Standard 17(43):9

Wilson D R, Feringa G 2011 The image of nursing in Botswana. Beginnings 31(2):12–14

CHAPTER 5

Nursing care and nurse caring: issues, concerns, debates

Debra Jackson and Sally Borbasi

LEARNING OBJECTIVES

This chapter will:

- introduce caring as a professional concept that is entwined with understandings about nurses and nursing
- explore caring as a theoretical concept
- discuss perceptions of nurse caring from the perspective of patients/clients
- provide an overview of issues related to care and cure
- critique caring as the basis of the discipline of nursing
- consider threats to nurse caring
- contemplate opportunities for nurse caring.

KEY WORDS

Caring, clinical nursing, cure, work, patients/clients

NURSING AND CARING

The concept of caring is intertwined with nursing—some literature even states that caring and nursing are synonymous (Hayes & Tyler-Ball 2007, Wilkin & Slevin 2004)—and has been identified as central to the theory and practice of nurses (Papastravou et al 2012). For many years, nurse theorists have developed theories of nursing in which caring is positioned as a major foundational element (Leininger 1984, 1986, Watson 1985, Watson et al 2005). Efforts to theorise caring, and understand it as a concept that is able to be compatible with, and integral to, the practice of nursing, have occupied a lot of energy in nursing for a number of years, and continue to attract the attention of nurse scholars from all over the world (e.g. Finfgeld-Connett 2008, Sumner 2008, Papastravou et al 2012). The close relationship of nursing and caring is able to be seen in the many definitions and perspectives of nursing that position caring as inherent and central to the nursing role (e.g. Benner 1984, Leininger 1984, Sumner 2008, Swanson 1993, Watson 1988, Watson et al 2005, Papastravou et al 2012).

Initially, the concept of caring may appear to be simple and uncomplicated, and, indeed, general dictionary definitions of caring define it in simple terms. It is a generic word and one that is widely used in the general lexicon—meaning that it is not 'owned' specifically by nursing, nor does it apply only to nurses and nursing. However, when used in relation to nursing, the concept of care cannot be oversimplified. Terms such as *nursing care* and *nurse caring* carry certain meanings and understandings. In these contexts, care is a complex, multidimensional concept that is positioned as the characteristic that distinguishes nursing, and sets it apart from other health-related activities. Although a caring perspective is not unique to nursing, it is widely accepted that nursing has an essential role to care for the health of individuals, families and communities, and many believe the care given by nurses has the potential to restore health (Benner et al 1999, Watson & Foster 2003).

In this chapter we introduce caring as a professional concept, and acquaint you with some of the major arguments and viewpoints associated with caring in general and nurse caring in particular. In writing this chapter we have drawn on a substantial body of international literature that reflects some of the major perspectives of nurse caring that have been published over the past 20–30 years. It is necessary to cover literature over this long period in order to develop an appreciation of the longitudinal and international nature of the debates and discussions around caring. Furthermore, you will see that many of the issues remain unresolved, and that this is one debate that will continue into (and likely even beyond) your own nursing careers.

CARING AS A THEORETICAL CONCEPT

The complexity around such a seemingly uncomplicated and simple concept such as caring can be seen when one considers the plethora of literature devoted to it. Even a cursory database search on caring will generate copious literature on the subject. Try it! Upon examining this literature you will also see that this is a discussion that has spanned generations of scholars and that each generation builds on the work of previous scholars. You will also see it reveals a multitude of definitions, and various positions on the ways that caring can be conceptualised. Several theories of nursing have been developed from the standpoint of defining and describing caring practices. Leininger (1986) believes caring is the essence of nursing, but dismisses the idea of nurses' care motivated by a sense of duty. Rather, she considers caring as learned because it is an integral part of cultural life. However, factors within various cultures (e.g. gender) may either curtail or facilitate the use of care knowledge by nurses, and many fear that caring—and more especially compassion—are qualities that are fast disappearing in the contemporary healthcare environment.

REFLECTION

Do you agree that caring and compassion are under threat in the contemporary healthcare environment? If you like, visit the UK Health Service Ombudsman's report of the stories of ten people over the age of 65, from all walks of life and from across England. Issues are raised that may be a catalyst for your thinking about this http://www.ombudsman.org.uk/care-and-compassion/introduction

---

Watson (1988), another well-known luminary on the subject, writes of a science (and practice) of caring, and conceptualises caring as the ethical and moral ideal of nursing. In 1990, Rawnsley noted that caring:

> … has been proposed to be a philosophy and science, an ethic, an interactive set of client expectations and nursing behaviours, expert nursing practice, the hidden work of nursing and a synonym for nursing itself.
> (Rawnsley 1990:42)

If we look at feminist and nurse Falk Rafael's (1996:3–17) work, she suggested caring could be considered either 'ordered caring', 'assimilated caring' or 'empowered caring' (p 4). Ordered caring she proposed as problematic for nurses because it is about merely following orders: 'it allows only a severely limited scope of caring, one that is devoid of knowledge, power or ethics' (Falk Rafael 1996:11). To illustrate this point, she draws on the example of the kindness and gentleness shown by nurses towards psychiatric patients as they were led towards the Nazi gas chambers. Assimilated caring was described as a form of caring in which the feminine construct of caring is grounded in (male) scientific discourses. This appropriation of a male construct is proposed as giving legitimacy to the essentially female activity of caring. Falk Rafael positioned empowered caring as the most desirable and effective form of caring. This form of caring, she asserted, was grounded within a feminist perspective, and involves the use of power, knowledge and ethics. Falk Rafael (1996) proposes the acronym of CARE (credentials, association, research, expertise) to encapsulate the elements of this empowered caring.

REFLECTION

Do you think the work that Falk Rafael published in 1996 about caring is still relevant today?

Another theorist you may have found through your literature searching proposed holistic caring as a form of nurse caring (Williams 1997). Williams regards this as a global concept with four dimensions that she names physical caring, interpretive caring, spiritual caring and sensitive caring. No doubt known to you, holism is a concept crucial to the effective practice of nursing, and is a term used to describe the nurse's belief that a 'patient is a person with social, physical, mental, and spiritual components' (Williams 1997:61–62). Holism is positioned as central to notions of professional caring, and is so intrinsic to this, it is often taken for granted—viewed as a 'given'—and therefore often not described or examined in discussions on professional caring. The use of a holistic perspective is said to facilitate an ethos that recognises the uniqueness and value inherent in individuals, and allows for the provision of individualised nursing care. More recently, a theory of 'nursing as caring' has been offered by Boykin and Schoenhofer (2001) who consider human beings as a species to be innately caring, and that reaching one's full potential in terms of caring is a lifelong process.

Through the literature, there is general agreement about the difficulties associated with defining and positioning caring (Bassett 2002, Paley 2001, Sumner 2008). What is more, it has even been suggested that the task of rescuing the concept of caring from its elusivity is impossible, a situation Paley (2001) attributes to problematic suppositions about the nature of knowledge. Nevertheless, even accounting for the difficulties associated with defining caring, the importance of exploring how nurses have theorised and attempted to understand the elusive nature of a concept so central to their practice cannot be underestimated.

REFLECTION

Do you think these theories are relevant in today's world? If yes, why? If not, why not?

Let's look at more of the literature. Many nurses consider caring as being primarily a relationship between nurse and others, in which experiences are shared. Consider Pearson (1991:199), for example; he describes the broad, global human concept of caring as 'investing oneself in the experience of another sufficiently enough to become a participant in that person's experience'. Sullivan and Deane (1994) assert that nurse caring prizes human relationships, and is informed by principles of sharing, sincerity, concern and moderation. Wolf et al (1994:107) propose that nurse caring has several tangible dimensions, including 'respectful deference to others, assurance of human presence, positive connectedness, professional knowledge and skill, and attentiveness to the other's experience'.

In addition, caring is understood to have intellectual as well as emotional aspects (Kapborg & Bertero 2003), and in 1992 Pepin suggested two dimensions of caring: love and labour. Love is said to consist of affective (i.e. pertaining to feelings) concepts such as altruism, compassion, emotion, presence, connectedness, nurturance and comfort, and it is this aspect of caring that has dominated the nursing literature (Pepin 1992). Labour refers to the element of care related to toil and service, and encompasses roles, functions, knowledge and tasks. Though Pepin (1992) suggested that this latter dimension of caring has received much less attention in the nursing literature, a number of these issues are discussed in some depth in nursing discourses on topics such as competency and clinical expertise (e.g. Hardy et al 2002). When considering the concepts of emotion and labour it would be remiss not to mention the concept of 'emotional labour'. This term emanated from sociology and pertains to workers who are required to display emotions that are in keeping with organisational requirements, rather than how the person—the individual nurse—truly feels (Gray 2009, Mann & Cowburn 2005, Staden 1998). Research has shown this to be an under-appreciated and stressful (Henderson 2001, Mann & Cowburn 2005), yet essential aspect of nurses' caring work (Gray 2009).

EXPERIENCING NURSE CARING: WHAT DO PATIENTS SAY?

Upholding the theory that caring is a concept central to the practice of nurses is not only important for the profession, but is also highly significant for the recipients of that care. It makes sense that if nurses are to claim they are caring professionals, they are obliged to find out what nurse caring means to patients, and how nurses can demonstrate care for patients. Somewhat ironically it has been the more recent rise of quality improvement processes that has spearheaded the interest in patients' views about the care they receive in healthcare settings, and this movement has not been led by nurses, but economists. Another determinant of mounting interest in patients' satisfaction with care is the fact that patients are no longer ill-informed, passive recipients of health services, but increasingly informed and active consumers who expect a certain standard of care and are not afraid to litigate should their expectations not be met.

REFLECTION

- Have you ever been a recipient of a health service?
- What approach/es do you take if the 'care' you receive falls short of your expectations?
- What are your expectations of 'care'?
- Are you able to articulate them?
- If you have experienced being a patient, would you say that your perceptions of what constitutes caring were different from those you hold when you practise as a nurse or nursing student?

If we continue our literature searching, it can be seen that patients' views of professional caring may be very different from those proposed by nurses. Nurses often (but not always) embrace psychosocial models of caring, while studies of patients often (but not always) suggest that patients value caring that is more technical or task-orientated in nature. For example, one study exploring the caring behaviours of hospital nurses from patients' perspectives found physical caring behaviours such as 'monitoring' were ranked much higher than aspects of caring such as 'trusting relationships', which could be considered to be affective or psychosocial in nature (Greenhalgh et al 1998, similarly Webb 1996). Indeed in 1996, Webb cautioned nurses against placing too much emphasis on the psychological elements of care at the expense of physical or technical aspects of care. In light of burgeoning technological intervention, this advice appears sound. Yet, the difference in perceptions of caring between nurses and patients warrants consideration. Understandings of caring can vary across cultures, and a study of patient and nurse perceptions of caring that was undertaken in six European Union countries revealed some differences between patient and nurse perceptions (Papastravou et al 2012).

In Western industrialised societies, technological skills and expertise are viewed as high status, and the domain of 'professionals'. In times of vulnerability, such as when people are ill, people like to feel assured they are in the care of competent health professionals, and perhaps view technological proficiency as evidence of such competence and expertise. The interpersonal aspects of caring so highly idealised by nurses may be viewed by patients as 'non-professional' caring—the type of caring available to them within their own social worlds, and not something they necessarily seek within a context of professional caring.

Other factors may also play a part in how patients experience or view nurse caring. For example, a Norwegian study demonstrated a gender-related difference in satisfaction with the quality of nursing care between young female patients when compared to young male patients (Foss 2002). In this study, the young female patients perceived nurses to be less committed and caring, to have less time and to be less skilled than did the male patients.

Similarly, a Jordanian study (Ahmad & Alasad 2004) that surveyed patients for their opinions of nursing care discovered that male patients tended to have a more positive experience of nursing care than did their female counterparts. The most important predictors for satisfaction with care in Ahmad and Alasad's study, however, related to the nurse's ability to meet the patient's information needs, the amount of information provided and the time nurses spent with patients. Demonstrating respect and courtesy towards family and friends was considered another major predictor. Patients appreciated those nurses who 'told them what to expect in the next shift, took interest in them as persons, provided them with privacy and perceived them as friends'. The authors concluded that the best aspects of nursing care are a 'happy atmosphere, patients' privacy and individualised care' (Ahmad & Alasad 2004:239).

REFLECTION

- What are your views on the findings by Ahmad and Alasad (2004)?
- Would you tend to agree/disagree with them?

In Sweden a study was conducted into patient satisfaction with nursing care at night (Oleni et al 2004). A number of nurses and patients were surveyed for their opinions. The study found a significant difference between nurses' and patients' assessments of patient care requirements in terms of nursing intervention. The nurses' assessments of nursing care were more positive than patients' perceptions. Patients scored lower for the concepts of information and participation, observation and monitoring, and night rest. Again this study demonstrated the importance patients attach to nurses providing them with appropriate and adequate information in order to better place the patient to influence and take responsibility for the care they receive. Patients were less positive about nursing observation and monitoring, and almost a quarter of them were dissatisfied with their ability to rest at night.

If we look at the findings from a review of predominantly quantitative observational studies related to patient satisfaction with the care provided by nurses, patient satisfaction was revealed as contingent on a number of factors (Johansson et al 2002). These included technological competence, as well as being responsive, kind, attentive, calm and encouraging. Insufficient information was shown to be 'perhaps the most common cause of dissatisfaction' (Johansson et al 2002).

Even as we write this chapter, the world of healthcare is changing and the way patient care is organised and delivered is undergoing constant reformation. Because it is a commodity limited in resources yet high in demand, the healthcare arena and all who service it are under duress to do more with less. Nurses everywhere are experiencing heavy workloads, long hours and increasingly complex professional demands. This is not a context conducive to the provision of personalised care and considered information giving.

Yet in the world of healthcare today it would appear the pendulum is returning to nursing interventions based on feeling as being more important for patient satisfaction than medical–technical interventions (Johansson et al 2002). As a recent study of patient experience revealed, it is the ability of nurses being able to show that the patient is an important person and that nurses really care about them that epitomises the best nurse caring behaviours (Mok & Pui Chi Chiu 2004). Todres, Galvin and Holloway (2009) call for a more 'humanised' form of care and have written extensively about their humanising value framework as a model for guiding care.

Caring behaviour considered paramount to patient and family includes the creation of a natural and constructive relationship between nurse and patient—indeed, the capacity to 'feel kinship' with the patient is attributed to the best nurses and the value of physical contact, especially if it has a comforting effect, should never be underestimated (Johansson et al 2002). Hayes and Tyler-Ball (2007) undertook a study of trauma patients' perceptions of nurse caring, and found that the patients found it difficult to separate their care experiences into care received in different areas of the hospital. Rather, patients formed a picture or view of the hospitalisation experience, and this meant that overall perceptions of very good care could be compromised by a single negative episode of care.

To conclude this section, we would like to use the words of one of Australia's eminent leaders in nursing, Professor Judy Lumby, who at the beginning of this century stated: 'ultimately it is the patient who must judge whether we care' (Lumby 2001:144). In a technologised world that values profit over people, it is hard to imagine that a nurse who exhibits caring behaviour could fail to make a difference.

CARE AND CURE

As you are no doubt aware, in a relatively short space of time, rapid developments in medical science, nursing knowledge and related health technologies have acted to dramatically improve patient outcomes and prolong life. We are now told that the human genome project and similar advances in science will lead to predicted increases in human life expectancy by as much as 25 years, and living into our hundreds will become commonplace (BBC World Service 2000).

In most parts of the world, these same technologies have radically and permanently changed the face of healthcare, and this has been the catalyst for a discussion in nursing and health that has become known as the 'care/cure' debate (e.g. Baumann et al 1998, Graham 2008, Webb 1996). This is a debate that has raged for quite a number of years. Johnston and Cooper (1997) suggest that the healthcare system in the United States was designed to cure illness and disease, rather than care for people and their health. This is the case for many Western healthcare systems, and provides a challenge for those whose main imperative is to care.

Clearly, caring alone will not meet all the health needs patients have but, as Webb (1996) pointed out, curing strategies may be insufficient unless accompanied by a caring dimension. In recent times a number of nursing scholars have published work on the concept of nursing as a therapeutic activity in its own right and the need for effective therapeutic relationships if the patient is to be 'cured' (Ersser 1997, Freshwater 2002, Johns 2001, Ramjan 2004). Williams (1997) too has suggested caring is, in itself, essential to cure. She proposes that caring nurse behaviours have been demonstrated to have positive effects in terms of patients' wellness and, conversely, non-caring behaviours by nurses have been shown to negatively affect patient well-being and recovery.

Writing from a medical perspective, Graham (2008:310) highlights the importance and value of family-centred primary care models within service contexts, which he names as 'cult of cure' systems. However, the concepts of care and cure historically have been constructed as binary and oppositional. Moreover, the difference between the roles of nurse and physician is often centred on ideas of the nurse as caring and the physician as curing. Sullivan and Deane (1994; similarly, Caffrey & Caffrey 1994) suggest caring (as nursing) is viewed as a traditionally feminine activity, and has not been conferred the power and status of male-defined activities, of which the physician/curer may more easily lay claim.

Indeed, if we look back over time, we can see it was Florence Nightingale herself who appeared to reject the idea that nurses can have an essential curing role. In her book *Notes On Nursing* (Nightingale 1859–1946:74), she states 'nature alone cures', but goes on to say 'what nursing has to do is to put the patient in the best position for nature to act upon him [sic]' (p 75). More recently, in defining professional caring, several scholars have contended these two concepts are not truly antagonistic (e.g. King & Norsen 1994, Leftwich 1993). Nurses identify elements of both caring and curing, and certain science-based skills and knowledge are highly valued as essential to caring (Carper 1978, Wolf et al 1994). Furthermore, patients themselves expect nurses to have a high level of professional proficiency and technical skill, which are associated with 'cure', and construct these as key aspects of professional caring (Borbasi 1996, Ray 1987, Wolf et al 1994).

King and Norsen (1994) contend that notions of 'care/cure' as solely the domain of either nurse (care) or physician (cure) are not helpful or acceptable, as nurses and physicians have both curing and caring dimensions to their practice areas (see also Leftwich 1993). In a similar vein, Webb (1996) urges nurses to overcome the cure/care dichotomy between medicine and nursing, and argues it is no longer important to distinguish the care given by specific professional groups but to focus instead on establishing clear goals of care. Rather than regarding notions of care and cure as being polarised or at opposite extremes, then, it is more accurate to say the notions of care/cure are compatible and complementary. Both are acknowledged and accepted as key aspects of nursing's agenda, and both are reflected in the theories of professional caring constructed by nurses (Wolf et al 1994). Moreover, in today's health service we are seeing an increasing emphasis on multidisciplinary approaches to caring.

Having acknowledged that nursing is a composite of care and cure, it is perhaps ironic to note that the circumstances within which nurses find themselves working today probably mitigate against both. While some patients may be fortunate enough to be cured, technological and pharmacological advances have meant many are merely 'contained' in a state of chronic illness (Rizza et al 2008). Often these patients are aged with multiple co-morbidities, which makes caring for them extremely complex and, by the same token, nurses, because they are so occupied with administering medical treatments, may overlook the nurse caring behaviours so important to patient satisfaction and wellbeing. Have we perhaps reached a stage where neither cure nor care is winning out?

CARING AS THE BASIS OF THE DISCIPLINE OF NURSING

In addition to being complex and multidimensional, caring is also controversial, for among members of the profession, the debates about the centrality of caring to nursing continue (Cloyes 2002, Paley 2001, Sumner 2008). There are conflicting trains of thought and these challenge the relevance and appropriateness of caring as a foundational aspect of nursing. Stockdale and Warelow (2000) raise concerns about the inconsistencies around care and caring, and the ill-defined nature of caring. They point out the difficulties associated with adopting care as the essence of nursing, when there is not a universal accepted definition from which nursing can continue to develop.

All would agree that nurses do have a curative (as well as a caring) orientation, and in 1987 Kitson argued that if nurses choose to align themselves with care rather than cure, with the nurturing processes rather than with technology and treatment, then they will need to identify how to organise and put into operation those skills they possess. Successful execution of the caring role is, she believes, 'intimately bound up with having the necessary space to practice, sufficient room to manoeuvre and to be able to explore new areas of knowledge and expertise' (Kitson 1987:324).

In a very influential piece of work, Dunlop (1986) questioned whether a science of caring is even possible and resolves that, if it is, it will have to take a hermeneutical form (based on hermeneutics)—a 'form that in many ways does violence to our traditional ideas of science', but one that 'challenges the male hegemony of science' (Dunlop 1986:669). In a philosophical critique, Walker (1995) has also highlighted the problem of nurses' attempts to represent nursing as both a discourse of science and a discourse of caring.

The emergence of differing perspective(s) about the nature of nursing has not been without debate, and there are nurses who believe that an emphasis on alliance to concepts such as caring and holism, with their attendant rejection of the natural sciences, will do more harm than good to nursing's attempts to become a credible academic discipline. Indeed, in some quarters there is strident scepticism. Writing in 2002, Paley positions the ideology of caring as 'a slave morality', and goes on to state that:

> It represents an attack on the 'medical-scientific model', motivated by resentment, and designed to establish nursing's superiority. Its effects have been debilitating, and it has prevented nursing from becoming a 'noble' (that is, properly scientific) discipline.
> (Paley 2002:25)

However, meeting the demands of the caring imperative concerned with cure requires that nurses have considerable specialist knowledge of a range of scientific disciplines such as pharmacology, anatomy, physiology, biochemistry, immunology, microbiology and physics. A sound scientific knowledge base is undeniably essential for nursing, given the need for continued development of the discipline and the need to meet the demands of increasingly technological societies; none would argue that competency in the scientific disciplines is not an essential aspect of nursing knowledge and integral to the caring imperative claimed by nursing.

THREATS TO CARING

From much of what we have said so far, it can be seen that the concept of caring is inherently incompatible with the underlying objectives of many of the organisational structures in which nurses find themselves today. In many parts of the (Western) world, healthcare is not intrinsically altruistic; nor is it based on any real system of equity (Lumby 2001). Rather, healthcare tends to be resourced on a fee-for-service basis, and access to healthcare services is therefore linked very strongly with an individual's ability to pay for such services. Healthcare is increasingly looked at with entrepreneurial, rather than philanthropic, eyes. To investors, provision of healthcare services may represent an opportunity for profit, and even 'whilst appropriating the language and images of nursing for business purposes, many entrepreneurs treat professional nursing care as a commodity to be whittled away until it becomes impotent' (Jackson & Raftos 1997:38). Although, to be sure, nurses comprise the largest occupational/professional group within the healthcare system; the system itself is based on a set of values that directly challenges and compromises the very essence of nursing.

In the past it was thought that large, impersonal institutions, by their very nature, may devalue caring by providing little incentive or opportunity for nurses to demonstrate behaviours associated with caring, or failing to provide an environment where caring could be expressed (Morse et al 1990). Align that with today's healthcare system, shaped as it is by overarching economic influences such as cost containment and profit margins, and we have even less of a platform for caring work (Jarrin 2006). Economic imperatives have been the catalyst for reexamining the whole concept of 'patient care', and attempts have been made to reconceptualise traditional care delivery in order to come up with ways of doing more with fewer resources (Caplan & Brown 1997, Johnston & Cooper 1997, Ray 1989). These new approaches in provision of care are sometimes presented as strategies to improve patient care but, as Williams (1997) suggests, frequently they are more concerned with institutional cost saving than on quality patient care (similarly, Duffield & Lumby 1994, Lumby 2001).

This positioning of the wealth of an individual as a major indicator for allocation of (increasingly scarce) health resources is, by its very nature, incompatible with nursing's caring imperative, which places a high value on the individual (Chinn 1989, Morse et al 1990, Williams 1997). Care is most likely to be viewed by nurses as a resource to be allocated on the basis of need rather than ability to pay, and the challenge for us as nurses is to provide effective care in the context of ongoing resource constraints. These tensions are inherent in the working life of many nurses, and compromise the ability of nurses to provide care in the way idealised by the profession.

This key philosophical difference between nursing's caring imperative, and the underlying ethos of many (Western) healthcare systems, throws nurses and health administrators into a permanent state of possible conflict, and has the potential to become a source of professional tension for nurses (Jackson & Raftos 1997, Jarrin 2006, Johnston & Cooper 1997, Kralik et al 1997). As a result, many nurses leave nursing disillusioned with a 'system' that inhibits nurse caring behaviour. As we have experienced on an international scale, this contributes to critical shortages of nursing staff, which places the system, including patients and remaining staff, under even greater duress (Hinshaw 2008).

More than two decades ago Ray (1989) attempted to reconcile the seemingly irreconcilable by proposing a theory of caring compatible with the bureaucratic cultures existing within large organisations. She suggested it is essential that the discipline of nursing comes to terms with the corporatisation of healthcare, and that a failure to do this would be disastrous for nursing.

The transformation of American and other Western healthcare systems to corporate enterprises emphasising competitive management and economic gain seriously challenges nursing's humanistic philosophies and theories and nursing's administrative and clinical practices. The recent refocusing of nursing as a human science and the art and science of human caring places nursing in a vulnerable position. When pitted against the new goal of corporate advancement in healthcare delivery, nursing faces a loss of self-identity and an increased risk of alienation and confusion in this competitive arena (Ray 1989:31).

Using a grounded theory approach, Ray generated a 'theory of the dynamic structure of caring in a complex organization' (Ray 1989:31), and proposes this as a means by which nurses can practise within bureaucratic health structures without compromising nursing's caring imperative. This theory proposes several 'structural caring categories', which Ray names as political, economic, legal, technological/physiological, educational, social, spiritual/religious and ethical (Ray 1989). Caffrey and Caffrey (1994) suggest that caring will never be accommodated as a core value while profit remains a primary motive of healthcare systems. In the ensuing years since Ray's original work, concerns have continued to be raised and the fact that these comments are still so salient, and that many of these issues continue to confound us, shows the longitudinal and complex nature of the debate. The message from this lengthy discussion in the literature is that in meeting the current resource and organisational challenges there is a need to recognise the ways that caring is or can be enacted at the administrative and managerial levels of healthcare and the health professions (Erdmann et al 2011).

Insidiously, over the last few years, further threats to nurse caring have emerged, largely in the form of unregulated healthcare workers and the implementation of education and training programs for new breeds of healthcare practitioners. While nurses may have expanded and extended their roles at upper echelons in the health system, they need to be constantly on guard at the rear end: never more so than in a time of cost constraint and massive shortfalls in registered nurse numbers (Hinshaw 2008). It may well be that nursing, as we know it today, will shortly be overrun by workers who will do the job, but do it without any regard to caring as nurses have conceptualised it.

In some parts of the world this could already be the reality. A 2011 report of 10 investigations by the UK NHS ombudsman into the care of older persons in hospital found a 'casual indifference' to their dignity and welfare highlighting a definite lack of care and compassion in meeting the needs of these individuals and their families (http://www.ombudsman.org.uk/care-and-compassion/).

CONCLUDING THOUGHTS

Caring is proclaimed and understood as the basis of modern nursing and, as you are discovering, nurses have produced vast amounts of literature on aspects of care and caring, and how they may be applied in a nursing context. However, while the concept of professional caring is difficult to articulate, it is recognised as being a complex concept involving the development of a range of knowledge, skills and expertise. Professional caring has similarities with non-professional, or informal, caring and applies knowledge derived from various discipline areas to promote the health and wellbeing of people.

The major perspectives of caring recognise the importance of various types of knowledge and, with few exceptions, all allude to the expressive, artistic and scientific perspectives said to construct nursing. Other common themes that characterise the constructions of caring adopted by nurses are holism, compassion, empathy and communication. Evidence suggests that patients, too, view caring as a perceptible concept, and highly value it as an essential and healing aspect of their professional encounters with nurses. However, in contrast to the ways nurses view caring, reflection on what is known about patients' attitudes to nurse caring suggests that, above all, patients want a nurse who demonstrates caring through clinical and technical competence, as well as through interpersonal skills and, increasingly, a person who keeps them informed along each step of their illness trajectory, including informing family and friends.

Accepting caring as the basis of nursing practice and scholarship is not without problems. Issues of autonomy and power are ill at ease with the concept of caring. Servitude and altruism are intrinsically linked to caring, and these do not sit well with nursing's move to professionalism. To provide adequate care takes time and time costs money. Many nurses work within organisational structures whose primary motivation lies with the cost containment or the accumulation of wealth, rather than a mandate to heal—these economic factors may compromise or even be antithetical to nursing's imperative to care.

The caring imperative, therefore, represents a potential source of stress and occupational conflict for nurses. While it is argued that the need for nursing to place caring as a central concept has never been greater, there are concerns that the caring components of nursing are deemed unsophisticated and hence inferior to the therapeutic interventions of medicine and other allied health service providers. There is the potential for caring to become overlooked—to dissipate.

Despite the many creative theories of nurse caring, the tasks of establishing coherent and clear connections between caring and notions such as professionalism, scholarship and autonomy remain incomplete. Nurses are left with many issues to consider and debate. Even as the healthcare system as we know it today is shaped, reshaped and shaped again, in the years to come the conundrum of caring as the basis of nursing practice and scholarship will no doubt continue to captivate and confound nurses.

REFLECTIVE QUESTIONS

1 Think for a moment about why you chose nursing as a career. Did the desire to care for people have any role in your decision making?

2 Take some time to reflect on your experiences of caring for and being cared for. Based on your experiences to date, how would you define caring?

3   Think about some of the ways you show care to the significant people in your life. Do you think that any of these ways of showing care will be the same or similar to how you will show care to your patients/clients as a nurse?

4   Some people view nursing and caring as being synonymous. Do you think this is good for nursing? Why? Why not?

RECOMMENDED READINGS

Dunlop M 1986 Is a science of caring possible? Journal of Advanced Nursing 11(3):661–670

Hayes J, Tyler-Ball S 2007 Perceptions of nurses' caring behaviours by trauma patients. Nursing Administration Quarterly 14(4):187–190

Lumby J 2001 Who cares? The changing health care system. Allen & Unwin, Sydney

Papastravou E, Efstathiou G, Tsangari H et al 2012 A cross-cultural study of the concept of caring through behaviours: patients' and nurses' perspectives in six different EU countries. Journal of Advanced Nursing 68:1026–1037

Sumner J 2008 Is caring in nursing an impossible ideal for today's practicing nurse? Nursing Administration Quarterly 32(2):92–101

REFERENCES

Ahmad M, Alasad J 2004 Predictors of patients' experiences of nursing care in medical-surgical wards. International Journal of Nursing Practice 10(5):235–241

Bassett C 2002 Nurses' perceptions of care and caring. International Journal of Nursing Practice 8(1):8–15

Baumann A, Deber R, Silverman B, Mallette C 1998 Who cares? Who cures? The ongoing debate in the provision of health care. Journal of Advanced Nursing 28(5):1040

BBC World Service 2000 Who wants to live forever? Online. Available: www.bbc.co.uk/worldservice/people/highlights/000822_116.shtml 22 Aug 2000

Benner P 1984 From novice to expert: excellence and power in clinical nursing. Addison Wesley, Menlo Park, California

Benner P, Hooper-Kyriakidis P, Stannard D 1999 Clinical wisdom and interventions in critical care: a thinking-in-action approach. WB Saunders, Philadelphia

Borbasi S A 1996 Living the experience of being nursed: a phenomenological text. International Journal of Nursing Practice 2(4):222–228

Boykin A, Schoenhofer S O 2001 Nursing as caring: a model for transforming practice. Jones & Bartlett, Publishers, National League for Nursing Press, Sudsbury, Massachusetts

Caffrey R, Caffrey P 1994 Nursing: caring or codependent? Nursing Forum 29(1):12–17

Caplan G, Brown A 1997 Post-acute care: can hospitals do better with less? Australian Health Review 20(2):43–52

Carper B 1978 Fundamental patterns of knowing in nursing. Advances in Nursing Science 1(1):13–23

Chinn P 1989 Awake, awake. Advances in Nursing Science 11(2):1

Cloyes K 2002 Agonizing care: care ethics, agonistic feminism and a political theory of care. Nursing Inquiry 9(3):203–214

Duffield C, Lumby J 1994 Caring nurses: the dilemma of balancing costs and quality. Australian Health Review 17(2):72–83

Dunlop M 1986 Is a science of caring possible? Journal of Advanced Nursing 11(3):661–670

Erdmann A L, De Andrade S R, Ferreira De Mello A L, Klock P, Do Nascimento K C, Santos Koerich M & Stein Backes D 2011 Practices for caring in nursing: Brazilian research groups. International Nursing Review 58:379–385.

Ersser S 1997 Nursing as a therapeutic activity: an ethnography. Avebury, Aldershot

Falk Rafael A 1996 Power and caring: a dialectic in nursing. Advances in Nursing Science 19(1):3–17

Finfgeld-Connett D 2008 Qualitative convergence of three nursing concepts: art of nursing, presence and caring. Journal of Advanced Nursing 63(5):527–534

Foss C 2002 Gender bias in nursing care? Gender-related differences in patient satisfaction with the quality of nursing care. Scandinavian Journal of Caring Sciences 16(1):19–26

Freshwater D (ed) 2002 Therapeutic nursing: improving patient care through self-awareness and reflection. Sage, London

Graham R 2008 Medicine and children with special health care needs: conflict with the cult of cure. Journal of Developmental and Behavioural Pediatrics 29(4):309–310

Gray B 2009 The emotional labour of nursing – Defining and managing emotions in nursing work, Nurse Education Today, 29(2):168–175 (http://www.sciencedirect.com/science/article/pii/S0260691708001056) Keywords: Emotional labour; Nursing

Greenhalgh J, Vanhanen L, Kyngäs H 1998 Nurse caring behaviours. Journal of Advanced Nursing 27(5):927–932

Hardy S, Garbett R, Titchen A, Manley K 2002 Exploring nursing expertise: nurses talk nursing. Nursing Inquiry 9(3):196–202

Hayes J, Tyler-Ball S 2007 Perceptions of nurses' caring behaviours by trauma patients. Journal of Trauma Nursing 14(4):187–190

Henderson A 2001 Emotional labour and nursing: an under-appreciated aspect of caring work. Nursing Inquiry 8(2):130–138

Hinshaw A S 2008 Navigating the perfect storm: balancing a culture of safety with workforce challenges. Nursing Research 57(1) Supplement 1:S4–S10

Jackson D, Raftos M 1997 In uncharted waters: confronting the culture of silence in a residential care institution. International Journal of Nursing Practice 3(1):34–39

Jarrin O F 2006 Results from the nurse manifest 2003 study: nurses' perspectives on nursing. Advances in Nursing Science. Philosophy and Ethics 29(2):E74–E85

Johansson P, Oleni M, Fridlund B 2002 Patient satisfaction with nursing care in the context of health care: a literature review. Scandinavian Journal of Caring Sciences 16(4):337–344

Johns C 2001 Reflective practice: revealing the [he]art of caring. International Journal of Nursing Practice 7(4):237–245

Johnston C, Cooper P 1997 Patient-focused care: what is it? Holistic Nursing Practice 11(3):1–7

Kapborg I, Bertero C 2003 The phenomenon of caring from the student nurse's perspective: a qualitative content analysis. International Nursing Review 50(3):183–192

King K, Norsen L 1994 The care/cure, nurse/physician dichotomy doesn't do it anymore. Image: Journal of Nursing Scholarship 26(2):89

Kitson A L 1987 Raising standards of clinical practice—the fundamental issue of effective nursing practice. Journal of Advanced Nursing 12(3):321–329

Kralik D, Koch T, Wootton K 1997 Engagement and detachment: understanding patients' experiences with nursing. Journal of Advanced Nursing 26(2):399–407

Leftwich R 1993 Care and cure as healing processes in nursing. Nursing Forum 28(3):13–17

Leininger M 1984 Care: the essence of nursing and health. Slack, New Jersey

Leininger M 1986 Care facilitation and resistance factors in the culture of nursing. Topics in Clinical Nursing 8(2):1–12

Lumby J 2001 Who cares? The changing health care system. Allen & Unwin, Sydney

Mann S, Cowburn J 2005 Emotional labour and stress within mental health nursing. Journal of Psychiatric and Mental Health Nursing 12:154–162

Mok E, Pui Chi Chiu 2004 Nurse–patient relationships in palliative care. Journal of Advanced Nursing 48(5):475–483

Morse J, Solberg S, Neander W et al 1990 Concepts of caring and caring as a concept. Advances in Nursing Science 13(1):1–14

Nightingale F 1859–1946 Notes on nursing. Harrison Book Company, London

Oleni M, Johansson P, Fridlund B 2004 Nursing care at night: an evaluation using the Night Nursing Care Instrument. Journal of Advanced Nursing 47(1):25–32

Paley J 2001 An archaeology of caring knowledge. Journal of Advanced Nursing 26(2):188–198

Paley J 2002 Caring as a slave morality: Nietzschean themes in nursing ethics. Journal of Advanced Nursing 40(1):25–35

Papastravou E, Efstathiou G, Tsangari H et al 2012 A cross-cultural study of the concept of caring through behaviours: patients' and nurses' perspectives in six different EU countries. Journal of Advanced Nursing 68:1026–1037

Pearson A 1991 Taking up the challenge: the future for therapeutic nursing. In: McMahon R, Pearson A (eds) Nursing as therapy. Chapman & Hall, London

Pepin J 1992 Family caring and caring in nursing. Image: Journal of Nursing Scholarship 24(2):127–131

Ramjan L M 2004 Nurses and the 'therapeutic relationship': caring for adolescents with anorexia nervosa. Journal of Advanced Nursing 45(5):495–503

Rawnsley M 1990 Of human bonding: the context of nursing as caring. Advances in Nursing Science 13(1):41–48

Ray M 1987 Technological caring: a new model in critical care. Dimensions in Critical Care Nursing 6(3):173–179

Ray M 1989 The theory of bureaucratic caring for nursing practice in the organizational structure. Nursing Science Quarterly 13(2):31–42

Rizza R, Eddy D, Kahn R 2008 Care, cure and commitment: what can we look forward to? Diabetes Care 31(5):1051–1060

Staden H 1998 Alertness to the needs of others: a study of the emotional labour of caring. Journal of Advanced Nursing 27(1):147–156

Stockdale M, Warelow P 2000 Is the complexity of care a paradox? Journal of Advanced Nursing 31(5):1258–1264

Sullivan J, Deane D 1994 Caring: reappropriating our tradition. Nursing Forum 29(2):5–9

Sumner J 2008 Is caring in nursing an impossible ideal for today's practicing nurse? Nursing Administration Quarterly 32(2):92–101

Swanson K 1993 Nursing as informed caring for the well-being of others. Image: Journal of Nursing Scholarship 25(4):352–357

Todres L, Galvin K, Holloway I 2009 The humanization of healthcare: a value framework for qualitative research. International Journal of Qualitative Studies on Health and Well-being 4:68–77

Walker K 1995 Courting competency: nursing and the politics of performance in practice. Nursing Inquiry 2(2):90–99

Watson J 1985 Nursing: the philosophy and science of caring. Colorado Associated University Press, Boulder, Colorado

Watson J 1988 Nursing: human science and human care. A theory of nursing. National League for Nursing, New York

Watson J, Foster R 2003 The Attending Nurse Caring Model: integrating theory, evidence and advanced caring—healing therapeutics for transforming professional practice. Journal of Clinical Nursing 12(3):360–365

Watson J, Jackson D, Borbasi S 2005 Contemplating caring: issues, concerns, debates. In: Daly J, Speedy S, Jackson D, Lambert V, Lambert C (eds) Professional nursing: concepts, issues and challenges. Springer Publishing, New York

Webb C 1996 Caring, curing, coping: towards an integrated model. Journal of Advanced Nursing 23:960–968

Wilkin K, Slevin E 2004 The meaning of caring to nurses: an investigation into the nature of caring work in an intensive care unit. Journal of Clinical Nursing 13(1):50–59

Williams S 1997 Caring in patient-focused care: the relationship of patients' perceptions of holistic nurse care to their levels of anxiety. Holistic Nursing Practice 11(3):61–68

Wolf Z, Giardino E, Osborne P, Ambrose M 1994 Dimensions of nurse caring. Image: Journal of Nursing Scholarship 26(2):107–111

CHAPTER 6

The growth of ideas and theory in nursing

Sarah Winch and Amanda Henderson

LEARNING OBJECTIVES

At the completion of this chapter, the reader will be able to:

- define the term theory
- describe the terms modernity and postmodernity
- identify the dominant historical and societal trends within the nursing profession
- explain how these trends influence the practice of nursing and accompanying knowledge development.

KEY WORDS

Theory, modernity, postmodernity, knowledge, practice

INTRODUCING THEORY

This chapter aims to help you understand the relevance of theory to inform the ongoing development of nursing knowledge and the improvement of nursing practice. Clinical practice informed by theory gives nurses the necessary foundation to enlighten and restructure healthcare and improve quality of care at all practice levels. We begin with a brief overview of the philosophies, models and theories that underpin contemporary nursing theories. The next section emphasises nursing practice with a focus on knowledge utilisation, with theory and research as tools of practice.

Broadly, we can state that theory refers to any attempt to explain or represent a phenomenon, and ranges from the highly abstract and large scale to the specific. Theories act as a lens by which to view the world. If you change the thickness of the lens and its shape, then what is being viewed is seen differently, in more or less detail, or expanded or reduced in size. Theories also act like a kaleidoscope, where turning the end of the instrument creates different patterns forming from the same small elements that are present. Theory and the application of theory to human understanding and social phenomena results in key elements (we shall call them variables and ideas) that underpin our understanding of the person and society being emphasised in different ways. Likewise, key philosophical ideas such as the nature of truth, evil and justice may be viewed differently.

When we focus on the process and practice of nursing, the central phenomena that require explanation are the nurse, the nursed and the care setting, including practices, processes and organisation. Nursing theories help us make sense of processes and practices. They explain why and when nursing takes place, provide an understanding of how the practice of nursing proceeds and also assist with practice change through critique. In this way nursing theories help us understand the practice of nursing, how we interact with the nursed and how we structure our nursing actions to provide nursing care.

Examples of well-known nursing theorists (Tomey & Alligood 1998)

Patricia Benner: stress and coping in illness

Madeleine Leininger: theory of cultural care, diversity and universality/transcultural nursing model

Betty Neuman: nursing systems model

Florence Nightingale: environmental adaptation theory

Dorothea Orem: self-care framework

Hildegard Peplau: theory of interpersonal relations

Martha E Rogers: science of unitary human beings

Nancy Roper, Winifred W Logan and Alison J Tierney: the elements of nursing: a model of nursing based on a model of living

Jean Watson: theory of human caring

NURSING AS SOCIAL PROCESS: THE ROLE OF SOCIAL THEORY IN UNDERSTANDING NURSING

Nursing can be viewed as a social and cultural product of society. That is, nursing is an interactive process that always takes place within a social context. Our common understanding of nursing involves a nurse and the nursed (the patient, consumer or client) interacting within a socially and politically constructed system (healthcare facility or provider) that directs actions and responses.

Knowledge of the role of social theory is valuable when we seek to answer the 'how' and 'why' questions about nursing and the social context from which it arises. The field of social theory is comprehensive, as it spans all of the social sciences and the humanities. In the following section we provide an overview of two major ways that social theory contributes to nursing. These are: an analysis of modernity and its contribution to the type of world we live in; and a critique of the social milieu that constructs and defines nursing.

MODERNITY AND POSTMODERNITY: HOW SOCIAL THEORY INFORMS THE WAY WE THINK

Modernism, and postmodernism, are terms that hold a number of meanings in different contexts. For example, they may refer to specific styles of literature, art and architecture in the nineteenth and twentieth centuries. Or, as we explore here, they can elicit two different ways of thinking, both of which are fundamental to how we understand nursing.

First, we review modernity and postmodernity as a particular set of philosophical beliefs. These provide a useful framework that we can use to analyse practice-specific theories by tracing the traditions from which they emerge. Our second understanding relates to how nursing as a social process happens within the different time frames that represent the modern and postmodern eras. This provides a broad social and historical context that explains the nature of nursing and the transformations to nursing practice that are initiated through social change. Later, we examine modernism and postmodernism as broad cultural configurations that influence how society is organised.

Modernity and the Enlightenment

For many theorists, modernity encompasses a large historical period that emerged in Europe dating from the Renaissance to the present. Philosophical ideas on the nature of knowledge and modern method (René Descartes), science as power (Frances Bacon), the state and the science of human nature (Thomas Hobbes) and modern politics and power (Niccolo Machiavelli) construct the early basis of modernity. Later, in the eighteenth century, many of these ideas had their full intellectual flowering in a time known as 'the Enlightenment'. The goal of the Enlightenment project was to replace the ignorance, tradition and superstition present in the church-dominated societies of the Middle Ages, with knowledge that was based on science and reason. This far-reaching period of intellectual development is still prominent in much of contemporary thinking in nursing and other disciplines.

Ideas on the nature of human life that stem from the Enlightenment period reflect a particular belief about the self and the human condition. The modernist concept of 'the self' is a unified, rational, autonomous and essential entity. This means that 'the self' can be observed and studied. It is free, capable of thought and of independent action. This is a description of human beings as active agents doing things for reasons and shaping the world to their own ends. These core ideas about the nature of the self are central to many nursing theorists who see patients and nurses as autonomous beings who are able to be influenced in their behaviours to promote health and well-being or to address deficits caused by illness.

The Enlightenment period crystallised a belief in universal goals and human progress towards an ideal through the application of value-neutral knowledge. Knowledge derived from the empirical or natural sciences can be applied to society to increase human progress and happiness, while knowledge from the human sciences can be used to transform society into a scientific, rational culture. These ideas, which Yeatman (1991:3) terms 'rational utopianism', underpin modernist emancipatory politics; that is, the search for truth and progress through value-free, objective knowledge.

For researchers working within this framework (and this includes most nurses), it is important to select the correct research method, as this endorses 'truth' and provides theory that is an objective reflection of a securely grounded world (Hollinger 1994). Society and history are seen as a whole, able to be grasped through totalising methodologies and explained by grand and comprehensive explanations (meta-narratives). In nursing these would take the form of theories of caring or grand theories of nursing.

Research methods based on modernist assumptions promote the ideas of objectivity, and most importantly value neutrality. In this way a society based on science and universal values can be assumed to be truly rational and emancipatory. In this way, theory is viewed as an objective representation of social reality. Ideas from the Enlightenment period have led to positivism, scientism and an emphasis on technological reason. For example, although ideas about ageing have been present in the wider literature since ancient times, the Enlightenment constructed the idea of 'old age' through medicine, science and philosophy as an essential part of life. Modernity spawned practices of calculation, division and ranking of the population. It was then possible to separate older age as a distinct developmental stage (Katz 1995). Using these methods, all human institutions and practices, including hospitals and nurses, could be analysed by science and arguably improved. This is a core belief that is very much a part of healthcare and service provision today.

Modernity is also about order and rationality (logical thinking underpinned by science). This order and stability are maintained in modern societies through the means of 'grand or master narratives'. These are stories about the practices and beliefs present in a society. A 'grand narrative' in Australian culture may be that the family is a 'haven' and a 'central building block' of society. Generally if we support families to function well they will raise the next generation properly and care for their sick and elderly. Contemporary healthcare and social policy reflect this type of grand narrative. For example, aged care policy, such as home and community care, is based on supporting families (often aged spouses) to care for their partners. Likewise, early discharge policy and short stays in acute care hospitals rely on a well-organised, functioning family to provide supportive care.

Postmodernity

The central theme of modernity is a belief in the idea of progress in human life through the application of value-free knowledge gained in an objective way (science). However, as the German philosopher Jürgen Habermas and others have established, the twentieth century experience of the Holocaust and nuclear devastation shattered confidence and faith in scientific progress (Harvey 1989). Postmodernism (which in our discussion here includes the related although not identical category of poststructuralism) presents an altogether more pessimistic view of the world in general. It seeks to critique or deconstruct grand narratives to reveal the contradictions and instabilities that are inherent in any social organisation or practice. For example, in Australia, community nurses know that the grand narrative involving the family as a source of comfort and support is not always true. Postmodernism, while rejecting grand narratives, prefers 'mini-narratives', stories that explain small practices and local events, rather than large-scale universal or global concepts. These 'mini-narratives' are locally based on particular situations and do not claim to be universal or generalisable to other contexts. They have great application in promoting understanding of aspects of nursing practice.

Drawn from a complex mix of ideas from theorists such as Hegel, Nietzsche and Weber, the postmodern position is associated with concepts such as irrationality, play, deconstruction, antithesis and indeterminacy (Gillan 1988). In a sense these are the opposite of the science-based rationality that underpins modernism. Critics of the Enlightenment, such as the well-known philosopher Nietzsche, argue that truth, knowledge and rationality are not immutable and science itself may rest on faith (Hollinger 1994). Postmodernism, taken to its extreme, refutes all claims to truth and reduces theory to narrative or storytelling. Postmodernism abandons the dualism of facts and values, objectivity and subjectivity, descriptions and interpretations, and gives all methodologies a political emphasis, while contextualising all claims, methods and values. Moreover, postmodernism does not accord 'reason' a central and transcendental status.

From the Enlightenment onwards, the idea of the 'subject' has had a central place in thought about the special nature of humanity. For key Enlightenment thinkers, the autonomous subject was the central tenet of civil society. By stark contrast many postmodern thinkers dispute the concept of the sovereign individual or subject, viewing these ideas about the subject as a form of grand narrative that requires deconstruction itself. For postmodernists, individuals are subjects, constituted through a variety of practices and knowledges or discourses in society in which they are positioned at any one point in time. The modernist, humanist concept of a unified, rational, autonomous and essential self is seen as illusory and results from regular positioning within a common, frequently used discourse (Grosz 1993).

Postmodernity has influenced several thinkers and observers of nursing practice including Winch (2005), who argues that this type of analysis can provide a highly analytical view of nursing practice. This view links the minutiae of nursing work with formation of identity (of the subject), and the monitoring and fashioning of patient and nurse conduct within broader historical, social and political processes and institutions.

Characterising modern healthcare institutions

The second way by which we may understand modernism and postmodernism is to view them broadly as historical cultural configurations that influence how society is organised. In two to three centuries modern industrial capitalism altered earlier farming or rural societies and set the scene for the society we know in Australia today. In line with the massive social change from the modern to the postmodern, nursing as a social process or cultural product has also been transformed.

Jameson (1984) outlines three primary phases of capitalism in Western industrialised nations that have produced particular cultural practices associated with modernism and postmodernism. These provide a framework for how we may understand healthcare and nursing. The first predates both modernism and postmodernism and is termed *market capitalism*. This occurred in the eighteenth through to the late nineteenth centuries in Western Europe, England and the United States. This phase is associated with particular technological developments such as the steam-driven engine. It is in this phase that nursing began to emerge as a central form of healthcare responsible for cleanliness and hygiene, with the growth of the clinic and the asylum. The work of the nursing theorist Florence Nightingale is prominent in this period.

The second phase, termed *monopoly capitalism*, occurred from the late nineteenth century until the mid-twentieth century, and is associated with modernism, industrialism, the growth of cities, the nuclear family, democracy and social legislation. It is in this phase that we see the growth of particular institutions such as the modern hospital, the development of the health professions and the rise of medicine as the dominant and most powerful form of healthcare.

The third phase, the one that we currently occupy, is a form of multinational or *consumer capitalism*, a postindustrial or postmodern society. Developing after World War II, the third phase encompasses all of the second phase but emphasises new technologies, marketing, selling and consuming commodities, and the growth of the internet. It is in this era that multinational pharmaceutical companies have grown powerful, seeking to influence medical care and the consumption of particular drugs, ordered through medical practitioners and marketed in some countries, such as the United States, directly to the consumer. Modern managerialism has also crept into healthcare and influenced nursing work, with a focus on healthcare targets and clinical pathways. Health services are now managed as businesses, with patients as consumers (Winch & Henderson 2009).

Our consideration of the modern and postmodern has ranged over a wide number of issues, of which there is no clear agreement among social theorists, philosophers or nursing thinkers. Some argue that we live in truly postmodern times, and we must abandon the quest for truth and justice through the application of science. Others still believe that society is evolving to become a more logical and rational place, despite the odd setback. Over this period of time, nursing has ebbed and flowed with the dominant social and cultural practices of the time. What is clear is that the work that nurses do is essential in a civil society. What is less certain in a postmodern, postindustrial time is how that work may be fragmented or reorganised and what nursing may look like in the future.

IMPLICATIONS FOR THE DEVELOPMENT OF A BODY OF KNOWLEDGE

Social theory has influenced how nurses inquire into their profession. This inquiry has explored ways to study human beings, what counts as 'evidence', reflection on practice and analysing the profession itself. Prevailing ideas and theories have been instrumental in how nurses approach and conduct their practice and accordingly the development of professional knowledge. We now provide a brief overview of some of the more dominant ideas and theories that have influenced the discipline of nursing. These influences are significant determinants of how nursing is presently understood and practised.

The contribution of scientific inquiry

From the Enlightenment period onwards, science and reason were perceived to be methods to obtain value-free knowledge in a neutral manner. Prior to the Enlightenment, nursing work had been undertaken by untrained religious people and local women with experience of caring for family members or having babies (Ehrenreich & English 1973). A structured logical analysis of human behaviour was developed by John Locke (1690) in *An Essay Concerning Human Understanding*. Locke espoused the belief that all ideas originate in experience. The inherent premise was that a newborn infant must acquire his or her ideas of this world by observing what goes on around him or her. The limits of understanding are therefore set by the limits of sense and reason. This argument was readily adopted as the dominant philosophy on all aspects of intellectual life during the eighteenth century (Miller 1985). This argument was termed empiricism. It referred to the idea that what was known was only possible through sensory experience. Knowledge could therefore be validated (Mitchell 1987).

Florence Nightingale (1820–1910) gave shape and form to what was to become the discipline of nursing by using the scientific methods proposed from the Enlightenment period. Tutored in mathematics as a child, Nightingale systematically collected data and analysed this statistically (Cohen 1984). Nightingale's explanation of the phenomena of concern to nursing marks the beginning of systematic inquiry and the development of a knowledge base (Newman 1983). She applied 'scientific inquiry' to illness generally to derive specific nursing interventions. Nightingale is best known for her carefully collected information in relation to the environment, namely the concepts of ventilation, warmth, light, diet, cleanliness and noise (Tomey & Alligood 1998). Through careful observation, keen documentation and subsequent analysis of these factors, she sought insights into causal relationships on which nursing could make a difference.

Nightingale also needed to persuade influential politicians who championed her cause. She used the dominant method of the day to progress this, namely observation, to collect objective data and logic/reasoning instead of religion and superstition (Ehrenreich & English 1973). Since Nightingale, nurses have approached their practice in a structured and systematic manner. In order to expand an understanding of the discipline, nursing has sought theory in an attempt to describe, explain, predict and control. Nurses have borrowed theory from a range of other disciplines to assist in understanding the core phenomena inherent in nursing. In many situations nurses have modified and adopted theory from these disciplines in an attempt to develop a nursing-specific theory.

The dominance of empiricism in the practice of nursing

Physiological theories based in scientific methods of inquiry were well advanced by the second half of the nineteenth century and provided information about how the body functioned (Miller 1985). The biomedical model, the basis of contemporary acute medical practice, arose from this form of investigation. This model views people as biological beings, made of cells, tissues and organs that achieve homeostasis, an internal mechanism that keeps physical and chemical parameters of the body relatively constant. Consistent with the notions of reason and causality that accompanied modernity, how the body functioned could be likened to a machine (Benner & Wrubel 1989, Pearson et al 2005).

The biomedical model has continued to dominate healthcare during the twentieth century (Aronowitz 1998), and has become the dominant paradigm in many areas of practice—not only the medical profession but also for nurses (Pearson et al 2005). For example, during the initial establishment of intensive care areas, nurses frequently learnt with doctors about how the physiological body responded in situations of illness (Fairman 1992). Nurses, who had become responsible for the physical body, were learning more about the physiological responses that accompanied health problems. Potentially this knowledge was instrumental in assisting health restoration, nurses could act quickly using this information and interventions based on biomedicine could be appropriately administered.

Increasing knowledge of human physiology has resulted in a plethora of methods and tools to diagnose and prescribe treatment. These methods have largely been dictated by the medical profession. Nursing care that is related to supporting medical interventions follow this biomedical understanding. Accordingly, biomedical scientific knowledge generally assumes priority in nursing practice (Henderson 1994). This situation has arisen primarily because healthcare is directed by medicine and provision of care by nurses is largely organised to support interventions directed by the medical profession.

The extensive use of the biomedical model has similarly led to an emphasis on technical-related aspects of the nursing role. This can be partially explained by the observation that during clinical interactions the body is essentially objectified. In the physical interaction the patient experiences his or her body as a scientific object beneath the dispassionate gaze consistent with scientific investigation (Leder 1984). This has inadvertently led to a devaluing of assisting the individual through the experience of their illness (Pearson et al 2005). When disease is conceptualised as the aberrant dysfunction at the tissue, cellular or organ level, the biomedical model is an efficient theoretical framework to explore this function (Benner & Wrubel 1989).

This perspective has been contested by many contemporary nursing theorists working from a postmodern perspective. These theorists (e.g. Martha Rogers, Jean Watson and Patricia Benner) are interested in the non-technical, or more caring, relational aspects of the nursing role, which examine the minutiae of the daily practice of nursing work and the patient's experience of illness from their own perspective. They argue that this is more akin to the reality of nursing as it is actually practised. Nurses can make an important contribution to such dimensions of patient care. They have a capacity to recognise and explore individuals' spirituality, feelings, situated meaning and ethical concerns that accompany their (the individual's) journey through the illness trajectory that are lost in a purely biomedical or scientific approach. The work of these postmodern scholars has resulted in a growing appreciation of the experience of illness and also recognition of tacit nursing knowledge (Benner & Wrubel 1989).

THE META-PARADIGM OF NURSING: IDENTIFYING A DISTINCT BODY OF KNOWLEDGE

In line with the emergence of organised society and the modern-day hospital (Bullough & Bullough 1972), during the phase we have identified as *monopoly capitalism*, nursing knowledge grew through a complex mix of practice, science, social and behavioural theories and tradition. This resulted in a body of healthcare knowledge that is respected independently of medicine, although not necessarily seen as equal or as valuable. During the push to obtain professional status, nurses recognised the need to identify core proponents that would assist in the continuous debate and refinement of a unique body of knowledge. To assist with this, a meta-paradigm was sought by which to organise and direct the knowledge that would become nursing's unique focus.

A meta-paradigm of any discipline is a statement or group of statements identifying the relevant phenomena to the discipline (Fawcett 1984). It originates from the term 'paradigm', used to describe accepted practices and techniques through which a discipline accumulates and refines its knowledge base. According to Kuhn (1970), a paradigm assists in the articulation and refinement of the phenomena being explored. Exploration of the scholarly arguments, as they pertain to nursing, identifies four central recurring themes that can arguably be described as constituting a meta-paradigm for nursing. The components of the paradigm are identified as: nursing (as an action); client (human being); environment (of the client and nurse–client); and health. The nurse interacts with the client and the environment for the purpose of facilitating the health of the client (Fawcett 1984, Newman 1983).

These four components facilitate the description and explication of theories in nursing. For example, the model proposed by Roper et al (1990), that addresses clients' activities of daily living, is a development on earlier notions of understanding health. This model recognises the integral part of psychosocial wellbeing on health, and appropriately ensures consideration of environmental factors including communication and capacity to develop relationships. These components of the meta-paradigm are essential because what is meant by nursing is largely influenced by the meanings and the importance attributed to it (Newman 1983). Insights into potential meaning may be derived through an understanding of the shifts and developments in how two of these components, the client and the environment, are understood.

Understanding the client

Words referring to the person receiving the nursing care have changed in line with some of the broad cultural configurations that we mentioned previously. Historically, nursing language uses the term 'patient' to refer to the nursed. In modern times (i.e. the postindustrial age), we have exchanged this term for 'client' and, in some cases, 'consumer'. This interesting change of language is meant to confer an attitude of active participation of the person receiving care.

These changes in nomenclature about the person being nursed are, in part, related to how the individual being nursed is actually viewed—that is, how they are understood as a human being and a person. How the individual is approached and how nursing care is attended to has largely been influenced by how the human body has been conceptualised, which has in turn influenced what practices are perceived to constitute nursing.

According to the biomedical model, health was the maintenance of the body's biological functioning. However, with increasing knowledge about the human body, the conceptualisation of the individual, and accordingly health, has broadened. Methods of scientific inquiry have been used to describe not only the internal operation of the biological body, but also human behaviour. Consistent with empirical research, initially human behaviour was likened to a stimulus–response model—for example, if a person was hungry they sought food. Subsequent to these initial observations and experiments, it was recognised that there was a cognitive component to human behaviour. Individuals could think, plan and make decisions on remembered information.

Acceptance of the cognitive component of the individual has been very influential in broadening the scope of nursing work. The impact of psychological wellbeing on overall health status meant that nurses could have a sphere of influence apart from the technical interventions accompanying tests, procedures and other intrusions into the body.

Aspects of the human condition relating to stress and anxiety are core concepts repeatedly studied in nursing. These concepts frequently accompany deviations of health when experienced by clients, and they are an area in which nurses are readily able to make a difference (Devine & Cook 1986). Many nursing theories have been developed in response to the potential of psychological issues that affect individuals with deviations in their health condition. Theorists using this approach include Peplau and Travelbee (Tomey & Alligood 1998).

Consistent with postmodernity, the limitations of experimental psychological research in explaining the human condition have been exposed by Sigmund Freud. The work of Freud is powerful in challenging the notion of accepted empiricism. Freud, through recognition of the subconscious of individuals, exposed another form of knowledge that was not acquired through empirical studies (Miller 1985). Freud's work demonstrated the importance of the unconscious and instinctual forces in human conduct (Miller 1985). The recognition of this knowledge is influential in postmodernity—there is now acknowledgement that we can learn more about ourselves and how we function within the world apart from rigorous empirical methods. Meanings are understood as specific to the individual or a small group of individuals as 'mini-narratives'.

Understanding the environment

From the inception of this chapter we have argued that the social and cultural environment produces nursing and structures nursing action. Nursing does not occur in a vacuum. Despite this fundamental premise, the various conceptualisations of the environment remain the most ill-defined of all the central concepts of the espoused meta-paradigm (Brodie 1984). Kleffel (1991) similarly reviews the perspective of the environment, and concludes that the concept of the environment is important as a domain of nursing knowledge, as it is the nature of the environment as it is conceived in global terms that impacts on nursing.

We have seen how the nature of nursing and transformation of nursing practice can be initiated through shifts in social thoughts and ideas that emerge from the global environment, such as the growth of science as an explanation (from the Enlightenment) or the different ways that nursing work has been produced across the broad epochs of monopoly and postindustrial capitalism. Let us now take a specific example that affects nursing practice and that has become prominent in the postindustrial era—that is, growth of the business model of healthcare.

Among the competing discourses involved in the complex production of healthcare in Western industrial nations, the strength of the business-model-driven healthcare system is paramount. The roots of modern managerialism with its stress upon healthcare targets, admissions, discharges and care pathways can be traced to the industrial revolution. This factory-style production of nursing work is a form of Taylorism (Lundy 1996). Taylorism involves taking a professional skill set and breaking it up into component parts, which can then be further classified according to a particular skill level. Workers with less training can participate in what is hitherto a complete professional activity. This provides definite economic benefits, as fewer of the more highly trained professionals are required. For the nurses working on the factory line, producing regimented segments of nursing care according to prescribed pathways, the scope of what we would term professional nursing practice is stymied. In a climate that Hofstadter (1963) has termed *unreflective instrumentalism*, there has been a loss of the complexity of nursing and the ability for the high level of analysis and reflection necessary for a practice-based profession to provide the highest level of care.

In this type of business-driven healthcare environment, Ackroyd and Bolton (1999) argue that while nurses do retain autonomy from managers, the context of nursing is controlled via the supply of patients. By increasing the number of patients, managers control the time that nurses have available to treat each individual patient. This means that nurses have to work harder if they want to give what they feel is an appropriate level of care. In this way, key parameters of nursing activity are gradually lost to the profession that may wish to control the quality of its work. Thus we can see that awareness of the environment in which nurses work is revealing—as the environment prescribes not only the conditions in which development of knowledge occurs, but also how that knowledge can be applied. Concomitantly, it is argued that the nursing profession is starting to mature and that professional nurses have started to examine their behaviours and how these have emerged, and are managing their situation to better suit the profession.

CONCLUDING THOUGHTS

Nursing has been informed and influenced by many different ideas and trends within modern society. These are evident in the education, practice and research of nursing. The involvement of nurses in understanding the foundations of their professional practice opens for scrutiny the basis not only for current practice but also for future directions.

The way you think about people and nursing have a direct impact on how you approach individuals, what questions you ask, how that information is processed and what nursing activities are included in the care offered. The challenge for nurses is to have a comprehensive understanding of ideas, and how they have contributed to contemporary practice. This platform can then be interrogated to derive the best outcomes for future practice and the strategic development of optimal practice and development of the profession.

REFLECTIVE QUESTIONS

1 To what extent is theory development crucial to nursing and nursing practice?

2 How does the Western industrial healthcare environment affect nursing work in the twenty-first century?

3 How does the conceptual shift of postmodernity affect the development of nursing knowledge in practice?

4 What local situations and conditions operate in your sphere of practice that influences the nursing care you provide?

RECOMMENDED READINGS

Alligood M, Marriner-Tomey A (ed) 2002 Nursing theory: utilization and application, 2nd edn. Mosby, St Louis

Hollinger R 1994 Postmodernism and the social sciences: a thematic approach. Sage, London, pp 169–177

Pearson A, Vaughan B, FitzGerald M 2005 Nursing models for practice, 3rd edn. Butterworth–Heinemann, London

REFERENCES

Ackroyd S, Bolton S 1999 It is not Taylorism: mechanisms of work intensification in the provision of gynaecological services in a NHS hospital. Work Employment and Society 13(2):369–387

Aronowitz R A 1998 Making sense of illness. Cambridge University Press, Cambridge

Benner P, Wrubel J 1989 The primacy of caring. Addison Wesley, Menlo Park, California

Brodie J A 1984 Response to Dr J Fawcett's paper. Image: Journal of Nursing Scholarship 16(3):87–98.

Bullough B, Bullough V 1972 A brief history of medical practice. In Friedson E, Lorber J (eds) Medieval men and their work. Aldine-Atherton, Chicago, pp 86–102

Cohen I B 1984 Florence Nightingale. Scientific American March:128–136

Devine E C, Cook T D 1986 Clinical and cost saving effects of psychosocial educational interventions with surgical patients: a meta-analysis. Research in Nursing and Health 9:89–105

Ehrenreich B, English D 1973 Witches, midwives, and nurses. Writers and Readers Co-operative, London

Fairman J 1992 Watchful vigilance: nursing care, technology and the development of intensive care units. Nursing Research 41:56–60

Fawcett J 1984 The meta-paradigm of nursing: present status and future refinements. Image: Journal of Nursing Scholarship 16(3):84–86

Gillan G 1988 Foucault's philosophy. In: Bernauer J, Rasmussen D (eds) The final Foucault. MIT Press, London

Grosz E 1993 Bodies and knowledges: feminism and the crisis of reason. In: Alcroff L, Potter E (eds) Feminist epistemologies. Routledge, New York, pp 187–216

Harvey D 1989 The condition of postmodernity. Basil Blackwell, Oxford

Henderson A 1994 Power and knowledge in nursing practice: the contribution to Foucault. Journal of Advanced Nursing 20(5):935–939

Hofstadter R 1963 Anti-intellectualism in American life. Alfred A Knopf, New York, pp 233–271

Hollinger R 1994 Postmodernism and the social sciences: a thematic approach. Sage, London

Jameson F 1984 Postmodernism: or the cultural logic of late capitalism. New Left Review 146:53–92

Katz S 1995 Disciplinary texts: rhetoric and the science of old age in the late nineteenth century and early twentieth century. Australian Cultural History 14:109–126

Kleffel D 1991 Rethinking the environment as a domain of nursing knowledge. Advances in Nursing Science 15:307–315

Kuhn T S 1970 The structure of scientific revolutions. University of Chicago Press, Chicago

Leder D 1984 Medicine and paradigms of embodiment. Journal of Medicine and Philosophy 9:29–43

Lundy C 1996 Nursing beyond Fordism. Employee Responsibilities and Rights Journal 9(2):163–171

Miller G A 1985 Psychology: the science of mental life. Penguin, London

Mitchell G D 1987 A new dictionary of sociology. Routledge & Kegan Paul, London.

Newman M A 1983 The continuing revolution: a history of nursing science. In: Chaska N L (ed) The nursing profession: a time to speak. McGraw Hill, New York, pp 385–393

Pearson A, Vaughan B, Fitzgerald M 2005 Nursing models for practice, 3rd edn. Butterworth–Heinemann, Oxford

Roper N, Logan W, Tierney A 1990 The elements of nursing, 3rd edn. Churchill Livingstone, Edinburgh

Tomey A, Alligood M R 1998 Nursing theorists and their work, 4th edn. Mosby, St Louis

Winch S 2005 Ethics, government and sexual health: insights from Foucault. Nursing Ethics 12(2):177–186

Winch S, Henderson A 2009 Making cars and making healthcare: a critical review. Australian Medical Journal, 191(1):28–29

Yeatman A 1991 Postmodern critical theorising: introduction. Social Analysis 30:3–9

CHAPTER 7

Becoming a critical thinker

Steve Parker

LEARNING OBJECTIVES

At the completion of this chapter, the student will be able to:

- describe the essential nature of critical thinking
- describe the significance of critical thinking to nursing practice
- describe the main characteristics of a critical thinker
- explain the basic structure of an argument
- apply the basic structure of an argument to various areas of nursing practice
- identify resources for further reading and the study of critical thinking.

KEY WORDS

Critical thinking, reflection, action, evaluation, argument, induction, premise, nursing process, decision making

WHAT IS CRITICAL THINKING?

There are a variety of definitions of critical thinking and no general consensus on any one of them (Riddell 2007). Scheffer & Rubenfeld (2000) conducted an international study to try to arrive at a consensus definition specifically for nursing. The large majority of participants in the study finally agreed that:

> Critical thinking in nursing is an essential component of professional accountability and quality nursing care. Critical thinkers in nursing exhibit these habits of the mind: confidence, contextual perspective, creativity, flexibility, inquisitiveness, intellectual integrity, intuition, open-mindedness, perseverance, and reflection. Critical thinkers in nursing practice the cognitive skills of analysing, applying standards, discriminating, information seeking, logical reasoning, predicting and transforming knowledge.

However, there continues to be ongoing discussion of what critical thinking actually is. This situation means we need to be careful about relying on any one definition. Paul and Elder (2002) provide a helpful general definition when they suggest that '[c]ritical thinking is the disciplined art of ensuring that you use the best thinking you are capable of in any set of circumstances'.

In essence, critical thinking refers to the activity of *questioning what is usually taken for granted*.

Whether we are aware of it or not, all behaviour is based on certain values, assumptions and beliefs. These form the basis for our decisions to act in certain ways. In a professional context such as nursing practice, everything that we think, say or do is the result of a complex web of beliefs, values and assumptions that have formed as a result of our life experiences. As we grow up in our family, attend school, participate in religious communities, associate with friends, watch television, read newspapers and work for various employers, we develop a 'pair of spectacles' through which we understand and interpret the world and all that happens in it. Just as a person who wears glasses eventually becomes unaware that they are even wearing them, so too each of us adjusts to our worldview 'spectacles' until, often, we are completely unaware what values, beliefs and assumptions are influencing us in a specific situation.

Critical thinking means stopping and reflecting on the reasons for doing things the way they are done or for experiencing things the way they are—focusing on what is frequently taken for granted and evaluating the values, beliefs and assumptions that are held, and asking whether or not what is done and thought is justifiable or not. These characteristics of critical thinking imply a self-consciousness of what, how and why we are thinking, with the intention of improving thinking. In short, 'critical thinking is thinking about your thinking while you're thinking in order to make your thinking better' (Paul 2008). Improving thinking is essential because it is intimately related to the many decisions that need to be made each day. The quality of our lives is determined by the quality of our decisions, and the quality of our decisions is determined by the quality of our reasoning (Schick & Vaughn 1995). In particular, '[i]f nurses are to deal effectively with complex change, increased demands and greater accountability, they must become skilled in higher level thinking and reasoning abilities' (Simpson & Courtney 2002:89).

The National Competency Standards for the Registered Nurse (2006) in Australia recognises the importance of critical thinking for nurses by including a domain of competency entitled *Critical Thinking and Analysis*. It states that this domain

... relates to self-appraisal, professional development, and the value of evidence and research practice. Reflecting on practice, feelings and beliefs and the consequences of these for individuals/groups is an important professional benchmark.

An important aspect of critical thinking is healthy scepticism. This scepticism is necessary because there are many attempts to persuade us to accept various claims. These attempts to persuade also occur in professional contexts. For example, research reports suggest changes to practice; peers argue that their way of acting is the right one; therapists promote various interventions; administrators argue that certain changes need to be made to the workplace; and so on. Often these claims are contradictory, so they cannot all be acceptable.

Practitioners need to sort through all these, often competing, claims. To accept them all without question will, at best, be highly confusing and, at worst, may endanger the lives of others if actions are based on wrong information or conclusions. To adopt an attitude of healthy scepticism means to cautiously listen to or read the claims that others make, carefully evaluate their legitimacy, and not rush to accept a conclusion without careful thought.

The same rigorous thinking needs to be done about our own nursing practice. We make decisions every moment that we assume are of benefit to our patients. Asking questions about the practices we engage in, including what evidence is available to support their efficacy, is essential if our nursing practice is to produce positive outcomes for those for whom we care.

It is possible, of course, to become too pedantic, resulting in inaction because we are not prepared to accept anything unless it is 100% proven. This is why the scepticism needs to be healthy. There is a limit to what can be known for certain. And part of critical thinking is knowing these limits and making the best evaluation under the circumstances.

THE RELATIONSHIP BETWEEN CRITICAL AND CREATIVE THINKING

Critical thinking is not the same as creative thinking. According to Miller and Babcock (1996:117), creative thinking is, among other things, more divergent, messy, unpredictable, provocative, spontaneous and playful than critical thinking. They describe critical thinking as selective, orderly, predictable, analytical, judgemental and evaluative.

Creative thinking, although different from critical thinking, is an essential, complementary process to critical thinking. As a practitioner, there are many situations that arise that do not fit with the ideal or that are not predictable. No individual person for whom nurses care ever fits the 'average' because each person and situation is unique. In order to solve problems for these unique situations and individuals, the practitioner needs to be able to develop new approaches and solutions so that all parties have their needs met. Miller and Babcock suggest that:

> Creative thinking is very useful when what we know and what we know how to do are not working, including the rules of reason, common sense, gravity, and routine. The creative thinker is willing to think wildly, without having any idea where her or his path of thinking may lead. Deliberative cognition is temporarily held in abeyance.
> (Miller & Babcock 1996:120)

Because creative thinking is so 'chaotic', it means that it needs to be evaluated to ensure that any conclusions that are reached are appropriate. In this regard, Ruggiero understands the mind to have two phases:

> It both produces ideas and judges them. These phases are intertwined; that is, we move back and forth between them many times in the course of dealing with a problem, sometimes several times in the span of a few seconds.
> (*Ruggiero* 1998:81)

In the past, critical thinking has often been presented apart from creative thinking. However, in practice, creative and critical thinking go hand-in-hand. Without creative thinking, critical thinking would be dry and mechanical. Without critical thinking, creative thinking would be chaotic and inefficient. As Ruggiero (1998:81) asserts, '[t]o study the art of thinking in its most dynamic form [where creative and critical thinking are intertwined] would be difficult at best'. Consequently, in practice, we need to consider them separately. However, although critical thinking and creative thinking are distinct from each other, they should never be separated.

THE CHARACTERISTICS OF CRITICAL THINKING

So what are the characteristics that a critical thinker will demonstrate? Jacobs et al (1997) have developed a set of observable skills that indicate the presence of critical thinking. These are grouped into categories, as described below.

First, a critical thinker needs the ability to integrate information from all relevant sources by being able to distinguish between relevant and irrelevant data, validate data that are obtained, recognise when data are missing, predict multiple outcomes, and recognise the consequences of actions.

Second, to think critically means to be able to examine assumptions by recognising them when they are present, detect bias, identify assumptions that are not stated, recognise the relationships of action or inaction, and transfer thoughts and concepts to diverse contexts, or develop alternative courses of action.

Third, it is important for the critical thinker to be able to identify relationships and patterns. This includes recognising inconsistencies or fallacies of logic, working out generalisations, developing a plan of action consistent with a model, and, where appropriate, seeking out alternative models.

Jacobs et al offer a definition of critical thinking that incorporates all these characteristics:

> Critical thinking is the repeated examination of problems, questions, issues, and situations by comparing, simplifying, synthesizing information in an analytical, deliberative, evaluative, decisive way.
> (*Jacobs et al* 1997:20)

Many more examples of various ways of describing the characteristics of critical thinking could be offered. One way of summarising these is to focus on critical thinking as reasoning. The heart of reasoning is the argument. In what follows, the nature of argument will be described, followed by a survey of the ways in which arguments 'appear' in nursing. Suggestions will then be offered regarding the way in which the principles of critical thinking might be applied in these areas. By doing so, the way in which this approach synthesises the skills of critical thinking will become obvious.

WHAT IS AN ARGUMENT?

In colloquial language the word 'argument' is often used for a shouting match between two people who are having a disagreement where the participants are very angry, abusive or physically aggressive. There may be shouting, pointing of fingers, threats, crying, name-calling, and so on.

However, in critical thinking, the term 'argument' does not apply to these situations. In fact, these situations are the very opposite of critical thinking. In critical thinking, an argument consists of a conclusion and one or more reasons that are intended to support the conclusion. Figure 7.1 shows the relationship between these parts of an argument. Each reason may or may not have evidence that is intended to support the reason or reasons.

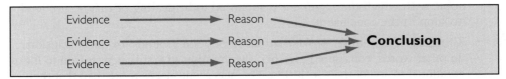

Figure 7.1
Components of an argument

Here is an example of an argument:

Every person has the right to choose how they live their lives. Therefore, a person has the right to choose to practise life-threatening behaviours if they wish.

This is an argument because it has a conclusion ('A person has the right to choose to practise life-threatening behaviours if they wish') and a reason intended to support that conclusion ('Every person has the right to choose how they live their lives'). At this stage, we are not concerned whether this is a good argument or not, only with what makes something an argument. If it were desirable, a person presenting this argument could provide some evidence for the first statement by drawing attention, for example, to various statements of human rights, the constitutions of countries or discussions about ethics. So an argument needs to have the following:

*   a conclusion, and
*   one or more reasons intended to support the conclusion.

What makes a sound argument?

For an argument to be sound, three criteria need to be met. First, the reasons need to be acceptable to the person evaluating the argument. Second, the reasons need to be relevant. And, third, the reasons need to provide adequate grounds for accepting the conclusion. Govier (1992) offers a useful way to remember these three criteria, which she calls the conditions of argument. If the first three letters of the word argument (ARG) are taken on their own, each letter stands for one of the conditions of argument. That is:

A   Acceptability
R   Relevance
G   Grounds

Govier's definitions of each of these conditions are also useful:

- Acceptability: The premises [reasons] are acceptable when it is reasonable for those to whom the argument is addressed to believe these premises. There is good reason to accept the premises—even if they are not known for certain to be true. And there is no good evidence known to those to whom the argument is addressed that would indicate either that the premises are false or that they are doubtful.

- Relevance: [Premises are relevant to the conclusion] when they give at least some evidence in favour of the conclusion's being true. They specify factors, evidence or reasons that do count towards establishing the conclusion. They do not merely describe distracting aspects that lead you away from the real topic with which the argument is supposed to be dealing or that do not tend to support the conclusion.

- Grounds: The premises provide sufficient or good grounds for the conclusion. In other words, considered together, the premises give sufficient reason to make it rational to accept the conclusion. This statement means more than that the premises are relevant. Not only do they count as evidence for the conclusion, they provide enough evidence, or enough reasons, taken together, to make it reasonable to accept the conclusion (adapted from Govier 1992:68–69).

The following example illustrates these criteria:

Nurses must have a practising certificate to be employed as a nurse.
Sue does not have a practising certificate.
Therefore, Sue is not permitted to be employed as a nurse.

Statements 1 and 2 are both reasons, which are intended to support the conclusion in Statement 3. If this is a sound argument, then the reasons must be relevant and acceptable, and they must provide adequate grounds for accepting the conclusion.

Statement 1 is certainly acceptable. Most countries have a requirement that nurses need to be licensed to practise. Statement 2 is hypothetical, so we will assume that it is true for the sake of the discussion. All the reasons, then, are acceptable. The two reasons are also relevant to the issue under consideration.

The next question is whether these reasons provide adequate grounds for accepting the conclusion. We can test this by asking:

Is it possible to reject the conclusion and still believe the reasons to be true? Or, in other words, even though the reasons are true, is there a legitimate way that we can escape accepting the conclusion?

So, could one believe that Sue could practise and still believe that the two reasons offered are true? In this case, the answer is no. If it is true that a nurse must have a practising certificate to practise, and Sue does not have one, we are 'compelled' to accept the conclusion that Sue cannot practise. This argument, then, is a sound one.

Another example will illustrate a poor argument:

Everyone's hair falls out when undergoing chemotherapy.
Jo is undergoing chemotherapy.
Therefore, Jo's hair will fall out.

First, are the reasons acceptable? Does a person's hair fall out when they are undergoing chemotherapy? Sometimes it does, but not necessarily everyone's. So this reason is not acceptable because, although some people's hair falls out, not everyone's does. For the sake of this discussion, the second reason can be accepted (that Jo is undergoing chemotherapy).

Both of the reasons are relevant, and so the final question is whether the reasons offered provide adequate grounds for accepting that Jo's hair will fall out. The answer is no because the first reason was false. Although it might be true that Jo's hair will fall out, it is not possible to predict it because not everyone's hair does when they are undergoing chemotherapy.

To summarise:

- An argument consists of a conclusion, with one or more relevant reasons that are intended to support the conclusion.

- Evidence may or may not be offered to support each reason.

- A sound argument is one in which the reason(s) are acceptable and provide adequate grounds for accepting the conclusion.

There are a few technical terms that need to be remembered in regard to what has been covered so far.

- A *reason* can also be called a premise.

- The question of whether reasons provide grounds for the conclusion is a question of *validity*. In everyday conversation, the word validity often has a broader meaning. In critical thinking, it is used to refer to the logical relationship between the reasons and the conclusion.

- When an argument has reasons that are acceptable and is valid (i.e. the reasons provide adequate grounds for accepting the conclusion), then the argument is said to be *sound*.

It is important to note that an argument can be valid but unsound. For example, the following argument is valid but unsound:

All nurses are female.
Jo is a nurse.
Therefore, Jo is female.

Statement 1 is not true, of course. Some nurses are male. Statement 2 can be assumed to be true. Because Statement 1 is false, we already know that this argument is unsound. But is it valid? Yes it is. If Statement 1 were true, the acceptance of Statement 3 would be unavoidable. This means that the argument is logically valid, but it is not sound—that is, it is not a sound argument.

CRITICAL THINKING IN NURSING

Critical thinking, in essence, means being able to identify the presence of an argument in any form and evaluate it. Once what makes a sound argument, and the questions needed to be asked to evaluate it, are known, it is possible to assess any argument that is encountered. Critical thinking means applying to this task thinking that has the characteristics discussed above.

This basic approach can be applied to many areas within nursing. In the following sections, some examples of these areas will be surveyed, how the basic framework introduced above applies to that area will be discussed and some guidelines for thinking critically about issues in the respective area will be offered. The overlaying of the structure of argument onto the various areas in nursing builds on the work of Mayer and Goodchild (1995) in their discussion of critical thinking in psychology.

Clinical practice

In clinical practice, decisions are constantly being made to act in certain ways for the benefit of clients. These actions can be beneficial or have serious consequences for the health and wellbeing of the people a nurse is working for or with. It is essential that these interventions be considered critically. Figure 7.2 illustrates the application of the basic argument framework to clinical practice.

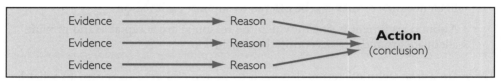

Figure 7.2
The basic argument framework applied to clinical practice

As can be seen, very little alteration is necessary. The equivalent of the conclusion is the particular action that has been, or will be, performed. Each of a nurse's actions should be able to be justified by appealing to an appropriate set of reasons. These reasons, in turn, must be based on high-quality evidence.

In the past, many of the actions and interventions of nurses have been based on tradition, folklore or no evidence at all. In recent years, however, the developing professional status of nursing has resulted in more concern about the basis for nursing action. There is a growing and strengthening movement called evidence-based practice, which promotes an attitude of thinking critically about what is done by nurses and asking on what basis actions can be justified.

The increasing interest of consumers in their own healthcare has also had an effect. People are no longer willing to allow health professionals to make all the decisions for them and are demanding higher quality care. The increasing incidence of litigation has also motivated a concern for basing nursing action on high-quality evidence.

On an individual level, a nurse should be able to justify any action performed on behalf of a client. The reasons need to be based on solid evidence. The source of this evidence may take many forms, including personal experience, traditions handed down between 'generations' of nurses and what is taught during nurse education. However, on their own, these sources of knowledge are not adequate. A formal process for exploring nursing knowledge is needed, which allows the testing of ideas and the validation of actions and interventions.

The activity of formal research provides this opportunity. Nursing research will be examined below from a critical thinking perspective. First, however, there are a number of questions that can be asked about practice, which will help nurses think critically about it. When reflecting on an action or intervention, ask the following questions:

- What are the reasons for acting or intervening in the way that is planned?
- What evidence is available that supports the reasons for acting in this way?
- Are the reasons relevant to the issue that is being considered?
- Are there other reasons that need to be considered?
- Is there any evidence that raises questions about the manner of acting or intervening?
- Do the reasons provide adequate grounds for acting in the planned way?
- Are there alternative actions or interventions that could be chosen and the reasons still be acceptable in these situations?

The nursing process

The nursing process is a common framework for making practice decisions in nursing; therefore, it will be briefly explored in relation to critical thinking. The steps of the nursing process are:

1. collection of subjective and objective data
2. arrival at a diagnosis of the client's problem(s)
3. planning of appropriate nursing interventions in response to the problem(s)
4. implementation of the planned intervention(s), and
5. ongoing evaluation of the effectiveness of the intervention(s) in relation to the client's problem(s).

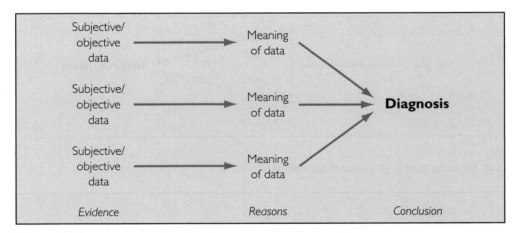

Figure 7.3
The three phases of nursing represented as an argument

The nursing process can be summarised in three 'phases':

1. diagnosis
2. intervention, and
3. evaluation.

Each of these three phases can be understood as an argument (remember the technical meaning of the term 'argument'). Figure 7.3 illustrates this.

The diagnosis is the equivalent of the conclusion in an argument. The data that are collected come from observations of the patient, as well as information provided by the client, relatives, friends, history, and so on. These raw data need to be interpreted and take on meaning in the context of developing a diagnosis. Finally, on the basis of the meaning of the data, a conclusion is arrived at in the form of a diagnosis.

Of course, the description here is somewhat simplistic. The actual process is much richer and more complex than this. However, understanding the process of diagnosis as an argument leads us to ask questions such as the following:

1. Are the data collected accurate? If not, how reliable are they?

2. Have the data been understood and interpreted correctly?

3. Are the data and their interpretation relevant to the diagnosis that has been chosen?

4. Does the interpretation of the data provide adequate grounds for arriving at the diagnosis?

5. Are there any other diagnoses that could possibly fit the data that have been collected? Are any of these more consistent with the data?

A similar process applies to the intervention and evaluation phases. Interventions and evaluation criteria must be justified to support claims of changes such as improvement or deterioration; or preservation of the status quo. Figures 7.4 and 7.5 illustrate the structure of argument related to these two phases.

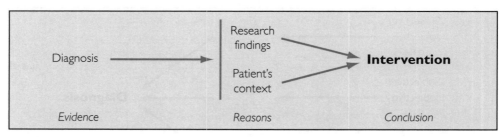

Figure 7.4
The structure of argument: intervention

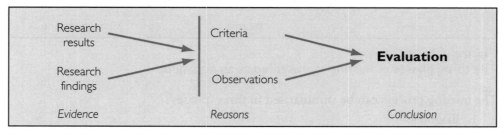

Figure 7.5
The structure of argument: evaluation

Thinking critically about research

The need for nursing research and the current focus on evidence-based practice has been described above. Nursing research provides the evidence nurses need to evaluate the appropriateness of nursing practice, helps to raise new questions for nurses to explore and provokes new ways of looking at what nurses do.

Nurses may relate to research in three ways. A nurse may be a 'consumer' of research, a researcher, or both. In this discussion, we will be focusing particularly on the role of research consumer.

It has already been argued that nurses must base their practice on high-quality evidence. The results of nursing research form the most significant source of this evidence for nurse practitioners. Nurses must avail themselves of the latest research in their area of practice, and this means that some understanding of the process is important.

Every research project suffers from limitations and flaws of some sort or another. So nurses cannot take a research report and automatically assume that it provides them with the best guidance for practice. The nurse needs to think critically about research reports. Understanding a research report to be an argument assists in thinking critically about the conclusions it draws (Mayer & Goodchild 1995). Mayer and Goodchild (1995) discuss the way in which any research can be understood as an argument. Figure 7.6 illustrates this approach.

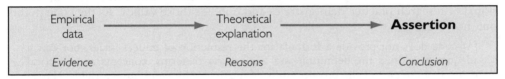

Figure 7.6
Understanding research as an argument

Given this understanding, it is possible to formulate a number of questions to help think critically about research:

- What is the assertion that is being made in the research report? What type of assertion is it? What type of evidence would be needed to be convinced of the truth of the assertion?

- What sort of evidence is offered to support the assertion being made? Is the evidence relevant to the assertion being made? Is adequate information provided to convince the reader that the evidence has been collected rigorously?

- Does the evidence offered provide adequate grounds for accepting the assertion that is being made? Is it possible to think of any other conclusions that could be drawn from the evidence offered? Are these alternative solutions more reasonable than the assertion made in the report?

- Does the theoretical explanation make sense? Are there alternative explanations that make more sense? Does the application of Occam's Razor (roughly this is the principle that the simplest explanation is most likely to be the right one) make any difference to the likelihood of the explanation being correct?

Asking these questions in relation to any research report heightens one's awareness that the conclusions of research are not always correct, nor is the process in arriving at that conclusion automatically sound. This promotes a careful assessment of new nursing practice proposals and consequent higher levels of safety in practice.

THINKING ABOUT ETHICS

Another essential area of which nurses need to be aware is ethics. Thinking ethically means to be able to justify what is done in terms of ethical principles. All behaviour needs to be ethical. Although there are high-profile issues such as euthanasia, abortion and organ transplantation that demand a great deal of attention, they are, perhaps, not the most important issues for nurses.

Issues such as the style of communicating with a patient, the facilitation of the signing of a consent form, communication with other professional colleagues and patients, the management of work rosters, the provision of childcare for employees, the influencing of clients in choosing treatment options—all need to be considered in ethical terms if the individual nurse is to practise with integrity and fulfil his or her obligations to clients.

Most professional bodies have documented codes of ethics and the nursing profession is no different. For example, the Code of Ethics for Nurses in Australia (Australian Nursing & Midwifery Council 2008) contains eight value statements for nurses to use as 'a guide when reflecting on the degree to which their clinical, managerial, educational or research practice demonstrates and upholds those values'. As the code points out, however:

> [A] code does not provide a formula for the resolution of ethical issues, nor can it adequately address the definition and exploration of terms, concepts and practical issues that are part of the broader study of nursing, ethics and human rights. Nurses have a responsibility to develop their knowledge and understanding of ethics and human rights in order to clarify issues relevant to their practice and to inform their response to the issues identified.

Because of this, nurses need to develop skills to be able to think through these issues and evaluate various options for practice. Understanding ethical thinking as an argument can help in this task. Figure 7.7 illustrates the components of an ethical argument. Each of these components will now be examined in relation to critical thinking.

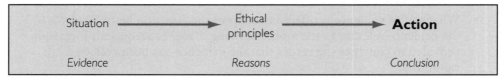

Figure 7.7
The components of an ethical argument

The situation

Ethical thinking is often taught using highly controversial case studies that involve an often unresolvable dilemma between competing principles. However, a number of false impressions may be gained from this. One possible false impression is that 'the continued use of controversial examples serves to exaggerate the extent to which morality, as distinct from moral theory, is controversial' (Coope 1996).

In reality, ethical thinking should pervade all activities, and ethical questions about practice should be continually asked. Ethical thinking should be an everyday activity, which may not always be about problems.

We usually find ourselves in situations where a decision needs to be made about how to act towards another person. These situations continually occur for nurses. For example, a patient might require a sponge in bed. This may not appear to be a situation where ethical thinking needs to take place. But, as this example is explored below, it will be seen that ethical thinking is fundamental to ensuring that the best care is provided.

The first thing to do when thinking ethically is to be aware of as much about the situation as is possible. Too often assumptions are made on the basis of past experience; but every person is different and has unique needs.

The principles

Everyone has a system of principles (values) that guide their lives and how they act. Some of these will be conscious; others may be unconscious. In healthcare, four principles have been identified as an essential starting point for ethical thinking. They are:

1. Autonomy: the right a person has to direct their own life and make their own decisions.
2. Beneficence: the responsibility of actively doing good.
3. Non-maleficence: the responsibility to actively avoid doing harm.
4. Justice: the responsibility to be fair in the way we treat others.

After gaining a knowledge of the situation, the next step is to ask which of the principles (values) are relevant to consider in the particular situation in which the nurse finds themselves. In the example of the person who needs to be washed in bed, the issue of autonomy is clearly relevant. How is autonomy to be ensured in this particular situation? How will the patient be empowered to make their own decisions about their hygiene and the way they wish to maintain it?

The principle of beneficence is also relevant. The whole reason for instituting the patient washing in bed is because it is believed it is good to promote hygiene. It is possible, however, that beneficence may spill over into a denial of the person's autonomy. When this happens, nurses are acting paternalistically—doing what they think is best for the patient—even if the patient does not agree with the nurse. Paternalism needs to be rigorously justified because it overrides a person's fundamental right to autonomy.

Many examples can be found of situations where paternalism occurs: imposing medication on a psychotic individual; or legally enforcing a blood transfusion for a child of a Jehovah's Witness parent. Unfortunately, on many occasions paternalistic attitudes prevail without adequate ethical justification.

Action

Once the situation is understood and the implications of the relevant ethical principles have been thought through, it is necessary to make a decision about how to act. Often this will not be easy. Sometimes, ethical principles conflict with each other (such as when beneficence and autonomy conflict). Nurses do not live and practise in an ideal world, and so it is necessary to be satisfied with the best decision that can be made under the circumstances. The point is not that perfect decisions have to be made; that is never possible. It is rather that whatever decisions are made and whatever actions are performed, they have been carefully thought through and can be justified by appeal to accepted ethical principles.

THE ETHICS OF CRITICAL THINKING

Often, when people learn the tools of critical thinking, they become highly critical of others. It is important that critical thinking be viewed primarily as a set of tools applied to one's own thinking. When evaluating the ideas of others, critical thinking skills are used to decide whether an idea is acceptable or should be rejected. Who the other person is is usually (but not always) irrelevant. When critical thinking skills undermine or attack other people, then the purpose of critical thinking is lost. One of the most important distinctions to remember is that between an idea and the person who presents the idea.

The critical thinker always needs to think critically within the framework of well-developed interpersonal relationship skills. Critical thinking skills are not weapons to be wielded to cut another person down to size. They are tools of personal growth, which allow one to travel through an often confusing landscape and keep one's bearings, while providing the best possible quality care for those to whom one is responsible and accountable.

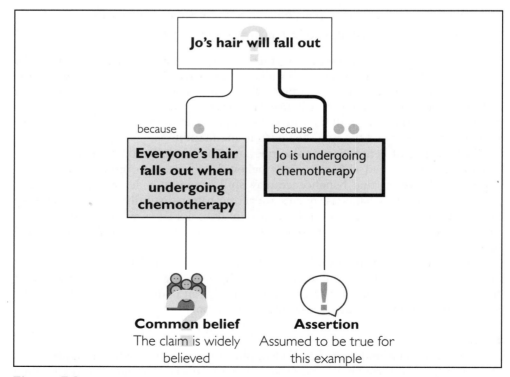

Figure 7.8
The argument about hair loss following chemotherapy

DEVELOPING CRITICAL THINKING SKILLS

There is no magical solution to actually developing critical thinking skills. An awareness of what critical thinking is and where it can be applied is an appropriate start. Like anything, it requires continual practice. Ultimately, it is about developing a conscious attitude of reflection during daily and professional life. Halpern (1998) suggests a number of attitudes and dispositions that support the development of critical thinking. They are: willingness to plan; flexibility; persistence; willingness to self-correct; being mindful ('the habit of self-conscious concern for and evaluation of the thinking process'); and consensus-seeking. As Halpern says:

> No one can become a better thinker just by reading a book. An essential component of critical thinking is developing the attitude and disposition of a critical thinker.

> Good thinkers are motivated and willing to exert the conscious effort needed to work in a planful manner, to check for accuracy, to gather information, and to persist when the solution is not obvious or requires several steps.
> (Halpern 1998:10–11)

Although it is hard work to develop new skills in critical thinking, the time and energy are well worth the rewards that come with the ability to think clearly.

You may also find using some software useful in helping you think critically. There are quite a few software packages available that can help visualise arguments and aid in the process of analysis. One of the best of these is Rationale, which allows you to create diagrams of arguments and your evaluation. Figure 7.8 shows a diagram, produced by Rationale, of the argument about hair loss following chemotherapy described above.

You can download a trial version of this software from http://rationale.austhink. com

CONCLUDING REMARKS

Critical thinking is a vital skill to have as a nurse. Nurses are engaged in providing care to people who have a right to high-quality professional conduct and health services. Nurses have a responsibility to make sure that their actions are based on rigorous evidence and can be justified with acceptable reasons. Although developing the skills to think critically may at times be difficult and demanding, thinking critically provides a greater level of confidence and satisfaction as nurses interact with colleagues, and it promotes high-quality, safe practice.

REFLECTIVE QUESTIONS

1 How has your understanding of thinking changed as a result of reading this chapter?

2 What areas of your professional life would benefit from applying the principles of critical thinking to them?

3 What will you do now to further develop your skill in critical thinking?

RECOMMENDED READINGS

Bandman E L, Bandman B 1998 Critical thinking in nursing, 2nd edn. Appleton & Lange, Norwalk, Connecticut

Browne M N, Keeley S M 2011 Asking the right questions, 10th edn. Longman

Miller A, Babcock D E 1996 Critical thinking applied to nursing. Mosby, St Louis (currently out of print but check your library)

Paul R G, Elder L 2002 Critical thinking: tools for taking charge of your professional and personal life. Prentice Hall, New Jersey

Rubenfeld M G 2006 Critical thinking in nursing: an interactive approach. JB Lippincott, Philadelphia

REFERENCES

Australian Nursing and Midwifery Council (ANMC) 2008 Codes of professional conduct and ethics for nurses and midwives. ANMC, Canberra

Coope C 1996 Does teaching by cases mislead us about morality? Journal of Medical Ethics 22(1):46–52

Govier T 1992 A practical study of argument, 3rd edn. Wadsworth, Belmont, California

Halpern D 1998 Critical thinking across the curriculum: a brief edition of thought and knowledge. Lawrence Erlbaum Associates, Mahwah, New Jersey

Jacobs P, Ott B, Sullivan B, Ulrich Y, Short L 1997 An approach to defining and operationalizing critical thinking. Journal of Nursing Education 36(1):19–22

Mayer R, Goodchild F 1995 The critical thinker, 2nd edn. Brown & Benchmark Publishers, Madison

Miller M, Babcock D 1996 Critical thinking applied to nursing. Mosby, St Louis

Paul R 2008 Critical thinking: basic questions and answers. Foundation for Critical Thinking. Online. Available: www.criticalthinking.org/aboutCT/CTquestionsAnswers.cfm 18 Oct 2008

Paul R, Elder L 2002 Critical thinking: tools for taking charge of your professional and personal life. Financial Times Prentice Hall, New Jersey

Riddell T 2007 Critical assumptions: thinking critically about critical thinking. Journal of Nursing Education 46(3):121–126

Ruggiero V 1998 The art of thinking: a guide to critical and creative thought, 5th edn. Longman, New York

Scheffer B K, Rubenfeld M G 2000 A consensus statement on critical thinking in nursing. Journal of Nursing Education 39(8):352–359

Schick T, Vaughn L 1995 How to think about weird things: critical thinking for a new age. Mayfield Publishing Company, Mountain View, California

Simpson E, Courtney M 2002 Critical thinking in nursing education: a literature review. International Journal of Nursing Practice 8:89–98

CHAPTER 8

Reflective practice: what, why and how

Kim Usher and Colin Holmes

LEARNING OBJECTIVES

After reading this chapter, students should have gained:

- an understanding of the importance and benefits of reflection to a practice-based discipline such as nursing
- insight into the nature of reflection and the ideas of its leading theorists
- an appreciation of the link between self-awareness and professional self-monitoring
- an understanding of the strategies that assist with reflection—for example, reflective writing, journalling, critical incident analysis, clinical supervision and forms of creative expression
- insight into the legal and ethical issues surrounding the keeping of professional journals.

KEY WORDS

Reflection, reflective practice, journalling, critical incident analysis, self-awareness

INTRODUCTION

The context in which nursing occurs has changed markedly in the last two decades. As a result of advances in nursing and medical knowledge, and reduced government spending (which has led to a reduction in hospital beds, shorter hospital stays and more rapid patient turnovers), workers in healthcare institutions are spending much more of their time dealing with acutely ill patients who require specialised care (Usher et al 2001). In order to function in these complex environments practitioners are required to constantly 'refresh and update their knowledge and skills, and frame and solve complex patient and healthcare problems' (Mann, Gordon & MacLeod 2009:595–6). This can cause feelings of concern or confusion, but it also offers us an opportunity to reconceptualise our profession by making it more responsive and reflective of the needs of society (Lauder, Meehan & Moxham 2004). The role of the nurse is also influenced by cultural, social, economic, historical and political constraints that all affect the ways in which nurses approach and react to certain situations (Taylor 2010). It is a given that society expects nurses to practise safely and to undertake what is necessary to keep up-to-date. Reflection helps us to self-correct where the notion of continuous improvement becomes habitual to our practice (Usher, Foster & Stewart 2012).

As a consequence of the changing healthcare arena, today's nursing graduates must not only be clinically competent practitioners, but also need to be adept at critical thinking in order to understand the complexities of the world and the rapidly changing practice arena, even though this can itself be challenging (Usher et al 1999, Johns 2009, Mann, Gordon & MacLeod 2009). Critical thinking, or the practice of questioning, is necessary so that practitioners integrate relevant information from various sources, examine assumptions and identify relationships and patterns (Parker 2010, Thompson & Pascal 2012). Reflective practice and critical thinking are often used interchangeably, but, while not identical, there is a reflexive relationship. After all, as Lumby (2000:338) explains, '. . . to adopt a critical approach to the world, it is necessary to reflect on the world and one's experiences in it'.

We begin this chapter by introducing you to the why of reflection, and explaining why reflection is a useful strategy for undergraduate nursing students, as well as registered nurses. We will also provide an overview of the related legislation that requires the use of reflective thinking in practice by registered nurses and makes it a requirement for all students exiting undergraduate university degrees. The next section of the chapter addresses the why and what of reflective practice, including an overview of the definitions of reflection.

WHY BE REFLECTIVE?

Every workplace presents a complex environment to the new recruit. It is often difficult to understand and appears to abound with multiple decisions, each coupled to a host of different ways in which the desired outcomes could be achieved. Nursing is no different. When you first enter a nursing context, perhaps during your first clinical placement, you will be confronted by discrepancies, such as those between 'ideal' and 'real' practice, and you will experience or witness difficult interpersonal relationships. It is important that these situations do not distract you from your nursing goals or from seeking to provide the best possible care. Although systematic reflection may at first seem difficult to undertake when you are working in a demanding clinical situation, it will help you to recognise and set aside the emotional content and enable you to learn from otherwise negative experiences (Mantzoukas & Jasper 2004). Reflection can take on an even more important role when you find yourself faced with difficult working conditions and environments (Usher et al 2012). Proposed as a way to make meaning out of complex situations (Mann, Gordon & MacLeod 2009), reflection will help you identify alternative ways you could react in the future, hopefully resulting in more positive outcomes. Importantly, reflection helps to ensure that our practice does not become so routine that our actions begin to contradict our values (Thompson & Pascal 2012).

Johns (1998) explains how reflection offers a way to bring to the surface the contradictions between what you intend to achieve in a situation and how you actually practise. In other words, being faced with contradiction opens the possibility for change and offers the practitioner the opportunity to achieve desired practice. One of the outcomes of reflection is thus a process of continuous monitoring and improvement of practice. It assists us to avoid taking situations at face value but rather to move beyond the taken-for-granted assumptions that may be informed by prejudice and discriminatory ideas (Thompson & Pascal 2012).

Regulatory authorities in Australia have embraced the need for practitioners who are reflective, and require that all nurses engage in some form of reflective activity. This is indicated by their adoption of the Australian Nursing and Midwifery Council (ANMC) competency standards for Registered Nurses (2006a). These are a set of competencies representing the minimum core standards for registration as a nurse in Australia. The competencies are organised into four domains: professional practice, critical thinking and analysis, provision and coordination of care, and collaborative and therapeutic practice. The domain of relevance to reflection includes self-appraisal, professional development, research for practice, reflecting on practice, feelings and beliefs, and the consequences of these for individuals. These competencies have been extended to apply to enrolled nurses and also specialty groups, such as critical care nurses and nurse practitioners. The National Competency Standards for the Midwife (ANMC 2006b) also has reflective and ethical practice as one of its four domains, and the codes of professional conduct for nurses and for midwives in Australia likewise require that they practise reflectively and ethically (ANMC 2008a, 2008b).

The Nursing Council of New Zealand has also incorporated reflection as a key competency for Registered Nurses. Reflection in the New Zealand registered nurse competencies comes under Competency 1.5: Practises nursing in a manner that the client identifies as being culturally safe (Nursing Council of New Zealand 2007). The Nursing Council of New Zealand also has competencies for enrolled nurses, midwives and nurse practitioners in which reflection plays a key role. Further information about these competencies is available from the following websites:

- Nursing and Midwifery Board of Australia competencies, and codes of professional conduct, for Registered Nurses: http://www.nursingmidwiferyboard.gov.au/Codes-Guidelines-Statements/Codes-Guidelines.aspx#codesofprofessionalconduct

- Competencies for the Registered Nurses' scope of practice in New Zealand: www.nursingcouncil.org.nz

Encouragement for reflection was also echoed in the education sector, in the *Review of higher education financing and policy (final report): learning for life* or the 'West Report' as it is commonly known (Department of Employment, Education, Training and Youth Affairs 1998), where reflection is listed as an expected attribute of graduates from all undergraduate university degrees in Australia. In other words, it is a requirement of your undergraduate education that you exit the program of study with the ability to reflect. As a result, all undergraduate degree coordinators are now charged with the responsibility of ensuring their graduates have been provided with the opportunity to develop the skill of reflection.

WHAT IS REFLECTION OR REFLECTIVE PRACTICE?

Reflection comes from the Latin verb *reflectere*, which means to bend or turn backwards. This infers that reflection is a process of going back over something after it has already occurred. This might include recalling thoughts and memories, in cognitive acts such as thinking or contemplation, or as a way of making sense of the situation so that necessary changes may be identified or made (Hickson 2011, Taylor 2010). We all reflect on what goes on around us to some extent. If you think about it, we do not generally just walk around in the world without noticing things or thinking about what has happened and how it has impacted on us. Similarly, we all reflect at some level on our practice, but it may only involve thinking about what happened rather than theorising about what happened and looking for ways to improve it in the future.

Thus, the type of reflection to be discussed in this chapter is actually a much more purposeful activity that leads to action that is better informed than that which occurred before the reflection took place (Francis 1995, Thompson & Pascal 2012). Rolfe et al (2001) argue that not all knowledge for practice comes from textbooks, research journals and lectures or other classroom activities. Rather, they claim that, in addition to what they call scientific knowledge, practitioners actually 'pick up' practical knowledge from their everyday experience, and reflection is the process of *theorising* about that knowledge. As a result, they claim that reflection provides the practitioner with access to the processes by which he or she makes clinical judgements, which can then be used to justify actions to others or pass on expertise to less experienced colleagues.

Taylor (2010) sees it as necessary to alert clinicians to the intricacies of nursing practice and the knowledge embedded in it, but Johns (1988) claims that being a reflective practitioner is more than just noticing things by chance in a situation. He suggests that it involves a deep sensitivity to what is happening around us, or '... a constant monitoring of self within the situation that ripples along the surface of conscious thought' (Johns 1988:14). It is also important not to assume that improved skill in reflective thinking equals learning, which in turn equals improved nursing practice. A study of reflective thinking in nursing by Teekman (2000) demonstrated that learning from reflection is not something that happens automatically. He identified the importance of coaching by a mentor, and a supportive environment, as ways to reduce the uncritical reinforcement of existing patterns of practice.

Much of the contemporary emphasis on reflective practice in nursing can be attributed to the work of the American educationalist Donald Schön (1983, 1987). Even though he was not the first to write about it, he actually coined the term 'reflective practice' (Teekman 2000), and has been very influential in the way nursing has embraced the notion. Schön (1983) argued that reflection is a strategy whereby professionals become aware of their implicit knowledge base. While he did not attempt to define reflection or reflective practice, he advocated two distinct types of reflection: *reflection-on-action* and *reflection-in-action*. The former, reflection-on-action, occurs after the event or action where details are recalled and analysed in some way with the aim of reviewing practice. It has been referred to as a type of cognitive 'postmortem' or an act of looking back at practice (Burton 2000).

Reflection-in-action occurs simultaneously or at the same time as practice. That is, reflection-in-action is said to occur when the practitioner engages in practice and makes adjustments as a result of relevant feedback. Rolfe (2001) claims that reflection-in-action is a more advanced form of reflection and leads to more advanced practice. He describes it as a process whereby the nurse is constantly testing theories and hypotheses in a cyclical process while simultaneously engaged in practice—what he termed 'nursing praxis' in an earlier paper (Rolfe 1993).

Boud et al (1985), however, noted an additional step in the reflective process, that of pre-reflection. In other words, they recognised the importance of reflection in anticipation of events. Greenwood (1998:1049) explains how preparing for experience involves the learner becoming aware of what they bring to the event and what they want from it (the personal), the constraints and opportunities the event provides (the context) and how they may acquire what they need from the event (the learning strategies). In fact, anticipation of challenging events is thought to stimulate reflection (Mann, Gordon & MacLeod 2009).

THE ROOTS OF REFLECTIVE PRACTICE

The ancient Greek philosopher Plato declared that the unreflective life was a life not worth living. Plato was drawing attention to the view that reflection is a distinctively human activity and without it we would be no more than unthinking automatons, our lives governed by our biological instincts and forever subject to those forces, human and natural, exerting power over us. Plato saw reflection, in other words, as vital to our identity as human beings and to our having a mind of our own, and thus to our personal freedom. We are free, he concluded, only to the extent that we are reflective beings.

This idea resurfaced and drove the huge change of thinking that occurred in seventeenth- and eighteenth-century Europe, which became known as the Enlightenment. Enlightenment philosophers such as John Locke in England and Jean-Jacques Rousseau in France argued that human beings are free to think and decide for themselves rather than simply accept the prevailing norms, largely imposed by those in power and notably by the Christian churches. Today we just accept this as natural and probably do not think twice about it, but in those days it was a radical and rather dangerous claim.

This history reminds us of several important principles concerning reflection. First, reflection is not an artificial technique that is being imposed by regulatory authorities or universities; rather, it is the refinement of a natural process that is part of being human, and which needs to be nurtured and encouraged. Second, we should always reflect upon, and if necessary challenge, prevailing ways of thinking and acting, even if it occasionally means being unpopular or thought foolish. When it involves 'big issues', this may be hard to do, but reflection and action working together (i.e. 'praxis') is the impetus for change, and ultimately for improvement. This applies in all arenas of human activity, including your local healthcare setting.

Although there are many ways of conceiving reflective processes, even within the same discipline, reflection as we refer to it here is not simply thinking, but rather thinking deeply, systematically, logically and deliberately. Political theorists have emphasised the role of reflection in challenging the status quo, and it plays an important part in the teachings of some political radicals and revolutionaries. Educationalists, such as the American John Dewey, have emphasised the role of reflection in learning and problem solving and have explored how reflection is related to experience. Dewey observed that 'we learn by doing and realising what came of what we did'; this 'realising' is the result of reflection.

Reflection also played an important part in the development of psychology as a discipline during the nineteenth century, in the form of 'introspection'—that is, reflection focused upon oneself. Until the rise of scientific psychology in the 1880s, introspection was the primary source of data for the elucidation of human psychology. An especially important figure, who brings the political and educational aspects together, is the Brazilian Marxist, Paulo Freire. His work is widely cited as the basis for the development of reflective processes in nursing, although nurses have mostly shied away from acknowledging the political revolutionary aspects of his work. Freire's concept of reflection was developed as part of a strategy for educating and politicising the impoverished and largely illiterate peasants of Brazil, and has an explicit emancipatory intent. The key idea, which makes it 'emancipatory', is that reflection and action should work together (as praxis), in order to generate new, enlightened and empowering ways of thinking and behaving.

This is an important way for you to think about reflection because, as a nurse, you will work in complex systems where you may feel powerless and unable to express your concerns and opinions; in this sense, you too may feel 'illiterate'. In order to create a sense of control and of having a worthwhile part to play, you can begin by engaging in reflective processes, and out of these should arise constructive courses of action which constitute 'praxis', an idea discussed further by Holmes and Warelow (2000).

Nursing's descriptions and adaptations of reflective processes have been clearly explored in a series of chapters in the classic text edited by Gray and Pratt (1991), and you should read these as part of your continuing education as a nurse (Cox et al 1991, Crane 1991, Emden 1991, Gray & Forsstrom 1991, Lumby 1991). The authors explain how reflective processes bring theory and practice together, what forms they can take and how they can be used by nurses in clinical, educational and research contexts.

The opening remark in Carolyn Emden's brilliant contribution nicely captures the spirit behind these chapters: 'Reflective practice is of pre-eminent interest to nurses,' she says, and '[t]o be a *reflective practitioner* suggests professional maturity and a strong commitment to improving practice—a reasonable aspiration for every Registered Nurse' (Emden 1991:335). The pioneering work of Boud and his colleagues (1985), which was mentioned earlier, plays an important role here. Emden (1991) explains how Boud's three phases of reflective learning—preparatory, experiential and processing—can be undertaken in your workplace, and provides actual examples of nurses' 'field notes', or written reflections. Like most nurse authors, Emden (1991) considered reflective processes to be inextricably tied to the 'critical social science paradigm'— that is, the politically informed approach we have noted above, which is interested in identifying and changing irrational, oppressive or counterproductive beliefs and practices.

Perhaps the most important exemplars of this approach in Australian nursing were at the School of Nursing at Deakin University, where reflective processes and critical social theory were used as the basis for the undergraduate nursing curriculum from 1988, and subsequently formed part of the Master of Nursing Studies degree;

and the Flinders University of South Australia, where they formed part of the Master of Nursing degree from 1991. The groundbreaking role of Deakin's nurse scholars has been acknowledged in the historical analysis by Nelson (2012), and most nurse scholars who have written about these topics are in some way linked to these two schools.

Emden (1991) summarises the ways in which reflective processes have the effect of 'educating the emotions'. Reflective processes should be mutually encouraged, and there is an educative element as you help others by recognising and responding to their needs and sensitivities, as well as your own; reflective processes also help you come to terms with the uncertainty of clinical practice and with its inevitable injustices and inadequacies. Clinical practice is never perfect; it is always constrained by resource shortages and by the failings of the system and those who work in it. It is part of the human condition that we cannot do everything right all the time, and that things sometimes go wrong. Reflective processes enable us to face up to this reality, but at the same time challenge us to overcome the obstacles and aspire to the best possible standards of practice. They contribute to our development as thinkers, practitioners and as people; that is why Emden (1991) referred at the outset to them being the hallmark of the mature professional.

THE BENEFITS OF REFLECTION

We have already noted some of the benefits which derive from reflective processes, but let us now discuss these in more detail. Freire (1972) insisted that action and reflection must work together, and we can agree with Emden when she describes action as a 'key outcome' of reflection. 'Action' can take many forms. For example, when you reflect upon your practice world and become sensitive to its inadequacies and injustices, you are most likely to want to do something about them, especially as you consider them in relation to individuals' rights. In contrast, action might involve improving your own clinical skills; your reflections having alerted you to shortcomings in your attitudes or skills, and you take action to bring them to a higher standard.

Another benefit of reflection is that it can help you elucidate the theory–practice relationship. Critical social theory insists that this relationship is 'reflexive'; in other words, theory feeds into your practice and practice informs your theory. This supports the suggestion by nurse theorists Walker and Avant (1983) that reflective processes can be used to help develop clinical practice by helping you to recognise, evaluate and refine your personal nursing theories (i.e. your beliefs about nursing and clinical practice). Indeed, much of Emden's (1991) chapter is about how to use reflection to help elucidate and develop your own theory of nursing. Since critical social theory is closely tied to these conceptions of reflection, it is widely argued that any theory of nursing developed in this way should be consistent with critical social theory, and many nursing scholars have attempted to show how this can work. Good places to begin exploring this topic include Holter (1988) and Crane (1991). This link has become more difficult to sustain, however, as critical social theory has been the subject of criticism in light of alternative ways of thinking about social structures and processes, including 'post-structuralism' and 'postmodernism' (Holmes 1995).

Another positive outcome of reflection, which follows on from its role in the 'education of the emotions' noted above, is that it sensitises us to the plight of less fortunate and marginalised people in society. We become more sensitive to the suffering, courage and determination of people who are faced with serious illness and to the problems faced by those who are oppressed, such as mentally disordered and intellectually disabled people and people who belong to ethnic and religious minorities. This increased sensitivity impels you towards greater engagement with such people, and a willingness to become involved in their problems. Not only are you aiming to improve your clinical performance with all your patients, but also to act as their support and advocate. You are not only motivated to question inadequate practices, but also to generate possible strategies for improvement. Even though it may be challenging, you will find that you cannot do otherwise, and you will enjoy increased levels of job satisfaction because this heightened level of engagement is intrinsically rewarding. A careful review of research supporting the use of reflective processes in nurse education (Epp 2008), concluded that a reflective practitioner has improved personal attributes and is better positioned to provide excellent patient care.

Once again, it is Carolyn Emden who sums up this aspect so accurately. She says:

> The outcomes of reflection are so profound, and so personally enlightening, that you are unable to let them go, or to return to former unquestioning ways. Increasingly, you are likely to recognise, and challenge, those political, social, and historical forces which are unjust, irrational, and oppressive in your professional life: together with colleagues and clients, you will wish to create and implement strategies of empowerment that lead to informed choice and fulfilling forms of action.
> (Emden 1991:352)

We might add that these benefits accrue not just in the context of your work, but also in your life generally. The big claim being made here is that reflection, because it educates your emotions and impels you to action, helps make you a better person and not just a better nurse. Let us now turn to consider the 'how' of reflection.

STRATEGIES FOR REFLECTION

Many strategies can be used for reflection, including writing (e.g. journalling and critical incident analysis), photography, drawing and other forms of creative expression.

Writing

Reflective writing has been advocated as a technique to aid reflection (Usher et al 1999, Rolfe et al 2001, Jasper 2006, Johns 2006). It involves the use of writing as a strategy to assist us to learn from experiences and involves engaging in the reflective process using writing as an instrument. It differs from other forms of writing in that it is undertaken primarily for the purpose of learning and to assist us to develop a deeper understanding of the subject of our reflection (Rolfe et al 2001). Van Manen (1990) says that writing is a reflective activity where we come to know and understand the way in which we know what we know. This can be achieved by writing and rewriting, so that we come to understand something in greater depth, in ways not previously open to us and in new or more intimate ways. Further, the '... act of writing forces a coherence and anchors thinking in a way that permits revisiting and reworking' (Usher et al 1999).

Journalling and *critical incident analysis* are two well-known types of reflective writing, but clinical supervision, poetry, letter, story- and group-writing activities are also examples of reflective writing.

Journalling

Journal writing has long been advocated as a strategy for the development of reflective practice (e.g. Boud et al 1985, Cox et al 1991, Heath 1998, Holly 1984, Usher et al 1999). By the term 'journal' we mean what is commonly referred to as a diary or log. Writing a journal involves the writing of accounts of practice experiences after they occur and allows the writer to take ownership of the content—for example, using the first person and writing about themselves. A simple format for writing a reflective journal in conjunction with a professional diary is available in a pocket-sized, spiral-bound format (Elsevier 2009).

However, journal writing offers the practitioner more than the opportunity to recount an experience; it provides an opportunity to return to the experience in its written form and then theorise about the experience from which conclusions are drawn. This type of reflective writing provides for many returns for analysis (Owens et al 1997), and the writer can add, delete or change entries as often as they wish. As a result, it becomes an ongoing critique of the practitioner's thoughts about an experience. Journals have also been described as cathartic because they offer an opportunity to 'work through' problems or difficult situations (Davies & Sharp 2000). The box below lists some journalling techniques, which are taken from Owens et al (1997).

Journalling techniques

Write a short biography to begin.
Select a quiet environment where you will not be interrupted.
Write vividly and as close to the event as possible.
Include your initial thoughts, but leave space where you can add comments at a later time.
Where possible, make use of diagrams, illustrations, photographs and drawings to aid your memory.
Make use of a book and use one side for writing and leave the other for later reflections.

Some students find starting a reflective journal a difficult task, but you should remember that there is no right or wrong way to do it. Cox et al (1991:380–1) identify three challenges that face the newcomer to journalling:

1 valuing journalling so that time and effort are allocated appropriately;

2 removing the 'censor' that inhibits us from writing honestly and accurately; and

3 reviewing the journal critically in order to identify areas of strength and weakness, and new ways of thinking and acting.

The use of a framework or model as a prompt for reflection has been advocated (Heath 1998, Jasper 2006, Johns 1998, Rolfe et al 2001) and you may find this useful. Have a look at the model proposed by Rolfe et al (2001) in Figure 8.1, and think about how you might use it to aid your reflection.

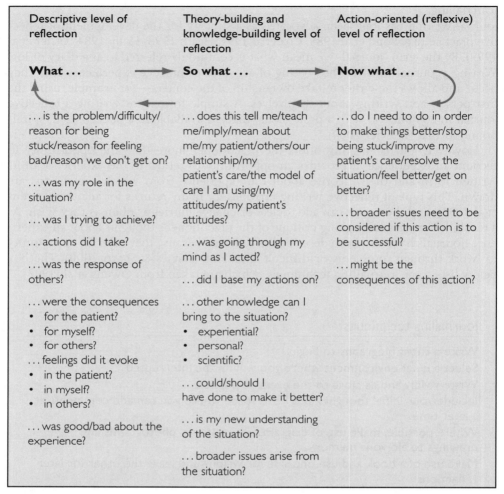

Figure 8.1
Framework for reflection
Source: Gary Rolfe, Dawn Freshwater and Melanie Jasper, *Critical Reflection for Nursing and the Helping Professions*, published 2001, Palgrave New York, reproduced with permission of Palgrave Macmillan.

Taylor (2010) offers a number of hints that may also be helpful: be spontaneous; express yourself freely; remain open to ideas; choose a time to suit you; be prepared personally; and choose a reflective method. It is also important to avoid the use of abbreviations, and resist the temptation to censor your writing, as this is more likely to assist with the exposure of the 'isms' we hold as an individual.

A further strategy that may also be helpful is the notion of a *critical friend*. Sharing with others opens reflective journal entries to a different perspective. The other person may offer alternative actions that could have been taken or might challenge you to think more deeply about a particular issue (Heath 1998). It is important that the critical friend is someone you trust, as they will be reading your entries and discussing them with you. The role of a critical friend is to support and guide you in your reflection, while posing questions and offering alternatives in a non-judgemental way (Taylor 2010). Duke describes how critical friends have:

> ... acted as a sounding board for my ideas and thoughts, sometimes they have given me an 'expert' view of an area of knowledge new to me, and sometimes they have stimulated a thought that I have then gone on to explore.
> (Duke 2000:152)

Ethical and legal issues related to journalling

One aspect of journalling that became a problem in the early 1990s, when reflective processes were still considered strange and dangerous by those in authority in health services, concerns their ethical and legal status. In short, these concerns were:

- whether journalling required the consent of institutions and individuals to whom they refer;
- whether journalling was appropriately conducted in work time or in the clinician's own time;
- who owned the journals, and who had a right of access to them; and
- what status the journals had in law; whether they could, for example, be used as evidence in the court room.

With the formal recognition that clinicians generally, and registered nurses in particular, are required to be 'reflective practitioners', it is now widely accepted that they should be journalling, and that this is part of their clinical work. Intellectual property is a vexed issue in law, and there does not appear to be any precedent set in either Australian or New Zealand law as to the obligations of clinicians in relation to journals, but there does appear to be general acceptance that they belong to their authors, and that employers therefore normally have no right of access. You should, however, be able to reassure managers that your reflective journal conforms to the usual ethical standards that apply in healthcare situations—namely, that they are securely stored and accessible only to authorised individuals (such as your supervisors or educators), that you use pseudonyms when referring to particular patients or colleagues, and that they are strictly for your private professional use. Existing privacy provisions in Australia and New Zealand require that no information is gathered from patients beyond what is required for the appropriate management of their health problem, and so you should not obtain additional information simply for the purposes of your journal.

Like all documents, journals may be ordered to be submitted as evidence in courts of law. Although this is extremely unlikely, and most of what appears in a journal may only have the status of 'hearsay evidence', it is wise to bear this possibility in mind. Another principle you should adopt, therefore, is that your journal should always refer to your colleagues and patients in a professional and respectful manner, even though it may express criticism. Your journal is, after all, not a vehicle for catharsis—that is, unrestricted emotional expression—rather, it is the professional documentation of your deeply and carefully considered thoughts.

Critical incident analysis

A critical incident is usually an event that is remembered as important to an individual or one that is provided to a learner for the purpose of reflection. The notion of a critical incident is considered problematic by some (Griffin 2003, Rolfe et al 2001, Thompson & Pascal 2012) who outline how the term is negative because it brings to mind something unfortunate or life threatening, something we certainly found in a study that utilised critical incident analysis with nursing students (Usher et al 1999).

Critical incidents, however, should be thought of as events that are meaningful or significant in some way; they need not necessarily be large or major occurrences (Rolfe et al 2001), and they can be negative or positive experiences (Davies & Sharp 2000). Critical incident analysis is thought to lead to:

> ... a deeper and more profound level of reflection because it goes beyond detailed description of an event that attracted attention, to analysis of and reflection on the meaning of the event.
> (Griffin 2003:208)

A study by Usher et al (1999) found that writing critical incident analyses offered undergraduate nursing students an opportunity to distance themselves from an event and, as a result, come to understand it in new ways.

The box below provides a framework for a critical incident analysis, which has been taken from Davies and Sharp (2000:67–8).

Framework for critical incident analysis

1 Give a concise description of the incident (which relates to the learning outcomes).
2 Outline the rationale for choice of incident and its significance and relevance to you.
3 Identify pertinent issues related to the incident.
4 Reflect on and analyse the key issues focusing on: your own involvement; feelings and decision making; the involvement and role of others; identification of any dilemmas or ethical elements; and the rationale for action, drawing on relevant theory evaluation of the situation and the implications for practice and personal learning.
5 Conclusion.

Photography, drawing and other forms of creative expression

Taylor (2010) describes how reflection can be facilitated by creative expression. She explains that it is unclear whether the awareness of the creative expression precedes or follows the reflection, but that it occurs sufficiently to include it as a way of reflective thinking. Some have been inspired to draw or write poetically as a result of events they have experienced, while others have used art forms, such as photography, drawing, painting or music in an attempt to express their reactions. Rolfe et al (2001) explain that these techniques are described as creative because they involve using the imagination to transform experience away from the more accepted ways of analysis to the use of metaphor as a way of creating insight and facilitating learning.

Self-awareness and clinical supervision

In essence, self-awareness is the foundation skill upon which reflective practice is based. It offers individuals the opportunity to see themselves in certain situations and to observe how they affected the situation and the situation affected them (Atkins 2000). In fact, this is what differentiates reflection from other types of mental activity such as logical thinking or problem solving (Boud et al 1985). Reflection is also a very personal experience, as it opens the self up to scrutiny (Johns 1998, 2006). As a result, reflection can be disconcerting to the individual, as taken for granted competence and ways of coping are exposed as inadequate.

Self-awareness is also an essential skill for professional monitoring. As a professional you are required to be aware of yourself, and the influence you have on patients and the healthcare context. Consequently, constant and vigilant self-monitoring is an important skill that every nurse needs to develop. Registered Nurses need to come to an understanding of their racist, sexist and ageist attitudes, for example, and identify how these impact on their practice. An awareness of your own frailties and susceptibilities is crucial to maintaining high standards of practice.

Many nurses do not care adequately for their own psychological and physical well-being, and yet are under pressure from their work and their domestic lives. It is important to consider whether you are going to work tired and distracted; whether you are overanxious, depressed or angry; whether you are going to work with a hangover and suffering the effects of too much alcohol. Many nurses find that the stress of their lives leads them to overuse medications, smoke heavily or resort to illicit drugs. The reflective practitioner is aware of these tendencies and will take remedial action, seeking appropriate advice and support.

A similar argument applies to any tendency that may ultimately lead to professional misconduct, including inappropriate sexual thoughts, feelings of aggression and racist, sexist, ageist or other prejudiced attitudes. A reflective practitioner becomes aware of these possibilities, takes action and thus maintains high standards of practice. This self-monitoring role leads us almost seamlessly into the issue of clinical supervision.

Reflective processes have been linked by many authors to the process of clinical supervision. Marrow et al (1997), for example, outlined ways in which supervision could help develop reflective nursing practice among both supervisors and supervisees, through group supervision sessions, diary writing and so on. More recently, Severinsson (2001) has described how clinical supervision in nursing can be based on a 'reflective practitioner model', citing the work of Schön and Johns, both authors we have mentioned in this chapter. She sees reflective processes as integral to the analysis and understanding of the theory–practice relationship, which is one of the goals of the supervisee, and the consequent development of 'know-how'. She also sees reflection as essential to self-awareness, emotional education and the development of 'know-what'. Supervision should be 'centred on enhancing the practitioner's ability to "reflect-in-action"' (Severinsson 2001:40)—that is, on the care being provided. She explains that:

> Clinical supervision demands reflection on what care is being provided. Reflection can result in a better understanding of oneself. There is a difference between concentrating on the dissatisfaction within oneself and striving not to repeat what caused it (e.g. feelings of guilt). It is important to find answers to questions such as:

Why did I make this mistake? Why did I fail to observe factors of relevance in caring for this patient? A deeper insight into patient needs may thereby be developed. (*Severinsson 2001:43*).

When you think about Severinsson's statement, it is not difficult to see how reflection could become a powerful tool in the supervisory process, and lead to real improvements in patient care.

PROBLEMS, CRITICISMS AND RESPONSES

Despite their endorsement by regulatory authorities and encouragement by educators, the use of reflective processes in nursing is not without critics. Some have argued that the evidence for their effectiveness, in increasing critical thinking, promoting learning and improving practice, remains weak (e.g. Burton 2000). However, there are several counterarguments:

- although little research has been conducted on its value to nursing, the concept of reflective practice is supported by empirical research conducted and elaborated over many years, notably in education, and the accumulated evidence as to its value in a variety of disciplines (e.g. science, social work, medicine, law, education) cannot be ignored;

- the research results, although limited, are favourable, and there is no evidence that clinicians taking time to engage in critical reflection has any detrimental effects;

- there are strong *a priori* (logical) arguments in its favour, such as the argument that a problem is unlikely to be acted upon unless it is recognised as a problem, and that learning entails reflection, and not merely experience or the absorption of facts;

- reflective processes acknowledge the value of the experiences and beliefs of all members of a discipline in contributing to its knowledge base and practice development; the alternative is that the views of a privileged group are allowed to dominate; and

- reflective processes happen naturally, and one cannot simply stop them without denying an integral part of one's personal identity; the alternative is to be robotic.

Oncology nurses, for example, reported reflective practice to be an important aspect of their work and of their support structures (Loftus & McDowell 2000), while the study by Johns (2001) showed that reflective practice serves to reveal the ways in which nurses care.

Finally, for the sake of balance, we should add that there are also a number of theoretical arguments that can be levelled at reflective processes in nursing. Cotton (2001) brought attention to some of these, notably:

- despite its championship by many nursing authorities, reflection remains ill-defined and elusive; she notes Johns' (1998:2) observation that 'it seems an academic pastime to try and define exactly what it [reflective practice] is';

- reflection is a strategy for scrutinising private thoughts, a form of policing or surveillance by oneself on behalf of others; this complaint derives from the work of the French philosopher Michel Foucault (1972);

- reflection only masquerades as radical; in reality it is aimed at imposing a standardised way of thinking and acting; and

- not enough attention is paid to the negative effects of reflection and the problems that arise in trying to be a reflective practitioner.

We believe these are important issues that need to be considered by those who champion reflection, but we do not regard any as fatal to that cause. Our response to these criticisms is, in short, that:

- the meaning of words is a matter of convention, and agreement takes time to emerge;

- self-scrutiny is a positive feature of professional life; indeed 'profession' is often characterised by such self-regulation;

- the aim is to open up the practitioner's mind to possibilities, not to impose rules, and reflective practitioners are therefore more likely to be creative, to challenge the status quo and to be independent thinkers; and

- the problems of reflective practice may have been underestimated, but they are increasingly acknowledged; in any case, this means only that we need to be better at reflective processes, not that they should be abandoned.

You should consider carefully, and reflect upon, the claims we have made in this chapter, and come to a reasoned and practical personal arrangement for your own development as a reflective practitioner. To help you do this, consider the questions overleaf, and undertake some further reading on the subject.

CONCLUSION

In summary, reflection is a useful learning and professional development strategy that helps the practitioner to monitor their practice, recognise the link between practice and theory, remain in touch with their values, develop awareness of their impact on their work and on relationships with others and remain in touch with the needs of the vulnerable in society. Reflective practice, while still considered to be a developing area by some scholars, is now considered of sufficient importance to be mandated by the regulatory authorities that oversee the practice of nurses and midwives. There are many strategies to enhance reflective practice such as writing, journalling, critical incident analysis, creative techniques and clinical supervision. Most importantly, continue to reflect on your practice and develop reflection as a routine part of your day as indicated by Hickson (2011:836):

> I continued to ask 'why' each thought and reflection was important and relevant, and from where these assumptions had come. I wondered about my experiences, my values, my gender, my influences, and how I influence other people around me. I thought about the binary language that I use and the dichotomous thinking that shapes the way I understand my interactions with other people. I enjoyed taking time to step away from the busyness of the workplace and have a helicopter view of myself being able to sit comfortably with the uncertainty.

REFLECTIVE QUESTIONS

1 How would you use pre-reflection to prepare yourself for the challenge of clinical practice?

2 Write a paragraph about how you will use reflective processes during your clinical practice. In the paragraph address the following:

(a) the technique you think would be best suited to you and why;

(b) whether a framework would help you; and

(c) the benefits you might receive.

3 How will you use reflective processes to enhance your self-awareness and ensure you practise at the highest possible standard?

4 Why is it important for you as a reflective practitioner to understand the theoretical background of reflection?

RECOMMENDED READINGS

Howatson-Jones L 2010 Reflective practice in nursing. Learning Matters, Exeter

Johns C (ed) 2010 Guided reflection: a narrative approach to advancing professional practice, 2nd edn. Wiley-Blackwell, Oxford

Koivu A, Irmeli S, Hyrkäs K 2012 Who benefits from clinical supervision and how? The association between clinical supervision and the work-related well-being of female hospital nurses. Journal of Clinical Nursing 2:2567–2578

Rolfe G, Jasper M, Freshwater D 2010 Critical reflection in practice – generating knowledge for care, 2nd edn. Palgrave Macmillan, New York

Severinsson E, Sand A 2010 Evaluation of the clinical supervision and professional development of student nurses. Journal of Nursing Management 18:669–677

Taylor B J 2010 Reflective practice for healthcare professionals, 3rd edn. Open University Press, Maidenhead

REFERENCES

Atkins S 2000 Developing underlying skills in the move towards reflective practice. In: Burns S, Bulman C (eds) Reflective practice in nursing: the growth of the professional practitioner, 2nd edn. Blackwell Science, Oxford, pp 28–51

Australian Nursing and Midwifery Council 2006a National competency standards for the Registered Nurse. ANMC, Canberra

Australian Nursing and Midwifery Council 2006b National competency standards for the Midwife. ANMC, Canberra

Australian Nursing and Midwifery Council 2008a Code of professional conduct for Registered Nurses in Australia. ANMC, Canberra

Australian Nursing and Midwifery Council 2008b Code of professional conduct for Midwives in Australia. ANMC, Canberra

Boud D, Keogh R, Walker D 1985 Reflection: turning experience into learning. Kogan Page, London

Burton A J 2000 Reflection: nursing's practice and education panacea? Journal of Advanced Nursing 31(5):1009–1017

Cotton A 2001 Private thoughts in public spheres: issues in reflection and reflective practices in nursing. Journal of Advanced Nursing 36(4):512–519

Cox H, Hickson P, Taylor B 1991 Exploring reflection: knowing and constructing practice. In Gray G, Pratt R (eds) Towards a discipline of nursing. Churchill Livingstone, Melbourne, pp 373–389

Crane S 1991 Implications of the critical paradigm. In: Gray G, Pratt R (eds) Towards a discipline of nursing. Churchill Livingstone, Melbourne, pp 391–411

Davies C, Sharp P 2000 The assessment and evaluation of reflection. In: Burns S, Bulman C (eds) Reflective practice in nursing: the growth of the professional practitioner, 2nd edn. Blackwell Science, Oxford, pp 52–78

Department of Employment, Education, Training and Youth Affairs 1998 Review of higher education financing and policy (final report): learning for life (DEETYA Publication No. 6055HERE 98A). Australian Government Publishing Service, Canberra

Duke S 2000 The experience of becoming reflective. In: Burns S, Bulman C (eds) Reflective practice in nursing: the growth of the professional practitioner, 2nd edn. Blackwell Science, Oxford, pp 137–155

Elsevier 2009 Diary and reflective journal for nurses and midwives, 2010–2011. Baillière Tindall, Oxford

Emden C 1991 Becoming a reflective practitioner. In: Gray G, Pratt R (eds) Towards a discipline of nursing. Churchill Livingstone, Melbourne, pp 335–354

Epp S 2008 The value of reflective journaling in undergraduate nursing education: a literature review. International Journal of Nursing Studies 45:1379–1388

Foucault M 1972 The archaeology of knowledge (translated by Sheridan Smith AM). Tavistock, London

Francis D 1995 The reflective journal: a window to pre-service teachers' practical knowledge. Teaching and Teacher Education 11(3):229–241

Freire P 1972 Pedagogy of the oppressed (transl. by Myra Bergman Ramos). Penguin, Harmondsworth

Gray G, Pratt R eds 1991 Towards a discipline of nursing. Churchill Livingstone, Melbourne

Gray G, Forsstrom S 1991 Generating theory from practice: the reflective technique. In Gray G, Pratt R (eds) Towards a discipline of nursing. Churchill Livingstone, Melbourne

Greenwood J 1998 The role of reflection in single and double loop learning. Journal of Advanced Nursing 27:1048–1053

Griffin M L 2003 Using critical incidents to promote and assess reflective thinking in preservice teachers. Reflective Practice 4(2):207–220

Heath H 1998 Keeping a reflective practice diary: a practical guide. Nurse Education Today 18:592–598

Hickson H 2011 Critical reflection: reflecting on learning to be reflective. Reflective Practice: International and Multidisciplinary Perspectives, 12(6):829–839

Holly M L 1984 Keeping a personal professional journal. Deakin University Press, Geelong

Holmes C A 1995 Postmodernism and nursing. In: Gray G, Pratt R (eds) Scholarship in the discipline of nursing. Churchill Livingstone, Melbourne, pp 351–370

Holmes C A, Warelow P J 2000 Nursing as normative praxis. Nursing Inquiry 7(3):175–181. Reprinted with comments in: Reed P (ed) 2003 Nicoll's perspectives on nursing theory, 4th edn. Lippincott, Williams & Wilkins, Philadelphia

Holter J M 1988 Critical theory: a foundation for the development of nursing theories. Scholarly Inquiry for Nursing Practice: An International Journal 2(3):223–232

Jasper M 2006 Reflection, decision-making and professional development. Blackwell, Oxford

Johns C 1998 Opening the doors of perception. In: Johns C, Freshwater D (eds) Transforming nursing through reflective practice. Blackwell Science, London, pp 1–20

Johns C 2001 Reflective practice: revealing the [he]art of caring. International Journal of Nursing Practice 7:237–245

Johns C 2006 Engaging reflection in practice: a narrative approach. Blackwell, Oxford

Johns C 2009 Becoming a reflective practitioner, 3rd edn. Wiley-Blackwell, Oxford

Lauder W, Meehan T, Moxham L 2004 Preface: Changing the face of mental health nursing. Journal of Psychiatric and Mental Health Nursing 11:1–2

Loftus L A, McDowell J 2000 The lived experience of the oncology clinical nurse specialist. International Journal of Nursing Studies 37:513–521

Lumby J 1991 Threads of an emerging discipline: praxis, reflection, rhetoric and research. In: Gray G, Pratt R (eds) Towards a discipline of nursing. Churchill Livingstone, Melbourne, pp 461–483

Lumby J 2000 Theory generation through reflective practice. In: Greenwood J (ed) Nursing theory in Australia: development and application, 2nd edn. Pearson Education Australia, Sydney, pp 330–348

Mann K, Gordon J, MacLeod A 2009 Reflection and reflective practice in health professions education: a systematic review. Advances in Health Science Education, 14:595–621

Marrow C E, Macauley D M, Crumbie A 1997 Promoting reflective practice through structured clinical supervision. Journal of Nursing Management 5:77–82

Mantzoukas S, Jasper M 2004 Reflective practice and daily ward reality: a covert power game. Journal of Clinical Nursing 13:925–933

Nelson S 2012 The lost path to emancipatory practice: towards a history of reflective practice in nursing. Nursing Philosophy 13:202–213

Nursing Council of New Zealand 2007 Competencies for the registered nurse. Nursing Council of New Zealand, Wellington

Owens J, Francis D, Usher K, Tollefson J 1997 Risks and rewards of reflective thinking. James Cook University, Townsville

Parker S 2010 Becoming a critical thinker. In: Daly J, Speedy S, Jackson D (eds) Contexts of nursing: an introduction, 3rd edn. Churchill Livingstone Elsevier, Sydney, pp 249–264

Rolfe G 1993 Closing the theory–practice gap: a model of nursing praxis. Journal of Clinical Nursing 2:173–177

Rolfe G 2001 Reflective practice: where now? Nurse Education in Practice 2(21) 21–29

Rolfe G, Freshwater D, Jasper M 2001 Critical reflection for nursing and the helping professions: a user's guide. Palgrave, New York

Schön D A 1983 The reflective practitioner: how practitioners think in action. Basic Books, New York

Schön D A 1987 Educating the reflective practitioner: towards a new design for teaching and learning in the professions. Jossey-Bass, San Francisco

Severinsson E I 2001 Confirmation, meaning and self-awareness as core concepts of the nursing supervision model. Nursing Ethics 8(1):36–44

Taylor B J 2010 Reflective practice: a guide for healthcare professionals, 3rd edn. Open University Press, Maidenhead

Teekman B 2000 Exploring reflective thinking in nursing practice. Journal of Advanced Nursing 31(5):1125–1135

Thompson N, Pascal J 2012 Developing critically reflective practice. Reflective Practice: International and Multidisciplinary Perspectives, 13(2):311–325

Usher K, Francis D, Owens J, Tollefson J 1999 Reflective writing: a strategy to foster critical inquiry in undergraduate nursing students. Australian Journal of Advanced Nursing 17(1):7–12

Usher K, Tollefson J, Francis D 2001 Moving from technical to critical reflection in journalling: an investigation of students' ability to incorporate three levels of reflective writing. Australian Journal of Advanced Nursing 19(1):15–19

Usher K, Foster K, Stewart L 2012 Reflective practice for the graduate nurse. In: Chang E M, Daly J (eds) Transitions in Nursing, 3rd edn. Churchill Livingstone, Sydney, pp 289–304

van Manen M 1990 Researching lived experience. State University of New York Press, New York

Walker L, Avant K 1983 Strategies for theory construction in nursing. Appleton Century Crofts, Norwalk, Connecticut

CHAPTER 9

Research in nursing: concepts and processes

John Daly, Doug Elliott, Esther Chang and Kim Usher

LEARNING OBJECTIVES

Upon completion of this chapter, readers should have gained:

- an understanding of the role of research in the development of contemporary nursing
- an appreciation of the need for a range of approaches to research in nursing
- basic knowledge and understanding of research processes in nursing
- an appreciation of the contribution of research to the development of knowledge and clinical practice standards in nursing
- a beginning understanding of research critique and research dissemination processes in nursing.

KEY WORDS

Quantitative research, qualitative research, mixed methods research, dissemination, critique, evidence

RESEARCH IN NURSING

This chapter introduces you to basic concepts and processes of research in nursing. Research has assumed a position of significance in Australian nursing, and there continues to be advances in knowledge development and the sophistication of research approaches (McKenna et al 2012).

The concept of research in nursing is not new in the Western world (D'Antonio 1997, Mulhall 1995). In Britain, Florence Nightingale was active in research in nursing in the nineteenth century, though it was not until 1940 that further progress occurred and it was 1963 before the first government-funded post to facilitate research in nursing was established in the Ministry of Health (Mulhall 1995).

Following initial government support for nursing research in the United States in the 1950s (D'Antonio 1997), specific research and education centres were established in universities by the 1970s. During this period, many universities had nursing degree courses at undergraduate and postgraduate level, as well as a significant number of nurse researchers with doctorates who were able to demonstrate research leadership for the profession.

For Australia and New Zealand, nursing was established as an academic discipline in the tertiary education sector in the 1980s, following transfer of courses from hospital schools of nursing. With the subsequent development of doctoral and research master courses in nursing, there continues to be growth in appropriately prepared researchers who can provide research leadership, disciplinary scholarship and contribute to the ongoing professionalisation of nursing throughout Australia and the Asia-Pacific.

The discipline of nursing, through various professional bodies, has highlighted the important role of research in the continued development of nursing as a practice discipline with a research-based body of knowledge (e.g. Australian Nursing and Midwifery Council 2006, Council of Deans of Nursing and Midwifery (ANZ) 2006). The Australian Nursing and Midwifery Council (ANMC) competency standards for the registered nurse (Australian Nursing and Midwifery Council 2006) clearly identify the importance of research to the registered nurse role, particularly in the following competency standards 3.1 to 3.4:

3.1 Identifies the relevance of research to improving individual/group health outcomes,

3.2 Uses best available evidence, nursing expertise and respect for the values and beliefs of individuals/groups in the provision of care,

3.3 Demonstrates analytical skills in accessing and evaluating health information and research evidence, and

3.4 Supports and contributes to nursing and health care research.
(*Australian Nursing and Midwifery Council 2006:4*)

WHAT IS RESEARCH?

Research is a rigorous and planned process of inquiry designed to provide answers to questions about phenomena of concern within an academic discipline or profession. It is defined as 'the systematic study of materials and sources to establish facts and reach new conclusions' (Compact Oxford English Dictionary 2004:1). Research is a complex subject and field comprising a number of well-established but diverse traditions. In a chapter such as this, we present only broad brushstrokes to familiarise you with key underpinnings of research processes in nursing. To develop in-depth knowledge and understanding of any one or a range of research traditions, processes and/or methods, further study and reading from a variety of sources will be necessary.

Research traditions can be investigated in relation to their philosophical underpinnings, and in the course of your reading of research you will encounter a number of essentially different paradigms. A research paradigm is an overarching framework that is based on values, beliefs and assumptions (Parse 1987). This framework contains theory about the nature of reality and guidelines for the methods to be used in carrying out research using (or within) the paradigm (Parse 2001). In addition, the ideas within the paradigm have implications for the type of knowledge being sought in a research study, the way in which the study will be carried out and the way in which outcomes from the work will be used.

As nursing is a complex field, researchers access a range of approaches, including positivist, feminist and interpretive paradigms. Quality research is labour, skill and resource intensive; therefore, a number of important decisions need to be made before embarking upon a research project. Not least, all research must be ethical, requiring adherence to strict guidelines (National Health and Medical Research Council 2007) and obtaining the necessary approval from institutional human research ethics committees (HRECs).

Research has the potential to serve a number of purposes in a practice-based discipline:

- test commonly held knowledge or assumptions
- widen understanding of a subject
- stimulate self-action/study
- develop best practice (i.e. evidence-based practice)
- explain behaviours
- allow predictions, and
- assist in the formation of a body of nursing knowledge.

Importantly, the use of research knowledge in practice is the most common contact professional and student nurses have with research. This contact will be through reading, reviewing and critiquing research studies published in the literature. Levels of research use and understanding can be described by the '4 As of research' (Crookes & Davies 2004:xiii):

1. Awareness of and access to the research literature
2. Appreciation (or ability) to understand and critique the language of research
3. Application of research findings to local practice settings, and
4. Ability to conduct original (primary) research independently or in a team.

The aim of the first three As of research is not to produce research workers, but to cultivate and nurture nurses to:

- accept research as a normal and integral aspect of nursing practice
- read and understand research reports
- apply research findings to clinical practice (i.e. evidence-based practice)

- influence colleagues on the use of research data, and

- accept responsibility for their own professional development (Crookes & Davies 2004:xii).

That is, not all nurses need to undertake research, but *all nurses* should *use research* in their practice. Some nurses will also undertake original research (the fourth 'A').

WHERE DO WE FIND RESEARCH?

Thousands of research journals, dissertations, reports and books are published each year. From a nursing perspective, outcomes of original research are disseminated primarily through journal articles and professional conference presentations.

One of the most important initial steps in the research process is conducting a thorough literature review. You will need to develop a search strategy to find relevant journals that shed light on the research area. Such a strategy needs to be both systematic and thorough to identify your research area (Wood & Ross-Kerr 2011). Working with the librarian is often a good start to the process. Students are often faced with the dilemma of how extensive a review is necessary. There is no formula to determine that 20 or 120 articles will provide the necessary background for the study. The number of references will depend on how familiar you are with the area under investigation, and the scope of the review will depend on how much research is available for that topic. Checking the reference list at the end of recent articles can often assist in the process. Experienced researchers know that maintaining an up-to-date review of the literature is an ongoing process throughout any research activity.

To begin, it is important to differentiate between primary and secondary sources (this is equivalent to primary and secondary research approaches). A primary source is a report written by the study author/s themselves. A primary source includes information on the rationale of the study, its participants, design, methods of collecting data, procedure, results, outcomes, limitations, recommendations and references. Most research articles published in professional journals are primary sources. A secondary source is one that summarises information from primary sources presented by other authors (see Table 9.1). When an author cites a previous study in the review of literature section, it is a secondary source. Therefore, constructing a literature review is often called 'secondary research', while developing and conducting an original study is called 'primary research'.

Both primary and secondary sources are important in different circumstances. Secondary sources such as systematic reviews (SRs) are becoming increasingly common as the best available evidence when reviewing clinical practice issues. However, use of secondary sources should be limited when undertaking your own secondary research (i.e. a literature review), with all relevant primary sources reviewed being the aim.

Bibliographic databases

Libraries now provide online access to reference sources via electronic databases to assist students in locating references on a specific topic and to undertake their own literature searches. These searches generate complete bibliographic details, including abstracts, of literature sources published in a particular area of interest. It helps to be in the library to get assistance from the librarian when you run into problems in accessing the databases.

Table 9.1
Glossary of common research terms

Term	Meaning
Construct validity	The extent to which a measuring instrument measures a theoretical construct or characteristic
Descriptive statistics	Description of characteristics (e.g. frequency, percentages), but no inference of relationships between variables
Exclusion criteria	A list of characteristics that exclude an individual from being in a study (e.g. less than 24 hours admission in hospital, presence of other illnesses that may influence patient outcomes)
Explanatory variable	Independent variable; the intervention being manipulated to exhibit a change in the outcome variable
Inclusion criteria	A list of the characteristics required for a subject to be included in a study (e.g. patients admitted for cardiac surgery, 16 years or older, English language skills (reading and writing) sufficient to complete the study questionnaires)
Inferential statistics	Statistical procedures used to test a hypothesis about the relationships between two or more variables (e.g. t-tests, analysis of variance, regression modelling) and the application of study findings to the population being studied (generalisability)
Integrative review	A style of literature review that combines findings from quantitative and qualitative studies, theoretical and methodological literature using narrative analysis
Measuring instrument	The tool used to measure the concept of interest (e.g. questionnaire, biochemical test)
Normal distribution	Distribution of scores for a particular variable follow a bell-shape pattern around the mean score for the sample; required to use inferential statistics
Outcome variable	Dependent variable; measurement of the concept being studied
Primary research	Original research conducted with participants (e.g. patients, health professionals, students)
Primary source	A report of original research written by the study author/s that includes information on the study rationale, participants, design, methods of collecting data, procedure, findings, discussion, limitations and recommendations for practice and further research
Reliability	The consistency or stability of a measure or instrument on repeated uses

continues

Table 9.1—*continued*

Term	Meaning
Responsiveness	The ability of a measuring instrument to detect small but important differences of a dynamic characteristic
Sample	A selected group of participants who have similar characteristics to the population from which they were drawn (i.e. representative); allows for generalisation of results from the study sample to the wider population
Secondary research	A process where data from previous primary research studies are reinvestigated (e.g. literature review, systematic review)
Secondary source	A source of literature that summarises information from original research (primary source) presented by other authors
Systematic review	A style of literature review combining findings from quantitative studies with similar hypotheses and methods, to inform research and practice using narrative and/or statistical analysis

A variety of indexes and databases are available, providing bibliographic listings of articles, abstracts, conference proceedings and books. All indexes provide bibliography citations, giving the authors' names, publication date, article title, journal volume and issue number, and pages. Each academic discipline has an index to its collection of journals.

Common health sciences bibliographic databases include the Cumulative Index to Nursing and Allied Health Literature (CINAHL), which has journals from nursing and allied health disciplines listed; and Medline, a database of medical and health studies (Elliott 2007c). A related database, Pubmed, provides free public access to Medline studies (see www.ncbi.nlm.nih.gov/entrez). Other important databases that may include studies relevant to your topic are: Education Resources Information Centre (ERIC); Psychology Abstracts, Sociological Abstracts, Cancer Therapy Abstracts (CANCERLIT); and Dissertation Abstracts International.

Most databases use key words or medical subject (MeSH) headings, and a thesaurus function provides a structure for linked terms. When a topic is not found in the subject headings, you can search key words that have been adopted by most of the journal publishers. Many journals also publish key words with an article. Most university libraries hold extensive electronic collections of refereed journals across a range of disciplines. Many databases now provide links to online full-text papers, although this function may be restricted to journal subscribers (check with your professional library for access rights to specific journals).

Peer-reviewed journals

Peer-reviewed journals serve many important functions, including facilitation of expert review of manuscripts, reporting the findings of research studies or theoretical papers, dissemination of these manuscripts that have been approved for publication following peer review, and serving as a resource for students, scholars and researchers involved in compiling and/or developing knowledge in an area of nursing research or practice. Criteria that must be met before a paper is approved for publication in a refereed journal vary, but all editors will be concerned with maintaining a standard of excellence in regard to scientific merit and the literary standard of the work, the relevance of the paper in terms of its potential to contribute to knowledge development in the topic area and of interest to the readers and subscribers of the journal.

There are many peer-reviewed journals in nursing internationally. Each journal has its own aims, purposes and requirements, which must be followed by authors submitting their work for peer review with a view to being published in the journal. Professional journals from other health disciplines also publish relevant articles, depending on the topic. A number of journals in nursing and medicine follow the Uniform Requirements for Manuscripts (URM) editorial guidelines from the International Committee of Medical Journal Editors (ICMJE; www.icmje.org). See journal websites for further information for readers and authors.

DEVELOPING RESEARCH AIMS, OBJECTIVES OR QUESTIONS

Research ideas come from many sources; some are derived from theoretical aspects, while others arise from the need to solve practice problems or to improve the quality of care. Having a good idea is often not enough—you need to translate that idea into a specific, researchable and feasible topic. Depending on the study topic, the statement can be constructed as an aim, objective, question or hypothesis. Regardless of form and structure, the study statement is a concise description of a problem or issue that can be challenged to generate new knowledge. The way research questions are worded can influence the research design and methods that follow.

This section briefly discusses how to develop a research statement based on the amount of knowledge and/or theory about the topic, and describes the importance of a thorough review of the literature to identify relevant theory and research.

Developing the study statement (aim, objective, question) is an important initial step, requiring discussion of your topic with colleagues or experts in the field. This enables development and refinement into a narrow and researchable topic. Often the initial research topic is too broad to provide a feasible project in terms of timeframe and resources. Consider the following example: Do undergraduate students taught in a supportive environment increase their learning capabilities as graduates? Before this can be answered, a number of issues have to be clarified. What exactly is a supportive environment? What does it mean to increase their learning capabilities? How do we measure learning capabilities? How do we determine learning capabilities in graduates? Until you can define the terms and determine how to measure the variables they represent, you cannot answer the original question. Frequently, researchers have to narrow the topic area or, in some cases, the types and number of settings or the number of participants they include in the study. This process of narrowing the topic ultimately must also be consistent with the research design and methods of the study.

These statements can be classified based on the amount of knowledge and/or theory about the topic area. Questions may be exploratory and descriptive, through to testing or confirmatory. Once the question has been formulated, the type of study design becomes clear. Exploratory studies are used when there is little or no literature on either the topic or the population to be researched. Questions at this level are designed to explore the topic or a single population. For example, 'What is …?' or 'What are …?' the phenomena or concepts of interest.

Studies that build on exploratory studies have some existing knowledge and theory about the topic and population. Questions at this level often examine relationships between phenomena or measurable variables; for example, 'What is the relationship …?' between two or more concepts. These questions lead to correlation designs where statistical analysis is used to determine the significance of the relationship between the variables. Questions at a testing or confirmatory level require considerable knowledge about the topic. Research at this level begins at knowing the relationships between variables; therefore, questions at this level are designed to examine why this relationship exists, with a rationale and with an explanation. These questions lead to experimental designs.

Opinion leaders (Liberati et al 2009, PRISMA 2009) have suggested the PICOS structure to generate informative titles that make key information easily accessible to readers: Participants; Interventions; Comparators; Outcomes; Study design.

Reviewing the literature

Whether you begin with a vague idea of a study or a well-developed research plan, every project is considered an extension of previous knowledge. An appropriate review of the literature, in which students and researchers draw on evidence from multiple sources, is therefore a common beginning stage of a study. First, your research question may have been addressed and answered, or a review can be the initial source of ideas for a research question. Searches of the literature will be more successful if they have well-formulated questions. Librarians will often help to focus your question, to assist you in the search and to select databases appropriate to your topic.

By being familiar with the literature and understanding what is already known and not known with existing research and theory in an area, you can devise your research study to explore any newly identified questions. A review will also assist you to establish a theoretical context and rationale for your study. From a practical (methodological) perspective, the review can also reveal appropriate research strategies, measuring instruments, techniques and analysis. The review allows you to learn from the strengths and limitations of other researchers' work in regard to successful outcomes and assumptions, and keeps you current with the research work being undertaken in your area of interest.

NURSING RESEARCH PROCESSES

Research can use qualitative or quantitative approaches independently, or increasingly in combination as a mixed methods approach (Burke Johnson & Onwuegbuzie 2004). Each of these processes is outlined below.

Qualitative research

The term 'qualitative research', or 'qualitative inquiry', spans a range of theoretical perspectives, research designs and approaches. This evolving field of research has its origins in the humanities and social sciences (Erikson 2011). Denzin and Lincoln (2011) argue that qualitative research embraces an avowed humanistic and social justice commitment to study the social world from the perspective of the interacting individual. From this principle flow the liberal and radical politics of action that are held by feminist, clinical, ethnic, critical, queer, critical race theory and cultural studies researchers. While multiple interpretive communities now circulate within the field of qualitative research, they are all united on this single point (Denzin &

Lincoln 2011:xiii). It focuses therefore on human experiences, including accounts of subjective realities, and it is often conducted in naturalistic settings involving close, often sustained, contact between the researcher and research participants (Denzin & Lincoln 2011, Sarantakos 2012). Naturalistic research is often referred to as field research because it is conducted in the 'field' (Polit et al 2001, Sarantakos 2012). This label may be applied to a range of contexts—for example, a community health centre, an intensive care unit or a participant's home.

> Qualitative inquiry seeks to discover and describe in narrative reporting what particular people do in their everyday lives and what their actions mean to them. It identifies meaning-relevant kinds of things in the world—kinds of people, kinds of actions, kinds of beliefs and interests—focusing on differences in forms of things that make a difference for meaning.
> (Erikson 2011:43)

The purely qualitative researcher approaches a study with a particular set of values and beliefs, which is different from the purely quantitative researcher. These differences relate to the world view (ontology) of the researcher, notions about epistemology (ways of knowing) and research methodology (Parse 2001, Sarantakos 2012). For example, in the qualitative or interpretive paradigm, value is placed on individual subjectivity, multiple truths are accommodated and individuals who participate in the study are regarded as active participants and partners in the research (Sarantakos 2012). In the positivist paradigm, the opposite applies and concepts such as control, precision, objectivity, testing, one truth, prediction and cause–effect are valued, while individual perceptions are not considered or trusted.

Qualitative research methods are richly descriptive in nature (Sarantakos 2012) and allow exploration of a range of human experiences, which are of interest in a discipline such as nursing—for example, the experience of suffering for people living with terminal cancer, the characteristics of cultural groups, including their health beliefs, or the question: 'What is comfort for recipients of nursing?' It may be possible to study these phenomena using a quantitative approach, but this could be very limiting. Human interaction and intrapersonal and interpersonal communication processes may influence the experience of comfort for recipients of care. Qualitative research approaches would therefore produce richer, more in-depth accounts of this phenomenon.

Sampling approaches in qualitative research deliberately seek people who have lived the experience under investigation. Reasoning in qualitative research is inductive, but may involve a process of induction–deduction. The advantage of using a qualitative approach is that the phenomenon may be studied more holistically, taking account of individual and group perspectives (Nieswiadomy 2002), with a focus on the human experience; this is sometimes referred to as 'lived experience' (Parse 2001). In qualitative studies, the researcher's aim is development of a thick description of the experience under investigation—that is, 'a rich and thorough description of the research context' (Polit et al 2001:472).

Qualitative studies are commonly carried out with small numbers of research participants and involve in-depth inquiry into the phenomenon of concern. The data in qualitative research are presented in the form of words rather than numbers. The researcher may interview participants and audio-tape the conversation, which is later transcribed for data analysis. In this way, narrative text is often assembled by the researcher in working with the research participants. The text of the interview can be analysed and developed into themes to reflect core ideas or recurring features in the data (Miles & Huberman 1994). This process involves intensive reflection on the part of the researcher. The qualitative paradigm is often referred to as interpretive because:

> ... social interaction is a process of interpretation; social reality is constructed through interpretation of the actors; social relations are the result of a process of interaction based on interpretation; and theory building is a process of interpretation.
> (Sarantakos 1993:50)

A range of research approaches are available, depending on the aims or purposes of the study. Each approach incorporates a way of structuring the study, selecting the research participants and collecting and analysing the data. Some examples are provided below. Readers are also directed to nursing and social science research texts for amplification of the approaches to qualitative research described below (Denzin & Lincoln 2011, Sarantakos 2012, Schneider et al 2007).

Phenomenology is a philosophy and a descriptive research method designed to uncover the essence and meaning of lived experiences—for example, suffering or grieving (Parse 2001). 'The phenomenologist investigates subjective phenomena in the belief that critical truths about reality are grounded in people's lived experiences' (Polit et al 2001:214).

Ethnography is a qualitative, theory-building, holistic research approach that is applied to study of the culture of a group (Nieswiadomy 2002, Polit et al 2001).

> In ethnographic research, the researcher frequently lives with the people [being studied] and becomes a part of their culture. The researcher explores with the people their rituals and customs. An entire cultural group may be studied or a subgroup in the culture. The term *culture* may be used in a broad sense to mean an entire tribe of Indians, for example, or in the more narrow sense to mean one nursing care unit.
> (Nieswiadomy 2002:153)

The ethnographer sets out to uncover the insiders' (emic) view of the culture under study as opposed to the outsiders' (etic) view (Polit et al 2001). Grounded theory is a research process designed to lead to generation of theory through study of a particular human context. In grounded theory research studies, 'data are collected and analyzed and then a theory is developed that is "grounded" in the data' (Nieswiadomy 2002:360).

Quantitative research

The term 'quantitative research' refers to studies that seek to measure some concept or phenomenon of interest (e.g. physical function, pain or student attitudes to learning about research). This view of the world ('paradigm') also uses terms such as positivist, reductionist or empirical. Deductive reasoning is used, with thinking leading from a known principle to an unknown, and is used to test a particular research hypothesis.

Quantitative research encompasses a range of research designs and associated methods; the most common designs for healthcare research are listed in Table 9.2. Selection of an appropriate design relates to the research question being posed (Sackett & Wennberg 1997). The topic of interest may be framed as a question, objective or research hypothesis. Each design incorporates a number of variations; readers are

Table 9.2
Common research designs

Design	Purpose
Descriptive	Examines characteristics of a single sample; clarifies concepts; generates questions about potential relationships between variables (e.g. case study, cross-sectional analysis)
Correlation	Examines (describes, predicts or tests) relationships between two or more variables, but does not infer a cause-and-effect relationship
Quasi-experiment	Tests a cause-and-effect relationship, but without control or randomisation (e.g. case control, intervention only)
Experiment	Tests a cause-and-effect relationship using randomisation, manipulation of an intervention and control of other variables (e.g. randomised controlled trial (RCT), laboratory experiment)

directed to any number of nursing research texts for amplification of these designs (see recommended readings later in this chapter).

Quantitative studies have a range of common characteristics that are applied to the specific research topic, and documented in a research proposal, grant submission, report or journal article (see Table 9.3). These studies rely on sampling a smaller group of individuals who have similar (representative) characteristics to the overall population of interest. Inclusion and/or exclusion criteria (defined in Table 9.1) are developed, which guide the selection of participants. This commonly includes the use of random sampling to select eligible participants. In experimental studies, the explanatory (independent) variable (an intervention) is manipulated by random allocation of informed and consenting study participants to a treatment or control group, while the outcome (dependent) variable of interest is measured and other related variables are controlled (as for a randomised controlled trial or RCT).

Measurement of the concepts of interest is conducted using single or multiple 'measuring instruments' (or tools). These can be physiological (e.g. heart rate monitor, blood glucometer) or psychological/psychometric (e.g. anxiety scales, functional status, quality of life). Ideally, an instrument should exhibit characteristics that are valid, reliable and responsive. Development of new instruments is time-consuming and resource-intensive, as the validity, reliability and responsiveness must be tested, and modification of items (questions) may be required to improve the performance of the instrument. Established instruments generally have had their validity and reliability rigorously tested over time, and have been accepted as useful research tools.

Instrument (measurement) validity refers to whether the instrument actually measures what it is intended to measure. The aim is for an instrument to have appropriate construct validity—that is, the extent that an instrument accurately measures a theoretical construct or trait that is established over time, following repeated use and testing of the instrument in various studies. With any instrument there is the possibility of measurement error. The aim of a good study or instrument is to minimise the chance of that error. There are numerous subforms of construct validity that

Table 9.3
Common characteristics of research plans and reports

Heading / Section	Sub-heading / elements	Comments
Abstract	May use a structured format – introduction, methods, results, discussion	A clear and concise summary, commonly with a word limit (200–300 words)
Introduction	Background literature	Justification/significance of studying the research topic; relevant paradigm discussed or implied
Methods	Study aim	May be structured with specific research objective/s, question/s, hypothesis/es
	Design	Specific label or description, reflecting the paradigm
	Sample	Inclusion criteria; access to eligible participants; may describe study setting
	Sampling approach	Description and justification for selecting participants (random, non-random approaches)
	Data collection approaches	Participant involvement, description of technique (e.g. questionnaire, interview, focus group, observation, document audit) and instruments (e.g. audio-taping, case report form), reliability and validity issues (audit trail, instrument validity)
	Data management and analyses	Collection, collation, cleaning, data checking, data security, specific analytical procedures
	Ethical considerations	HREC approval/s; participant rights, information, consent, data collection requirements, burden
Results / Findings		Data presentation and interpretation in relation to research objective/s or question/s
Discussion	Major findings	Discussion of findings in relation to other literature; describes strengths and limitations of this study
	Implications for practice	Contribution of study findings to knowledge of practice
	Recommendations for further research	Related knowledge gaps highlighted for exploration
Conclusions		Summary of work, highlighting study contribution to discipline knowledge

have been used to describe increasing rigour for testing an instrument's performance (Elliott 2007a:214). For example:

- Content. The instrument items reflect all major elements of the concept. Initially, 'face validity' is commonly assessed by a panel of experts or stakeholders to examine whether, on the face of it, the instrument appears to measure the concept.

- Relationship. The instrument performance is compared with other variables or measures or the 'gold-standard' criteria or instrument.

- Hypothesis testing. Tests the relationships between concepts.

Reliability relates to the accuracy of the instrument measuring the concept being investigated. This is tested in terms of:

- Stability (test–retest: similar scores on repeated testing for a stable trait)

- Homogeneity (internal consistency: all parts of the instrument measure the same characteristics), and

- Equivalence (interrater reliability: consistency between observers using the same instrument with the same study participants).

There are a number of statistical tests for reliability, which are commonly expressed as a correlation coefficient, ranging from 0.0 to 1.0. A reliability of 0.80 is considered the minimal acceptable coefficient for a developed instrument.

Responsiveness is the ability of an instrument to detect clinically important changes in the variable of interest with a participant (Elliott 2007a:217). This is the opposite characteristic to stability, and relates to the precision of measurement for the instrument. Unfortunately, assessment of this performance characteristic has been minimal when compared with reliability and validity testing.

In addition to the 'Glossary' at the end of this book, Table 9.1 explains some common quantitative research terms used in this chapter. More detailed glossaries are available in specific nursing research texts (see recommended readings).

Another key characteristic of quantitative research is that data are managed in numerical form to answer the study questions. All information is therefore transformed to numbers prior to data management and analysis. Data analysis procedures can be descriptive or inferential, depending on the design and the levels of measurement for each variable (i.e. nominal, ordinal, interval, ratio). Categories must be mutually exclusive and collectively exhaustive:

- Nominal. Assigns nominal values to classify characteristics into non-ordered categories (e.g. sex, religion, diagnosis). The assigned numbers do not convey any relative order or weight between the values (e.g. 1 = male, 2 = female; in this instance, there is no implication that '1' is ordered higher than '2', or that '2' is twice the score of '1').

- Ordinal. Values are ordered in a logical way to provided a relative ranking (e.g. use of Likert scales—'strongly agree', 'agree', 'undecided', 'disagree', 'strongly disagree'). Example of variables include pain, levels of mobility, self-care.

- Interval. Values exhibit a rank ordering with equal distance between values (e.g. temperature, scores on a linear analogue scale from 1 to 10). For example, 'On a scale of 1 to 10, how would you rate your pain?'
- Ratio. Values have the above characteristics plus a meaningful baseline or absolute zero (e.g. weight, height, heart rate).

Note that temperature scales vary in their level of measurement. For the Celsius scale, 0 degrees (0°C) equates to the freezing point of water, but then has minus values so zero does not indicate an absolute baseline, with no or 'zero' temperature. This reflects an 'interval' level of measurement (see above). On the Kelvin scale, 0° equates to absolute zero temperature (−273° C) and reflects a 'ratio' level of measurement.

Data management and analysis are commonly undertaken using software packages (e.g. Statistical Package for the Social Sciences (SPSS) is a comprehensive analysis package; MS Excel spreadsheet software can also undertake certain statistical analysis procedures). Study designs and methods that provide findings using inferential statistics allow the researcher to 'infer' that results from a sample of participants (e.g. patients) can be applied to the wider population being investigated. Inferential statistics are further categorised into parametric or non-parametric procedures. Parametric tests are used when the following assumptions are met: the sample was drawn from a normal distribution; random sampling was used; and data were measured at least at interval level.

As beginning research consumers, students must consider the objectives of the study and the related purposes for the statistical tests performed. Table 9.4 can be used to support the critique of papers for consistency between the purpose, the level of measurement and actual statistical tests that are appropriate to answer those questions. More in-depth information regarding the actual statistical tests is beyond the scope of this chapter, but can be found in comprehensive research texts (see recommended readings).

Mixed method research

While mixed method research originated many years ago, it was the publication of the *Handbook of Mixed Method* in 2003 by Tashakkori and Teddlie that led to a proliferation of mixed method research (Creswell & Zhang 2009). The development of mixed method research has also been instigated by funding groups who want researchers to use a variety of approaches to address social issues, the proliferation of novel research approaches and the development of computer-based technologies capable of merging different data sets (Hesse-Biber 2010).

Mixed method research is a systematic approach to the incorporation of two or more research methods in order to answer a single research question (Morse & Niehaus 2009). Importantly, the two approaches within the mixed methods study must be applied following the techniques for and in keeping with the principles of good research for each individual approach. However, for the combination of two or more approaches to be considered a mixed method study, integration of the different data sets must occur. In fact, this is probably the least understood and least developed aspect of mixed method research (Onwuegbuzie et al 2009). To be more explicit, each study is undertaken and analysed as required in keeping with the particular approach; however, either during the conduct of the two studies or in the interpretation phase there must be an attempt to integrate the data. For example, the data can be integrated

Table 9.4
Statistical purposes and related parametric and non-parametric tests

Statistical purpose	Parametric test	Non-parametric test
Compares *mean scores* for two independent samples	Two sample (unpaired) *t*-test (*interval/ratio data*)	Mann-Whitney U test (*ordinal data*)
Compares *mean scores* for two sets of observations from the same sample	Paired *t*-test (interval/ratio data)	Wilcoxon matched pairs test (*ordinal data*)
Compares *mean scores* for three or more sets of observations	One-way analysis of variance (ANOVA)	Kruskall-Wallis ANOVA by ranks
Compares *proportions* from two samples	Chi-square (χ^2) test	Fisher's exact test
Compares *proportions* from a paired sample	No equivalent	McNemar's test
Assesses strength of straight line *association* between two variables	Product moment correlation coefficient (Pearson's *r*)	Spearman's rank correlation coefficient (r^s)
Describes *relationship* between two variables, allowing one to be *predicted* from the other	Simple linear regression	Non-parametric regression
Describes *relationship* between a dependent variable and several predictor variables	Multiple regression	Non-parametric regression

Source: Adapted from Burns N, Grove S K 2005; Greenhalgh T 1997; and Schneider Z, Elliott D, LoBiondo-Wood G, Haber J (eds) 2003.

at the end where each data set is examined and used to help explain the other. Alternatively, the integration can occur during the study where, for example, the findings from one phase help to identify the participants to sample or the questions to ask in the following phase.

Reasons for using mixed method research vary. The researcher may want to look for convergence of the data collected using various methods as a way to indicate credibility of the findings, or the aim may be complementarity where the researcher wants to gain a deeper understanding of the issue or clarify a particular result. In addition, the reasons for selecting a mixed method design may arise where the results from one study help develop or inform another, or because the findings of a study raise questions or contradictions leading to the initiation of a further study (Hesse-Biber 2010).

There are several types of mixed method designs. The *triangulation design* is a one-phase study in which the quantitative and qualitative components are conducted simultaneously and with equal weight. Each data set is collected and analysed concurrently but separately, and data sets merged for interpretation (Creswell & Plano Clark 2011, Hesse-Biber 2010). The *embedded design* occurs where one data set (the secondary data set) supports the other (primary data set) in order to help answer the research question. Both types of data are collected in this design; however, one always plays a minor role, which distinguishes the embedded design from others (Creswell & Plano Clark 2011, Hesse-Biber 2010). While the first two designs described occur concurrently, the next two are *sequential*; data is collected and analysed in a linear fashion. The *explanatory design* is a two-phase design used when qualitative data is collected to help explain the quantitative results (QUAN ➔ qual). Hence, in the explanatory design the quantitative data is always collected first (Creswell & Plano Clark 2011, Hesse-Biber 2010). Lastly, the other major approach to mixed methods research is the exploratory design. The two-phase *exploratory design* is appropriate where the researcher wants to test an emergent theory or explore a phenomenon in depth and then build on the qualitative results by developing an instrument, identifying variables or declaring propositions for future testing (QUAL ➔ quan) (Creswell & Plano Clark 2011, Hesse-Biber 2010). Mixed method researchers use capital letters to identify the primary study or what has been termed the theoretical drive of the overall study. The theoretical drive, which is driven by the research question and study purpose, guides the selection of the core or primary method (Morse & Niehaus 2009). If the research aims to explore or describe a phenomenon, it is inductively driven and supported by a quantitative supplemental component (indicated by the QUAL ➔ quan symbol).

How nurses use research in their practice

Nursing and other health professionals are concerned with improving the quality of patient care and establishing standards for best clinical practice by examining the current knowledge base of the discipline. Findings from research studies are disseminated at conferences and in professional journals. Some studies are designed to inform practice development by describing a clinical practice, or comparing two (or more) different ways of performing a practice. Other types of studies may shed light on patients' experiences of phenomena that are poorly understood, such as hope or suffering.

The ability to critique studies relevant to practice is therefore a fundamental skill for undergraduate nurses to master in preparation for professional practice as registered nurses. Current registered nurses also need these skills in terms of continuing professional development. These critiquing and evaluation skills are not, however, easily attained, and do not magically appear at the end of a single university research course. Rather, your ability and confidence is additive and experiential, as it relates to experiences, practice and reflections over time. In fact, it is an ability that relates to 'lifelong learning' where we can always learn and improve our skills.

Evidence-based practice

With evidence-based practice (EBP) a major currency in contemporary healthcare, one major aim is promotion of best clinical or community practice based on the best available evidence. This evidence is now commonly informed from systematic review of a collection of original studies focusing on a specific clinical question.

Currently, both a 'systematic review' (SR) and an integrative review are adaptations of the narrative literature review, addressing a well-defined question. This review approach has explicit and systematic steps, including formulation of the clinical question, search strategy, study inclusions, quality review and critique of the methods of the included studies, and synthesis of study findings to inform practice. The purpose of this approach is to minimise bias in the review process.

The question for an SR has a specific clinical focus, with four (or five) components forming the acronym PICO(T):

P Problem (patient-related or a health issue)

I Intervention

C Comparison of interventions and/or control practice

O Outcome (that is measurable)

T Timeframe (Elliott 2007b:53).

The search strategy describes the databases (e.g. CINAHL, Medline) used and any journals searched by hand. Selection of articles is by key words in the article title or abstract, as well as any other filters (e.g. English language, study design). A preliminary review of the abstract enables identification of the papers for inclusion in the SR. The excluded papers may also be noted, including the reasons for exclusion. Included studies are then assessed according to structured and explicit criteria. An SR may also include the pooling and analysis of data from the studies investigated; this process is called a meta-analysis.

Organisational resources

A number of international and national organisations have developed repositories of SRs to guide appropriate clinical practice (Cochrane 1972). The Cochrane Collaboration was one of the first to develop as an international multidisciplinary collaborative group to systematically review clinical research, and is now represented in many countries including Australia (see www.cochrane.org.au). The Cochrane Collaboration aims to develop, maintain and disseminate SRs of healthcare interventions, and includes a database of completed and in-progress reviews and a bibliography of SR abstracts and methodological articles (see Cochrane databases available through your library).

Systematic reviews were developed to examine studies of cause-and-effect relationships (i.e. does a 'new' treatment improve a patient outcome?). The most powerful and rigorous design (the 'gold standard') for examining cause-and-effect questions in clinical practice is the randomised controlled trial (RCT). The classification therefore developed for rating the levels of evidence (National Health and Medical Research Council 2000) regard the RCT as providing the best evidence to answer cause-and-effect types of clinical practice questions:

Level I: a systematic review of all relevant randomised controlled trials (RCTs)

Level II: at least one properly designed RCT

Level III—1: well-designed controlled trials without randomisation

Level III—2: well-designed comparative studies with concurrent controls (e.g. cohort, case-control)

Level III—3: well-designed time-series studies with historical controls (before–after)

Level IV: post-test, pretest/post-test

If there is no rigorous scientific evidence available, then the opinions of respected authorities, clinical experience, descriptive studies or reports of expert committees can then be used to support clinical practice (National Health and Medical Research Council 2000).

Note however that nursing uses a variety of research paradigms and methods to answer questions that cannot be appropriately investigated by RCTs. We therefore need to consider how to evaluate non-RCT observational studies of nursing practice so that these findings can also guide nursing care. The Joanna Briggs Institute for Evidence-Based Nursing and Midwifery (see www.joannabriggs.edu.au) and the Centre for Evidence-Based Nursing in the UK (see www.york.ac.uk/healthsciences/centres/evidence/cebn.htm) conduct SRs of specific clinical practices, which are of importance to nurses.

Development of these necessary frameworks continues to evolve, but they are not yet formed or developed to an adequate level nationally or internationally. The goal remains to foster SRs of relevant studies on clinical nursing so that quality nursing practice will be informed by the best available evidence, regardless of the research design.

CONCLUSION

An understanding of basic concepts and processes in research is central to professional nursing practice. Ideally, quality nursing care is based on the outcomes of quality research processes. It is envisaged that, in time, one of the hallmarks of the profession of nursing will be the utilisation of research evidence to inform the best, safest and most appropriate care for patients and their families. All nurses engaged in nursing practice require research utilisation skills in order to make judgements about how relevant and applicable research findings are to practice. Nursing is a complex, practice-based discipline in which researchable questions will always require answers in order to extend knowledge. A range of research paradigms and approaches are available to appropriately answer these questions.

In the course of your reading and learning about research processes in nursing, you will discover that in some instances researchers use 'triangulation' of both quantitative and qualitative research processes to study a particular area of interest. The evaluative criteria for establishing the scientific validity of qualitative research are the subject of continuing development and debate (e.g. Cesario et al 2002). Questions remain about how to incorporate findings from qualitative studies, which may have no generalisation to the patient group in question, but which may provide valuable insights of patient experiences in guiding quality nursing practice.

This chapter has provided an introduction to the rich and complex research traditions, paradigms and methods which will be explored further during your undergraduate education and beyond into professional practice.

REFLECTIVE QUESTIONS

1 What processes could be followed in formulating a research problem in nursing?

2 What are the critical features of a comprehensive review of the literature?

3 What are the factors that would guide you in using a particular research approach?

RECOMMENDED READINGS

Borbasi S, Jackson D, Langford R 2008 Navigating the maze of research: enhancing nursing and midwifery practice, 2nd edn. Elsevier, Sydney

Carper B 1978 Fundamental patterns of knowing in nursing. Advances in Nursing Science 1(1):13–23

Creswell J W, Plano Clark V L 2011 Designing and conducting mixed methods research, 2nd edn. Sage, Los Angeles

McKenna H, Daly J, Davidson P M, Duffield C, Jackson D 2012 RAE and ERA: Spot the difference. International Journal of Nursing Studies 9:375–377

Wood M J, Ross-Kerr J C 2011 Basic steps in planning nursing research: from question to proposal, 7th edn. Jones and Bartlett Publishing, Sudbury, MA

REFERENCES

Australian Nursing and Midwifery Council (ANMC) 2006 National competency standards for the registered nurse, 4th edn. ANMC, Canberra

Burke Johnson R, Onwuegbuzie A J 2004 Mixed methods research: a research paradigm whose time has come. Educational Researcher 7:14–26

Burns N, Grove S K 2005 The practice of nursing research: conduct, critique and utilization, 5th edn. Elsevier/Saunders, St Louis

Cesario S, Morin K, Santa-Donato A 2002 Evaluating the level of evidence of qualitative research. Journal of Obstetrics, Gynecology and Neonatal Nursing 31:531–537

Cochrane A L 1972 Effectiveness and efficiency: random reflections on health services. Nuffield Provincial Hospitals Trust, London

Compact Oxford English Dictionary 2004 Online. Available: www.askoxford.com/concise_oed/research

Council of Deans of Nursing and Midwifery (ANZ) n.d. See www.cdnm.edu.au

Creswell J W, Plano Clark V L 2011 Designing and conducting mixed methods research, 2nd edn. Sage, Los Angeles

Creswell J, Zhang W 2009 The application of mixed methods designs to trauma research. Journal of Traumatic Stress 22(6):612–621

Crookes P A, Davies S (eds) 2004 Research into practice: essential skills for reading and applying research in nursing and health care. Baillière Tindall, Edinburgh

D'Antonio P 1997 Toward a history of research in nursing. Nursing Research 46: 105–110

Denzin N K, Lincoln Y S 2011 (eds) The Sage Handbook of Qualitative Research, 4th edn. Sage, Thousand Oaks, California

Elliott D 2007a Assessing measuring instruments. In: Schneider Z, Elliott D, LoBiondo-Wood G, Haber J (eds) Nursing research: methods and appraisal for evidence-based practice, 3rd edn. Mosby, Sydney

Elliott D 2007b Reviewing the literature. In: Schneider Z, Elliott D, LoBiondo-Wood G, Haber J (eds) Nursing research: methods and appraisal for evidence-based practice, 3rd edn. Mosby, Sydney

Elliott D 2007c Searching the literature. In: Schneider Z, Elliott D, LoBiondo-Wood G, Haber J (eds) Nursing research: methods and appraisal for evidence-based practice, 3rd edn. Mosby, Sydney, pp 91–107

Erikson F 2011 A history of qualitative inquiry in social and educational research. In: Denzin N K, Lincoln Y S 2011 (eds) The Sage Handbook of Qualitative Research, 4th edn. Sage, Thousand Oaks, California

Greenhalgh T 1997 How to read a paper: the basics of evidence based medicine, BMJ Publishing, London

Hesse-Biber, S N 2010 Mixed methods research: merging theory with practice. Guilford Press, New York

Liberati A, Altman D G, Tetzlaff J et al 2009 The PRISMA statement for reporting systematic reviews and meta-analyses of studies that evaluate health care interventions: explanation and elaboration. Journal of Clinical Epidemiology 62(10):1–34

McKenna H, Daly J, Davidson P M, Duffield C, Jackson D 2012 RAE and ERA: spot the difference. (Guest Editorial). International Journal of Nursing Studies 49:375–377

Miles M B, Huberman M 1994 Qualitative data analysis: an expanded sourcebook, 2nd edn. Sage, Thousand Oaks, California

Morse J, Niehaus L 2009 Mixed method design: principles and procedures. Left Coast Press, Walnut Creek, CA

Mulhall A 1995 Nursing research: what difference does it make? Journal of Advanced Nursing 21:576–583

National Health and Medical Research Council (NHMRC) 2000 How to use the evidence: assessment and application of scientific evidence. NHMRC, Canberra

National Health and Medical Research Council (NHMRC) 2007 Joint NHMRC/ARC/AVCC national statement on ethical conduct in human research. NHMRC, Canberra. Online. Available: www.nhmrc.gov.au/publications/synopses/_files/e72.pdf

Nieswiadomy R 2002 (ed) Foundations of nursing research, 4th edn. Prentice Hall, New Jersey

Onwuegbuzie A J, Slate J R, Leech N L, Collins K M T 2009 Mixed data analysis: advanced integration techniques. International Journal of Multiple Research Approaches 3:13–33

Parse R R 1987 (ed) Nursing science: major paradigms, theories and critiques. WB Saunders, Philadelphia

Parse R R 2001 Qualitative inquiry: the path of sciencing. Jones & Bartlett, Boston

Polit D F, Beck C T, Hungler B P 2001 Essentials of nursing research: methods, appraisal and utilisation, 5th edn. Lippincott, Philadelphia

PRISMA 2009 Online. Available: www.prisma-statement.org/

Sackett D L, Wennberg J E 1997 Choosing the best research design for each question: it's time to stop squabbling over the 'best' methods (editorial). British Medical Journal 317(7123):1636

Sarantakos S 1993 Social research. Macmillan Education Australia, Melbourne

Sarantakos S 2012 Social research, 4th edn. Palgrave Macmillan, London

Schneider Z, Elliott D, LoBiondo-Wood G, Haber J (eds) 2003 Nursing research: methods, critical appraisal and utilisation, 2nd edn, Mosby, Sydney

Schneider Z, Whitehead D, LoBiondo-Wood G, Haber J (eds) 2007 Nursing and midwifery research: methods and critical appraisal for evidence-based practice, 4th edn. Mosby, Sydney

Tashakkori A, Teddlie, C. (eds) 2003 Handbook of mixed methods in social and behavioral research. Sage Publications, Thousand Oaks, CA

Wood M J, Ross-Kerr J C 2011 Basic steps in planning nursing research: From question to proposal, 7th edn. Jones and Bartlett Publishing, Sudbury, MA

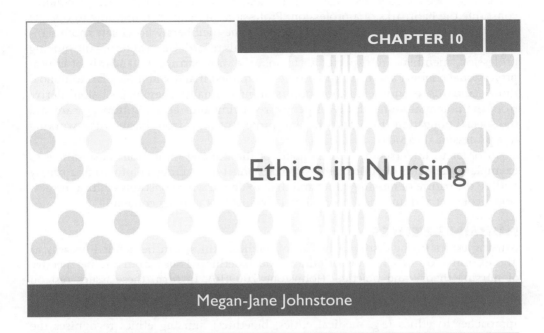

Megan-Jane Johnstone

LEARNING OBJECTIVES

This chapter will:

- define nursing ethics
- distinguish between ethical and unethical professional conduct in nursing
- explore the notion of 'everyday' ethics in nursing
- critique the development of patient safety ethics
- explore the risk of possible unintended consequences of implementing a regulatory as opposed to discretionary approach to patient safety ethics
- examine the relationship between patient safety and nursing ethics
- discuss critically whether nursing ethics has the capacity to improve and protect the moral safety of patients.

KEY WORDS

Ethics, nursing ethics, ethical and unethical professional conduct, patient safety, moral safety, patient rights, cultural considerations

PROFESSIONAL ETHICS

It has long been recognised that ethical standards and exemplary ethical conduct constitute the hallmarks of a profession. Professions are expected not only to operate under strict ethical standards but also to discipline members who violate those standards. Nursing as a profession is no exception in this regard. Upon entering the nursing profession, members are expected to uphold the most stringent standards of ethical professional conduct and can expect to be disciplined if and when they fail to uphold those standards, even if a violation occurs unintentionally. These expectations derive from the potential vulnerability of people requiring and receiving nursing care and the special obligation that nurses have to protect patients from harm when working in a professional capacity.

In order to understand why members of the nursing profession must adhere to exemplary standards of ethical professional conduct it would be helpful to first briefly outline the nature of nursing ethics and then to define what constitutes ethical professional conduct and unethical professional conduct in a nursing context.

NURSING ETHICS

Nursing ethics (to be distinguished from medical ethics) can be defined broadly as 'the examination of all kinds of ethical and bioethical issues from the perspective of nursing theory and practice' (Johnstone 2009:16). In turn, these issues rest on the agreed core concepts of nursing: person, culture, care, health, healing, environment, and nursing itself (i.e. what it is and what its end and purpose is). Unlike other approaches to ethics (e.g. medical ethics, bioethics), nursing ethics recognises the 'distinctive voices' that are nurses' and emphasises, as a starting point for systematic ethical inquiry, the importance of nurses' *actual experiences* as opposed to hypothetical examples or the experiences of members from other disciplines, which are not always relevant to nursing or to advancing moral wisdom in the practice of nursing.

Ethics works by providing an authoritative action guide on how to think about, understand, examine and judge how best to 'be moral' and live the moral life. When applied in professional practice contexts, ethics functions in two key ways:

- by ascribing moral values to things (e.g. 'it is wrong to cause harm to patients')

- by prompting us to consider and re-consider *what* we have judged to be 'right' and 'wrong' as well as the *justifications* we have used to support and defend those judgements (e.g. 'this action is morally wrong *because* it violates the moral principle of "do no harm"').

Authoritative action guides to ethical decision-making and conduct are found in the principles and standards expressed in the commonly accepted theories of human rights, ethical principlism (autonomy, beneficence, non-maleficence, justice) and virtue ethics—all of which have informed the development of nursing ethics and which have been comprehensively discussed in the nursing literature and expressed variously in nursing codes of ethics (Johnstone 2009).

Some nurses might think it unnecessary to appeal to 'high-brow' theoretical approaches (e.g. human rights, ethical principlism, virtue ethics) in their practice, preferring instead to draw on their own personal moral values, beliefs and experiences when dealing with ethical issues. While such a stance might serve them well when caring for their own loved ones, its application in a professional context is limited—especially when caring for people whose lifeways are unfamiliar to them. Not only might a reliance on personal ethics lead to moral mistakes being made, but, worse, to errors of moral judgement that result in morally harmful and even catastrophic outcomes.

ETHICAL AND UNETHICAL PROFESSIONAL CONDUCT

As stated in the opening paragraph to this chapter, exemplary ethical conduct is an important hallmark of a profession. But what is exemplary ethical conduct?

Exemplary or prototypical ethical professional conduct can be broadly defined as conduct or behaviour that complies with the agreed and expected ethical standards of a profession. Because the ethical standards of a profession tend to require a level of behaviour and demeanour that is above that ordinarily expected of lay people or 'the ordinary person on the street', it is also deemed to be 'ideal', 'typical' and hence 'exemplary'. By this view, ethical professional conduct in nursing can be defined as conduct by a nurse that complies with the agreed ethical standards of the nursing profession and, by virtue of being characteristic of the ideals that the nursing profession 'professes', is exemplary.

The exemplary ethical standards that registered nurses are expected to uphold are contained in various formal codes and guidelines relevant to the profession and practice of nursing. Notable examples include the *Australian Code of Ethics for Nurses* for nurses in Australia (NMBA 2008a), *Code of Professional Conduct for Nurses in Australia* (NMBA 2008b) and *National Competency Standards for the Registered Nurse* (NMBA 2006) (to access these and other documents visit http://www.nursingmidwiferyboard.gov.au/) and the New Zealand *Code of Conduct for Nurses* (Nursing Council of New Zealand 2012) (to access this code and other documents visit: http://www.nursingcouncil.org.nz/index.cfm/1,255,0,0,html/Code-of-Conduct-and-Guidelines).

These and related standards work by setting the 'ethical baseline' against which a nurse's conduct can be measured and evaluated. Thus, if a nurse engages in conduct that breaches the agreed standards of the profession (fails literally to 'measure up' to the standards in question) this may be deemed as unethical professional conduct and may result in a notification being made, in the case of Australian nurses, to the Australian Health Practitioner Regulation Agency (AHPRA) and, in the case of New Zealand Nurses, to the Nursing Council of New Zealand (NCNZ). If a notification is received by AHPRA the nurse may be investigated by the Nursing and Midwifery Board of Australia (which works in partnership with AHPRA) to 'ensure that appropriate action is taken, if required, to protect the public' (Johnstone 2012). Likewise in the case of notifications received by the NCNZ, which also has regulatory authority to investigate a nurse's conduct.

Unethical professional conduct is more complex than a mere failure to comply with agreed ethical standards, however. Unethical professional conduct may be more comprehensively defined as an umbrella term that incorporates the following three related although distinct notions: (i) unethical conduct, (ii) moral incompetence and (iii) moral impairment (Johnstone 2012). Here, *unethical conduct* may be defined as 'any act involving the deliberate violation of accepted or agreed ethical standards' and can encompass both 'moral turpitude' and 'moral delinquency' (Johnstone 2012). *Moral turpitude*, a legal concept that originates from the United States, refers to 'conduct that is considered contrary to community standards of justice, honesty or good morals' (Wikipedia—accessed 7 August 2012). *Moral delinquency*, in turn, refers to any act involving moral negligence or a dereliction of moral duty. In professional contexts, moral delinquency entails a deliberate or careless violation of agreed standards of ethical professional conduct.

Moral incompetence (analogous to clinical incompetence) pertains to a person's lack of requisite moral knowledge, skills, 'right attitude' and soundness of moral judgements (Johnstone 2012). The specific moral competencies expected of registered nurses in Australia are outlined in the *National Competency Standards for the Registered Nurse* and, for nurses in New Zealand, in the *Competencies for Registered Nurses* (NCNZ 2007). *Moral impairment* meanwhile is generally distinguished from moral incompetence. Unlike moral incompetence (attributable to a lack of moral knowledge, skills, etc.), moral impairment entails a disorder; for example, psychopathy, that interferes with a person's social and moral reasoning and hence capacity to behave ethically. More specifically, because of their impaired moral reasoning, they are unable to engage in the competent discharge of their moral duties and responsibilities towards others. Accepting the notion of moral impairment (a notion which has received little attention in the nursing literature), a nurse could be judged morally impaired when, because of their disorder, they are unable to practise nursing in an ethically just and morally accountable manner (Johnstone 2012).

'EVERYDAY' ETHICAL ISSUES IN NURSING

It is important to understand that ethical issues in nursing and healthcare contexts do not only involve the so-called 'big' or 'exotic' issues (e.g. abortion, euthanasia); they also involve fundamental questions about the nature and quality of professional–client relationships. This includes examining the more fundamental day-to-day practical ethical concerns relating to the precise impact that nurses' decisions and actions (or non-actions) have on the lives and welfare of other human beings, and the capacity of nurses to do harm to others while acting in a professional capacity.

The kinds of ethical issues faced by nurses today are as complex as they are varied. While in the past attention has tended to be focused on the better known bioethical issues such as abortion, euthanasia, organ transplantation, reproductive technology, genetic engineering and the like, over the past two decades there has been a significant shift in attention towards examining the other kinds of ethical issues faced by nurses. These issues include:

- 'everyday' practical ethical issues faced by nurses
- a genuine *nursing* perspective on common mainstream bioethical issues, and
- (the otherwise neglected) broader social justice issues associated with promoting the welfare, wellbeing and significant moral interests of highly vulnerable, stigmatised and marginalised groups of people.

The nursing ethics literature has borrowed heavily from bioethics to shape nursing ethics discourse. As a result the nursing ethics literature does not always represent or reflect the reality of the 'everyday' problems that nurses face. Some examples of the ethical issues that nurses may commonly encounter during the course of their practice include:

- *the moral boundaries of nursing* (e.g. nurses as carers being 'in relationship' with others, as opposed to being what the North American philosopher John Rawls

(1971) describes famously as 'detached observers choosing from behind a veil of ignorance')

- *catalysts to moral action* (e.g. 'experiential triggers' such as 'the look of suffering in a patient's eyes', as opposed to abstract moral rules and principles)

- *operating moral values* (e.g. sympathy, empathy, compassion, kindness, human understanding and a desire 'to do the best we can', rather than an obsession to 'do one's duty')

- *ethical decision-making processes* (which tend to be collaborative, communicative, communal and contextualised, rather than independent, private, individual, solo and decontextualised)

- *barriers to ethical practice* (which tend to be structural rather than knowledge-based—for example, organisational norms forcing compliance with the status quo, and negative attitudes and a lack of support from co-workers and managers) and

- *need for cathartic moral talking* (e.g. 'talking through' moral concerns in a safe and supportive environment to help relieve the distress that so often arises as a result of trying to be moral in a world that appears to be growing increasingly amoral) (Johnstone 2009:127).

What talking with nurses often reveals is that it is not the so-called paramount ('exotic') bioethical issues that trouble them, but the more fundamental issues of:

- how to help a patient in distress in the 'here and now'

- how to stop 'things going bad for a patient'

- how to best support a relative or chosen carer during times of distress and when the 'system' appears to be against them

- how to make things 'less traumatic' for someone who is suffering

- how to reduce the anxiety and vulnerability of the people being cared for

- where nurses can get help for their own distress, and

- how to make a difference in contexts where indifference to the moral interests of others is manifest (Johnstone 2009:128).

The above and other related concerns are all issues worthy of attention and consideration within and outside of the nursing profession. They are also issues that deserve to be recognised as being an integral part of a sound moral framework and approach that might be appropriately described as 'nursing ethics'.

PATIENT SAFETY ETHICS

Over the past decade increasing attention has been given to ethical issues concerned with the promotion of patient safety. The new and emerging field of patient safety ethics takes as its starting point recognition that all people requiring or receiving healthcare have a *right to be safe*—that is, the right to be kept free of danger or risk of injury while in healthcare domains (Johnstone 2007). The patient's right to be safe entails a correlative duty on the part of health service providers to ensure that people who are receiving care are kept free of danger or risk of injury while receiving that care. These moral prescriptions are unremarkable in that they reflect the well-established principle in healthcare of 'do no harm' and the associated moral duty on the part of all healthcare providers to avoid commissions and omissions that could otherwise result in preventable harm to patients (Beauchamp & Childress 2009).

In 2011, the Australian Commission on Safety and Quality in Health Care (ACSQHC) released its much anticipated *National Safety and Quality Health Services Standards*. These standards were developed after extensive public and stakeholder consultation to assist health service organisations to deliver safe and high-quality care and thereby 'protect the public from harm' (ACSQHC 2012:3). Of particular relevance to this discussion is the standard concerning Governance for Safety and Quality in Health Service Organisations (Standard 1) and the requirement for processes to be in place to ensure that 'patient rights are respected' and that patients be supported to be engaged in decisions about their care, including informed consent (ACSQHC 2011:21). In a consultation draft of guidelines for implementing the standards, actions are prescribed for implementing through organisational policies and practices:

- a patient charter of rights that is consistent with the current national charter of healthcare rights

- processes to enable partnership with patients in decisions about their care, including informed consent to treatment (these processes are to encompass provisions for 'Open Disclosure' when things go wrong, and advance care planning)

- procedures that protect the confidentiality of patient clinical records without compromising appropriate clinical workforce access to patient clinical information (these procedures are to encompass systems design that will restrict inappropriate access to and dissemination of patient clinical information)

- valid and reliable patient experience feedback mechanisms for use in evaluating the health service's performance (ACSQHC 2012:53–62).

Making patient rights the subject of a quality and safety regulatory mechanism is innovative and interesting. Whether this approach will achieve its intended outcomes, however, remains open to question (see, for example, Pronovost & Faden 2009, Wachter 2010). Given the profound cultural diversity of Australia's population and the diverse ultimate values and beliefs about health and healthcare that different cultural groups hold, there is a risk that some of the implementation strategies proposed in the guidelines might, paradoxically, cause rather than prevent moral harm. This risk is particularly high in instances where health service providers become too focused on complying with the prescribed 'actions required' at the expense of using their discretionary judgement and taking into account the culturally contextual nature of patient needs.

The ACSQHC guidelines recommend that 'language, sensory and cultural needs' are taken into account when implementing the proposed strategies (ACSQHC 2012:54). Unfortunately these provisions do not go far enough to ensure that a culturally competent and morally safe approach is taken when implementing such mechanisms as informed consent, confidentiality and advance care planning. If morally as well as clinically safe outcomes are to be achieved, then much greater attention will need to be given to recognising the critical missing link between culture, language and patient safety (Johnstone & Kanitsaki 2006); to ensuring a culturally appropriate approach to engaging patients as safety partners (Johnstone & Kanitsaki 2009); and, in the case of informed consent, confidentiality of clinical information and advance care planning, to upholding recognised cultural imperatives that have the capacity to guide the delivery of meaningful, morally safe and therapeutic care at the end of life (Johnstone & Kanitsaki 2008).

It is important for nurses to follow and participate in public policy development concerning healthcare delivery (such as the ACSQHC policy initiative just discussed) and develop a critical awareness that even the most well-intended and scrupulously designed public policy can have undesirable unanticipated consequences—that is, 'side effects discovered only after the policy is implemented, and which undermine the policy's effect or create new, complex problems' (Bridgman & Davis 2004:7). Unanticipated consequences (also referred to as *The Law of Unintended Consequences*) are generally thought to be caused by the complexity and rapidly changing nature of the world, human arrogance and self-interest, stupidity, self-deception and cognitive and emotive biases.

In a classic article on the subject, Merton (1936) outlines what he regards as the 'five most obvious limitations to correct anticipation of consequences of action':

- *Ignorance* (a lack of adequate knowledge, resulting in decisions being made on the basis of opinion and estimates);

- *Error* (an erroneous appraisal of a present situation and the inference that it will hold for a future situation, without recognising that while a procedure may have been successful *in certain circumstances*, it need not be so *under any and all conditions*);

- *Immediate interest* (an agent's paramount and immediate concern, which excludes consideration of other further and future consequences of the same act);

- *Basic values* (because of being enjoined by 'certain fundamental values' an actor feels no need to consider other further and future consequences);

- *Self-defeating prophecy* (because of fearing certain conditions and consequences before they occur, an actor devises solutions that may result in a social movement developing in an 'utterly unanticipated direction').

When applying a regulatory as opposed to a discretionary framework for managing ethical issues in healthcare, nurses have a moral responsibility to consider the possible unanticipated consequences of their actions. Regardless of their level or area of practice, nurses are obliged to take steps to help mitigate the kinds of limitations identified by Merton in the interests of protecting and upholding the moral safety of patients (i.e. ensuring that their significant moral interests are not harmed) throughout the trajectory of their care.

NURSING ETHICS AND PATIENT SAFETY

There is a strong theoretical as well as practical relationship between nursing ethics and patient safety. The standards and principles of nursing ethics have long required nurses to protect and promote the welfare, wellbeing and other significant moral interests of people in their care, and to 'take appropriate action to safeguard individuals when their care is endangered'. Over the past decade, however, both national and international professional nursing codes and statements of ethical professional conduct have made the issue of patient safety ethics more explicit by emphasising the responsibility of nurses to promote a 'culture of safety' in healthcare and to play an active role in reducing the incidence and impact of preventable adverse events in healthcare. An instructive example of this can be found in the *Code of Ethics for Nurses in Australia* (NMBA 2008a). Under Value Statement 6 of the *Code*, the following explanatory statement is provided:

> Nurses recognise that people are vulnerable to injuries and illnesses as a result of preventable human error and adverse events while in health care settings. Nurses play a key role in the detection and prevention of errors and adverse events in health care settings, and support and participate in systems to identify circumstances where people are at risk of harm. Nurses act to prevent or control such risks through prevention, monitoring, early identification and early management of adverse events. Nurses contribute to the confidential reporting of adverse events and errors, and to organisational processes for the open disclosure of these events to persons affected during the course of their care. (NMBA 2008a:12)

Deciding *that* action needs to be taken, as well as *what, when, where, how* and by *whom* are, however, all matters that require careful consideration. It is here that nursing ethics as a discipline and formal field of inquiry can be most helpful.

CONCLUSION

It is important to understand that ethics neither emerges from nor operates in a cultural or contextual vacuum, and that its processes (thinking, reasoning, doing) are vulnerable to all sorts of corrupting influences, including politics, prejudice and personal needs. These influences can result in decision making that is arbitrary, biased, capricious, self-interested and precariously based on personal preferences. It is for this reason that proper 'checks and balances' need to be in place that, in turn, are supported by an appropriate infrastructure (policies, processes and procedures).

Whether nursing ethics is 'up to the task' of guiding sound ethical decision making in healthcare contexts will depend ultimately on its capacity to:

- offer moral insight
- foster moral wisdom
- inform 'good policy'
- provide 'real' solutions to complex problems
- warrant principled dissent against questionable policies, decisions and actions by others
- enable foresight
- guide the prevention of future problems (preventative ethics)
- redress the harms caused by past problems (restorative ethics) (Johnstone 2008).

There are numerous complexities involved in building the capacity of nurses and nursing ethics to meet the inherent challenges that nurses can and do face during the course of their work. In order to meet these challenges responsibly and effectively, nurses have a professional obligation to advance their knowledge and understanding of what they can do to ensure that their decisions and actions are morally justified and will achieve their intended moral outcomes. Fulfilling this obligation will enable nurses to achieve the best possible position from which to practise and lead as ethical professionals.

REFLECTIVE QUESTIONS

1   Nurses are faced with ethical issues every day. In your view, what are the most pertinent and pressing ethical issues facing nurses today? How might nurses best deal with these issues?

2   How, if at all, might the study of nursing ethics assist nurses to practise nursing in a morally wise, just, effective and responsible manner?

3   What should a nurse do if she or he witnesses an instance of unethical professional conduct by either a nurse or other health professional? How would you assess that the conduct in question was, in fact, unethical? Would you report the matter to an appropriate authority? How would you approach this responsibility?

4   Is nursing ethics 'up to the task' of guiding sound ethical decision making in healthcare contexts and protecting the moral safety of patients? On what basis do you justify your answer?

RECOMMENDED READINGS

Beauchamp T, Childress J 2009 Principles of biomedical ethics, 6th edn. Oxford University Press, New York

Fry S, Veatch R, Taylor C 2011 Case studies in nursing ethics, 4th edn. Jones & Bartlett Learning, Sudbury, Mass

Johnstone M 2009 Bioethics: a nursing perspective, 5th edn. Churchill Livingstone/ Elsevier, Sydney

REFERENCES

Australian Commission on Safety and Quality in Health Care (ACSQHC) 2011 National Safety and Quality Health Service Standards. ACSQHC, Sydney

Australian Commission on Safety and Quality in Health Care (ACSQHC) 2012 National Safety and Quality Health Service Standards: Safety and Quality Improvement Guide, Consultation Draft July. ACSQHC, Sydney

Beauchamp T, Childress J 2009 Principles of biomedical ethics, 6th edn. Oxford University Press, New York

Bridgman P, Davis G 2004 The Australian policy handbook, 3rd edn. Allen & Unwin, Sydney

Johnstone M 2007 Patient safety ethics and human error management in ED contexts Part II: accountability and the challenge of change. Australasian Emergency Nursing Journal 10:80–85

Johnstone M 2008 Questioning nursing ethics. Australian Nursing Journal 15(7):19

Johnstone M 2009 Bioethics: a nursing perspective, 5th edn. Churchill Livingstone/ Elsevier, Sydney

Johnstone M 2012 Unethical professional conduct. Australian Nursing Journal 19(11):34

Johnstone M, Kanitsaki O 2006 Culture, language and patient safety: making the link. International Journal for Quality in Health Care 18(5):383–388

Johnstone M, Kanitsaki O 2008 Ethics and advance care planning in a culturally diverse society. Journal of Transcultural Nursing 20(4):405–416

Johnstone M, Kanitsaki O 2009 Engaging patients and safety partners: some considerations for ensuring a culturally and linguistically appropriate approach. Health Policy 90(1):1–7

Merton R 1936 The unanticipated consequences of purposive social action. American Sociological Review 1(6):894–904

Nurses and Midwifery Board of Australia (NMBA) 2006 National Competency Standards for the Registered Nurse. NMBA, Canberra

Nurses and Midwifery Board of Australia (NMBA) 2008a Code of Ethics for Nurses in Australia. NMBA, Canberra

Nurses and Midwifery Board of Australia (NMBA) 2008b Code of Professional Conduct for Nurses in Australia. NMBA, Canberra

Nursing Council of New Zealand 2007 Competencies for Registered Nurses. NCNZ, Wellington

Nursing Council of New Zealand 2012 Code of Conduct for Nurses. NCNZ, Wellington

Pronovost P, Faden R 2009 Setting priorities for patient safety: ethics, accountability, and public engagement. JAMA 302(8):890–891

Rawls J 1971 A theory of justice. Oxford University Press, Oxford

Wachter R 2010 Patient safety at ten: unmistakable progress, troubling gaps. Health Affairs 29(1):165–173

Wikipedia 2012 Moral turpitude. Online. Available: http://en.wikipedia.org/wiki/Moral_turpitude 7 August 2012

CHAPTER 11

An introduction to legal aspects of nursing practice*

Judith Mair

Upon completion of this chapter, the reader will have gained insights into:

- the basics of the Australian legal system
- basic principles of law applicable to nursing practice
- the legal rights of patients
- the role of the criminal law in nursing practice
- legal rules governing the registration and discipline of nursing.

KEY WORDS

Litigation, common law, precedents, legislation, assault, safety, negligence, duty of care, consent

---

* The author acknowledges that material for this chapter was drawn from a previously published work: Mair J, Blackmore K 1992. In: Cuthbert M, Duffield C, Hope J (eds) Management in nursing. WB Saunders/Baillière Tindall, Sydney.

INTRODUCTION

Today, more than ever, nurses have to consider the legal implications of their practice. Litigation against healthcare professionals has increased as healthcare consumers become more aware of their legal rights and, as the law develops, to acknowledge more factual circumstances that can give rise to a legal action. Operating alongside these changes is a higher patient expectation of a good outcome from the delivery of healthcare services. Whilst an employer of a nurse may be held to be vicariously liable for the tort of the nurse which occurs during the course of their employment, this does not absolve the nurse from responsibility for their actions. Nurses working independently or employed nurses acting outside of the scope of their employment who cause harm to patients can be held to be fully liable for their actions. Likewise, an employer may not be held vicariously liable for criminal acts committed by their employees in the course of their employment.

This chapter serves as an introduction to law relevant to nursing practice. This introduction is necessarily brief, and does not cover all aspects of law that affect nursing practice. The law evolves over time and changes are made as required, particularly statute law. Nurses should keep up to date and develop a deeper understanding of the legal system in which they practise, and the laws that govern clinical practice, through lectures and further reading. The aim of this chapter is to alert nurses to legal issues that may arise in the course of their nursing career and to assist them to understand the law relevant to those issues.

THE COMMON LAW BASIS

The common law was developed in England from the fourteenth century and became the basis of the legal systems of countries that were colonised by England.

The primary source of law in common law countries is a combination of common law, equity and legislation. Common law consists of the application of legal principles developed in past cases to determine the outcome of present cases. Common law is based upon the doctrine of precedent (i.e. by looking at how cases have been decided in the past and applying the principles developed in those cases to the present). Cases that have an important impact on the common law are reported in law reports relevant to particular courts. Less important cases are unreported but can still be accessed.

The common law remains a major source of law covering clinical practice. For example, the law relating to assault, false imprisonment, negligence and negligent advice is found within cases in which relevant principles of law recognising the right of a person to individual autonomy and bodily integrity have been developed. A court exercising equity can provide an alternative remedy where a common law remedy is insufficient to redress the wrong complained of. A court exercising equitable jurisdiction can issue an injunction to require another to desist from doing something, or can make an order for specific performance to a defaulting party under a valid contract to cause them to perform their part of the contract.

The second type of law is *legislation*, or statutory law, which is law developed by parliamentarians through the parliamentary process. An individual piece of legislation is referred to as a statute or an Act of parliament. Legislation is important in that valid legislative provisions prevail where there is any inconsistency with the common law. Thus parliamentary law can be used to change the law where it is considered that the common law is deficient or to govern new circumstances that have arisen. A new statute can be promulgated (enacted), or an older one can be repealed, in which case the common law is the governing law unless a new statute replaces the older statute. Statutes can also be amended which means that some provisions can be deleted, changed or new provisions added. Increasingly, statutory law is being applied to common law issues such as negligence.

Legislation can create new law that is not known at common law. An example of this is the statutory definition of brain death, which has enabled the removal of organs from a person whose brain has ceased to function but whose heart and lung activity is being sustained artificially.

Nurses practising in Australia need to be aware that, under the Australian system of Federation, the law can and often does differ from state to state or territory. As well as state-by-state and territory differences, the federal government has power, by virtue of the Constitution, to make laws that are binding on all states and territories (i.e. the Commonwealth of Australia Constitution Act). In some cases, this law-making power is exclusive to the federal government (e.g. the defence power). In other cases, the states and territories have a concurrent power to make law (e.g. taxation). However, in the latter case, a federal law will override a state/territory law where the federal law is intended to cover the field or there is an inconsistency between a valid federal law and a state/territory law (section 109 of the Constitution). The states and territories have residual power to make laws in all cases where the federal government has no power under the Constitution, express or implied, to do so. Most health law, such as the regulation of hospitals, falls within state/territory law.

Differences in law from state to state and territory are less obvious in common law cases. It is within parliamentary law that significant differences can arise. Legislation in one jurisdiction (state/territory) does not bind people in another jurisdiction unless the legislation has valid extraterritorial application. Even in this latter case, there must be some connection with the state/territory promulgating (proclaiming) the law. A person who commits an offence in one state and moves to another has to return or be extradited from the latter state if he/she is to stand trial in the state where the offence was committed.

Individual states/territories may enact parliamentary law to govern particular matters, while other states/territories may leave such matters to be covered by common law. For example, not all states/territories have legislated to control the reproductive technologies and those that have are not identical. When it is deemed desirable to do so, each state will enact uniform (identical) legislation to avert what can be regarded as forum-shopping (e.g. defamation laws).

Law is divided into civil and criminal. Civil *law* involves legal actions taken by a complainant (plaintiff) against another or others seeking a civil remedy for a legally recognised wrong—for example, a plaintiff seeking compensation for pain and suffering as a result of a nurse giving an injection incorrectly. The negligent practitioner is normally referred to as the defendant in the case. The task (onus) of proving the case rests with the plaintiff 'on the balance of probabilities'.

Other than Federal crimes, much criminal law is specific to a state or territory. Most criminal *law* consists of prosecutions brought on behalf of the state/territory to punish breaches of criminal offences, and a guilty verdict results in a fine and/or custodial sentence. The onus of proving a criminal offence lies with the prosecution, which must prove its case 'beyond a reasonable doubt'. The criminal law of murder and manslaughter, criminal assault and criminal negligence are some of the major criminal offences that can apply to nursing practice.

Legislation in all jurisdictions provides for limitation periods to apply for civil claims in the courts (e.g. Limitation Act 1969 (NSW)). An aggrieved party must commence an action within the specified limitation period; otherwise the claim will become statute barred. Limitation periods vary from jurisdiction to jurisdiction, but most are around three to seven years after the cause of action arises, or, in some cases, when the plaintiff first becomes aware that a cause of action exists. Notwithstanding that a limitation period has lapsed, it is usually possible to apply to a court to extend a limitation period in prescribed circumstances (e.g. a person who contracts HIV through a blood transfusion may not be aware that they have contracted the disease until some time after the expiration of a limitation period).

Whatever limitation period applies, most jurisdictions suspend the limitation period while an injured party is a minor. Therefore, a child who suffers an injury as a result of alleged negligence may not be affected by a limitation period until reaching majority. A person acting as 'tutor' for the child may take action on behalf of the child in the child's name prior to majority. If this is done, the evidence necessary to prove the case is more easily available sooner after the event than later.

Unless specifically stated, no limitation periods apply to most criminal offences. Thus, a nurse who causes the death of a patient intentionally or recklessly could be charged with murder or manslaughter many years after the event should evidence to support such a charge arise.

CIVIL LAW

As noted above, civil law involves legal actions taken by plaintiff(s) against another or others (defendant(s)) seeking a civil remedy for a legally recognised wrong. Nurses need to work within the context of civil law, as it relates to: patient safety; negligent advice; patient consent; patient freedom of movement; and patients' property.

Patient safety

By the very nature of their practice, nurses are engaged in close physical contact with patients. Some of the procedures performed by nursing staff pose risks to patients should the procedures be performed without due care and skill. If a patient suffers harm as a result of a nurse's failure to perform nursing duties at the standard to be expected of the nurse in the circumstances, then the patient has a right to sue in negligence to recover compensation.

Negligence is a *tort*, which means a civil wrong. The tort of negligence arises from the common law and is a means by which a person who suffers injury through a negligent act or omission can obtain compensation from the person responsible for the injury. To succeed in an action of negligence against a nurse, the plaintiff must prove, on the balance of probabilities, that the nurse was negligent. The plaintiff must prove that the nurse owed the patient a legal duty of care, that the nurse breached this duty of care and that the patient suffered harm as a result of that breach. The plaintiff must prove each and every one of these elements. Any act or omission that is not found to be negligent is referred to as an unavoidable accident or was caused by some other factor independent of the nurse's action.

In determining whether or not a legal duty of care exists, the courts resort to a test of foreseeability. Thus a duty of care can be shown to exist when a person can reasonably foresee that his or her acts or omissions are likely to place another at risk (see the case of *Donoghue* vs *Stevenson* [1932] AC 562). This is an objective test and the defendant's conduct is measured by a 'reasonable person' test. The fact that something is foreseeable is not sufficient—some foreseeable risks may be so remote they may be ignored. The test is 'reasonable foreseeability'. Thus it is reasonably foreseeable that a patient may suffer harm, such as nerve damage, if an injection is given incorrectly. On the other hand, it may not be reasonably foreseeable if the patient suffers some reaction to a drug which is idiopathic and could not have been foreseen with all proper care and history taking. Some risks are unknown and are therefore unknowable until such time as research and experience reveal them (e.g. the fact that giving Thalidomide to pregnant women to treat morning sickness can cause phocomelia in the unborn). Once known, the question arises as to whether the newly discovered 'foreseeable' risk is an 'unreasonable risk'. Unreasonable risks are those which a patient should not have to encounter.

The duty of care is to avoid unreasonable risk of harm to another. All people living in a society are expected to take some care for themselves and cannot complain if they suffer loss or injury from an accepted risk of harm. The law will often determine an unreasonable risk of harm by looking at the harm that is likely to be caused and/or the frequency of its occurrence. For example, if a particular harm is known to occur frequently as a result of particular acts or omissions, then the law is likely to hold that this will give rise to a duty of care. Likewise, the law will hold that a duty of care exists in any case where the foreseeable risk can result in serious disability or death, however infrequently such harm is likely to occur.

In some cases the law will hold that a particular risk, which may normally be considered 'unreasonable', may be taken to avoid a greater risk of harm. This is sometimes referred to as 'balancing the risks'. Thus it may be reasonable to do something that clearly poses a risk of harm to another, where the act is intended to avert a greater risk of harm. In one American case it was held that burns resulting from the application of hot water bottles in an emergency were not caused by negligence, as they arose from a calculated risk to avoid a grave risk of harm to the patient. The patient was suffering from severe shock caused by a postpartum haemorrhage and the hot water bottles had been applied as a part of emergency treatment (*McDermott vs St Mary's Hospital* 133 A 2d 608 (1957)).

Clearly, a duty of care will exist to avoid unreasonable risk of harm to patients receiving nursing care. However, the law does not require that there be an identified person in existence at the time that a negligent act or omission occurs. The law can impose a duty of care in circumstances where a 'class of persons' is likely to be affected now or in the future. This can include those not at immediate risk of harm at the time of the act or omission in question, but who come into the range of risk at a later point in time (e.g. a person who comes to the aid of another after an accident and is themselves exposed to a reasonably foreseeable risk by so doing).

A duty of care can arise to avoid harm to an unborn child, as well as to one that is not even conceived at the time of the negligent act or omission provided that there is a foreseeable risk of harm to them at the time of the act or omission complained of. In such a case, the child must be born alive and prove that any injury present at birth resulted from a breach of duty to take care not to injure it while it was unborn. A doctor was held to have had a duty of care to a child born with syphilis because he failed to submit a pregnant patient, whom he had cared for during a prior pregnancy, to syphilis testing. The doctor was held to owe a duty of care to the patient and any children later born to her (*X & Y (by her tutor) vs Pal and Ors* (1991) 23 NSWLR 27). The mother of a child who was injured as a result of the mother's negligent act whilst the child was in utero can be held liable to compensate for the child's injuries in some circumstances. A pregnant woman who caused an accident by negligently driving a motor vehicle on a country property was held to owe a duty of care to her unborn child. The child was born alive with injuries related to the accident and was awarded compensation for her mother's negligence (*Lynch vs Lynch (by Her Tutor Lynch)* (1991) 25 NSWLR 411).

Whether or not a breach of the duty of care has occurred requires consideration of the standard of care required in the circumstances. The standard of care is not perfect care, but reasonable care. It is an objective test and therefore is not dependent upon the particular skills and knowledge of the practitioner. The standard expected of the healthcare worker is that which is attributed to the class of healthcare workers to which the defendant belongs. Thus, the conduct of a nurse will be measured against that of the 'hypothetical reasonably competent nurse'. It is when the defendant's standard of care falls below that of the reasonably competent nurse that a breach of care is found.

Nurses who claim to have special skills will be required to exhibit a higher standard of care. Thus the clinical nurse specialist will be measured against the standard of the reasonably competent clinical nurse specialist, while the general ward staff will be measured against the standard expected of the reasonably proficient general ward nurse. An enrolled nurse's practice will be measured against that of the reasonably competent enrolled nurse. This test will apply whilst the practitioner is providing care within the realm of their expertise. Nurses undertaking tasks which are beyond their competence can be regarded as performing a negligent act.

The standard of care required can vary according to the condition of the patient and the patient's capacity for self-care. In considering the standard of care required, the nurse must take into account characteristics of the patient that may pose an additional risk for that person. Thus a higher standard of care will be required for a patient recovering from a general anaesthetic following surgery than for a patient who is fully conscious and has been returned to the ward. A higher duty of care will be required for a baby or child than for a competent adult patient.

The circumstances in which care is being provided can also be a relevant consideration in determining the standard of care required. A nurse involved in resuscitating a person at an accident site away from a well-equipped hospital where trained staff and proper equipment is at hand can only be expected to provide the standard of care that is reasonable in the circumstances. Provided the nurse exercises reasonable care and skill in the circumstances, there would be no breach of the duty of care.

Damage is the gist of the case in an action of negligence; a plaintiff must prove that foreseeable damage resulted from a breach of duty by the nurse. Damage may be physical, mental, financial or a combination of these. Once the plaintiff has proved that the nurse's breach of duty caused damage that was reasonably foreseeable, the defendant will be held liable to compensate for that damage and any further loss that flows reasonably and naturally upon the initial injury. Pain and suffering, loss of enjoyment of life, loss of expectation of life, loss of opportunity in life and financial consequences are examples of accepted heads of damage (categories of damage recognised by the courts) for which compensation can be sought in a negligence action. A young woman who suffered cerebral palsy due to the admitted negligence of an obstetrician at the time of her birth was awarded around $11 million which included a sum that would enable the plaintiff to finish her HSC and pursue some form of tertiary education (*Simpson vs Diamond & Anor* [No 2] [2001] NSWSC 1048). If no harm has been caused by the negligent act or omission then there can be no recovery of compensation.

There is a principle in law that a person must take his victim as he finds him. This is called the 'egg-shell skull rule'. What it means is that if the victim suffers greater harm because they have a particular disability, disorder or trait that renders them vulnerable to greater harm, then the tortfeasor must compensate for the full cost of the harm even though it is greater than that for other victims. A man who suffered a burn to his lip in a workplace accident later died when the injury turned cancerous. His employer was held responsible for his death (*Smith vs Leech Brain* [1962] 2 QB 405). An example would be harm caused by increased blood loss where the victim is a haemophiliac. In such cases it is irrelevant whether the tortfeasor was aware that the victim was particularly vulnerable.

If death occurs as a result of negligence, legislation provides that prescribed persons, usually close relatives, can bring an action against the person whose negligence caused the death (e.g. Compensation to Relatives Act 1897 (NSW)), provided the deceased would have been entitled to make a claim had they lived. For example, a man and his children may commence an action to be compensated for nervous shock suffered as a result of the death of the wife and mother caused by a negligent nursing act or omission.

Bystanders who witness an horrific incident may have a right to sue for compensation for nervous shock provided they satisfy a proximity test, that is that they were present at the scene of the incident in terms of time and space, and it was reasonably foreseeable that a bystander could suffer nervous shock. When the person involved in the incident is a relative, the next of kin may not be required to satisfy a proximity test. The wife of a police officer who was seriously injured in an accident developed a psychiatric illness because of what she saw and heard at the hospital where her husband had been admitted for treatment. She did not see or hear the accident or what happened afterwards at the scene of the accident. She suffered shock and fear that her husband might die and this was caused partly by what she saw and what she was told at the hospital the night of the accident and on the following day. She was able to recover compensation from the person who caused the accident even though she did not witness the accident and suffered the injury after the event (*Jaensch vs Coffey* (1984) 155 CLR 549).

Finally, the plaintiff must prove causation—that is, that the breach of duty caused the alleged harm. To prove a direct causal connection, the 'but for' test can be applied. But for the act or omission of the defendant, would the plaintiff have suffered the alleged harm? Even when an act or omission can be shown to have been negligent, a claim for damages will fail if the plaintiff cannot prove that the alleged harm was caused or materially contributed to by the defendant's negligent conduct. For example, a person who dies from a disease that they were suffering prior to the negligent act, and to which the negligent act was not an aggravating or contributing factor.

There are three main defences to an action in negligence. These are contributory negligence, *novus actus interveniens* and *volenti non fit injuria*. A defendant can claim contributory negligence where the plaintiff can be shown to have been partially responsible for what happened. The court will award damages in proportion to the extent it accepts that the plaintiff was negligent. A woman who successfully sued a doctor for his failure to refer her to an alternative specialist when she advised him she was unable to use the referral he had given her had her award reduced by 20% because of her subsequent failure to seek medical attention for four months despite suffering continued and severe vaginal bleeding (*Kalokerinos vs Burnett* CA 40243/95; CL11138/93).

Novus actus interveniens is applicable when a second negligent act results in increased harm to a person who has suffered harm from a prior negligent act and breaks the chain of causation. However, where the second negligent act is such that the chain of causation flowing from the first negligent act is not broken then the person who committed the first negligent act can be held liable for the consequences of both. For example, if a nurse's negligence caused brain damage to a child, necessitating intensive care, and the negligence of a second nurse in the intensive care unit exacerbated the harm to the child, then the first nurse could still be held liable for the increased harm as it was the original tortfeasor's act or omission which exposed the child to a subsequent foreseeable risk of harm. However, if the child were discharged from hospital following the maximum care that could be given, and then dies from other injuries sustained in a motor vehicle accident caused through another's negligence, then the first nurse is unlikely to be held responsible for the death.

Volenti non fit injuria applies when a plaintiff can be shown to have knowledge of risks and voluntarily undertakes those risks. As such, this defence has not been a major factor in cases involving the provision of healthcare services. Its main application is to cases involving sports and dangerous occupations. It cannot be argued that a patient voluntarily agrees to accept all known risks in healthcare.

When a plaintiff has suffered harm as a result of another's negligence, the plaintiff is required by law to minimise (mitigate) any loss. Thus an injured person is required to take reasonable steps to reduce the effects of (ameliorate) the harm caused. To the extent that there is an unreasonable failure to mitigate (e.g. undertake recommended physiotherapy which could improve their condition) a court will discount the amount of compensation that the plaintiff would have received.

In 2002, the New South Wales Parliament enacted the Civil Liability Act 2002, which modifies the law of negligence for New South Wales. In addition to statutorily providing the principles upon which claims for negligence may be made, which reflects the common law, the Act modifies the criteria for the awarding of damages in civil negligence cases. Insofar as professional negligence is concerned, the Act provides that, subject to exceptions:

> A person practising a profession ('a professional') does not incur a liability in negligence arising from the provision of a professional service if it is established that the professional acted in a manner that (at the time the service was provided) was widely accepted in Australia by peer professional opinion as competent practice (section 50).

Section 57 of the Civil Liability Act protects 'good samaritans' from personal civil liability in respect of their acts or omissions in providing emergency assistance to an injured person or a person at risk of being injured. This protection from liability does not extend to where the good samaritan's ability to exercise reasonable care and skill was impaired due to being under the influence of drugs or alcohol or when the good samaritan is impersonating a healthcare or emergency services worker or a police officer.

All other states and territories have introduced similar legislation to New South Wales. These Acts enhance or modify the common law, to a greater or lesser degree, and are variously called: Civil Liability (Queensland, South Australia, Tasmania and

Western Australia); Civil Law (ACT); Wrongs (Victoria); or Personal Injuries (Northern Territory) Acts. Some also provide protection from liability for persons rendering healthcare in emergency situations. Given that each of these Acts varies from state to state, nurses should source the relevant statute in the state in which they are practising.

Negligent advice

During the course of professional practice, patients ask nurses for advice on a whole range of matters such as diet and how to care for themselves after discharge from hospital. In giving advice, nurses must exercise a reasonable standard of care where the patient could suffer harm as a result of following the advice. Failure to exercise reasonable care in giving advice could leave a nurse open to an action of negligent advice.

The tort of negligent advice is a negligence action that is brought for damage caused by the giving of advice rather than by a defendant's act or omission. Liability for the tort is also applicable to the giving of information where the defendant has a sufficient interest to see that the information given is correct (e.g. providing an information sheet outlining dietary requirements).

For an action in negligent advice to be successful, the plaintiff must prove that the advisor is a professional (or claiming to have equivalent skills) and that the advisor was willing to use those skills to advise the plaintiff, in the knowledge that the plaintiff intended to make a decision in reliance upon that advice. It must be reasonable for the plaintiff to do so.

The plaintiff cannot succeed simply because the advice was wrong. The plaintiff must prove that the nurse owed a duty of care, failed to exercise reasonable care in the giving of the advice—according to the standards of a reasonably competent nurse— and that the plaintiff suffered harm following the advice (*Hills vs Potter* [1983] 3 All ER 716). It must be reasonable for the patient to rely upon the nurse's advice. A disclaimer of responsibility is effective; however, disclaiming responsibility for any advice given in the context of nursing care would be inappropriate given that a nurse's role involves giving advice to patients.

In order to avoid being sued for negligent advice, nurses should ensure that their nursing knowledge remains up to date and never give an impression that they have particular skills when they lack the capacity to give advice. When asked to give advice on a matter about which they lack knowledge, a nurse should either make it clear to a patient that they are not skilled in giving particular advice and consult with someone who can give appropriate advice, or not give the advice and refer the patient to another experienced and competent practitioner. In so doing, a nurse will be exercising an appropriate standard of care.

Patient consent

Most nursing practice involves touching patients. In accordance with common law principles, all persons have the right to determine what treatments or diagnostic tests they will be subjected to, unless there is some overriding law which allows treatment without consent. When a competent adult patient is treated without consent, that patient has a right to sue for assault. If a patient claims that treatment was carried out without sufficient information being given, then the patient must 'sue in negligence', the difference being in that in the latter case the patient must prove they suffered harm as a result of treatment carried out without 'informed' consent.

Assault is a tort, which serves to protect an individual's right to autonomy and self-determination. Assault consists of intentionally creating in another person an apprehension of imminent unwanted and unlawful contact. Although the actual touching of another without lawful authority is technically known as battery, the term assault is now in use to represent both the apprehension of and the unlawful contact itself.

Touching in anger, even if slight, is an assault, and can amount to criminal assault. Thus, even the slightest touching of a patient in anger can be regarded as a criminal assault. However, an assault may also be committed where a person is touched without consent and the touching is not an accepted incident of everyday life, for which a person is deemed to have given consent. Touching which occurs during medical examinations and diagnosis is not regarded in law as an incidental touching in society; therefore, for such touching to be lawful, it must be with the patient's consent or other lawful justification.

An assault is complete once touching has occurred without lawful justification; therefore, there is no need for a patient to prove that damage occurred as a result of the touching. It is not a defence to assault that treatment was carried out in good faith for the benefit of the patient when the patient is capable of giving consent and has not done so. A nurse may have intended to benefit the patient, but this issue will only go to mitigation and does not negate an assault if treatment was carried out without consent.

The law acknowledges that there are a number of ways in which consent can be sought. Consent may be obtained orally by asking the patient's permission before commencing treatment, and receiving an affirmative response. Consent may also be implied by the patient's overt physical response to suggested treatments. For example, the patient turns over and exposes a buttock when the nurse approaches with an expected injection. Consent in writing, and witnessed, is usually sought for major intrusions of the body, such as surgery. However, consent in writing cannot be taken to be absolute evidence of consent. A written and signed consent form comes under the best evidence rule but is not conclusive of a valid consent. In an emergency where a person is unable to give consent, a nurse is entitled to proceed to carry out measures that are aimed at saving life or avoiding severe injury while the emergency exists.

A patient's consent must be valid. A valid consent is one that is voluntarily given, covers the treatment to be carried out and is given by a legally competent person who has been given sufficient information about the procedure to be performed. A voluntary consent is one that is given freely by the patient in the absence of fraud or duress. Advising a patient of the benefits of treatment is part of a nurse's role but if the nurse becomes overbearing and the patient feels they have no choice, then the patient's consent is not voluntary. A patient who wanted a general anaesthesia for surgery gave up and agreed to a spinal anaesthesia at the insistence of a doctor and suffered injuries. It was held that her consent had been overborne by the insistence of the anaesthetist and others (see *Beausoleil vs Sisters of Charity* (1966) 53 DLR 2d 65). The consent must cover the treatment to be carried out, and any treatment that is related to the initial treatment. Any procedures carried out beyond that for which the patient consented (except in an emergency and the patient is incapable of giving or withholding consent) can result in a complaint of assault.

In order to give an informed consent, the patient must have a good understanding of what is to be done and the risks involved. Once the patient has been advised in broad terms of the nature of the procedure to be performed and agrees to it being performed, then there is no assault. However, any issue relating to the degree of information given regarding risks involved is a matter for the general law of negligence and is determined by what a patient should be told. In short, all patients should be told all 'material risks' inherent in a procedure, together with any risks that are of particular importance to the patient. What is a material risk is one if, in the circumstances of the particular case, a reasonable person in the patient's position, or the practitioner is or should be reasonably aware that the particular patient, if warned of the risk, would be likely to attach significance to it. A patient agreed to eye surgery on one eye without being advised that there was a remote risk she could become totally blind which was what happened. She was awarded compensation for the opthalmologist's failure to warn her of the remote risk (*Rogers vs Whitaker* (1992) 175 CLR 479). The concept of therapeutic privilege (withholding information from a patient) may still be applicable in very limited circumstances where the risk to the patient outweighs the responsibility to warn.

Legal capacity covers mental capacity and children. Mental health patients have issues involving consent to treatment covered by legislation in the various states/territories. Where a patient is unconscious or otherwise mentally incompetent, the defence of necessity applies and treatment may be carried out that is necessary to avoid a severe risk to the life of the patient or others (e.g. sedating a psychotic patient who is a risk to self and others). Legislation (e.g. the Guardianship Act 1987 (NSW) and its equivalent in other states) may provide for a guardian to be appointed to give consent for medical procedures on behalf of a person who is mentally incapacitated, or a court/tribunal may make such an appointment.

A combination of common law principles and legislation applies when treating children. At common law a child may consent to treatment that is therapeutic, provided he or she has sufficient mental capacity to understand the nature and consequences of the proposed treatment. The application of this principle requires a balance between the intellectual and emotional maturity of the minor and the complexity and seriousness of the proposed treatment (see *Gillick vs West Norfolk and Wisbech Area Health Authority* [1985] 3 All ER 402, approved by the High Court in the case of *Department of Health and Community Services vs JWB and SMB* [1992] HCA 15 'Marion's Case'). Presumably, a child of a quite young age could give a valid consent to a simple procedure that does not involve a great risk of harm. For example, a child who falls over and suffers a minor graze in the school grounds could be expected to have the capacity to consent to the wound being treated. In all other cases, parental or guardian consent should be obtained. A Family Court authorisation must be sought if consent is sought to carry out an elective procedure that will lead to an intellectually disabled person being made infertile. The parents of a 14-year-old girl who suffers from severe disabilities including mental retardation applied to the Family Court for an order authorising the performance of a hysterectomy and an ovariectomy on her. According to the Court the decision to cause a profoundly intellectually incapacitated child to be sterilised should not be within the ordinary parental power to consent but requires Family Court authorisation (see 'Marion's Case' *supra*).

Legislation can change or modify the common law. For example, legislation in New South Wales provides that consent to medical and dental treatment given by a parent or guardian of a minor aged less than 16 years, or by a minor aged 14 years or upwards, is a defence to an action for assault and battery in respect of that treatment.

Between the ages of 14 and 16, the consent can be a parent or the child, provided the child has sufficient maturity to understand the nature of the treatment and to give a valid consent. Below the age of 14 years, the consent of the parent or guardian is required (except in an emergency to save the life of the child). The definition of medical treatment includes treatment carried out by persons following the orders of a medical practitioner, and this would apply to nurses when they are carrying out a doctor's orders (see section 49 of the Minors (Property and Contracts) Act 1970 (NSW)).

When a parent or guardian has not given consent, or is refusing to consent to treatment that is for a child's benefit, most states/territories have legislation that enables doctors to perform life-saving treatments on children without parental consent (e.g. section 174 of the Children and Young Persons (Care and Protection) Act 1998 (NSW)). When a child needs treatment which is not immediately life threatening, the matter may be referred to the Supreme Court of a state/territory in its *parens patriae* jurisdiction, or the family law courts can make a decision consistent with the best interests of the child where parents or guardians refuse consent to non-urgent treatment for a child, or there is any dispute regarding consent (e.g. Blood transfusions: *Women's and Children's Health Network Inc vs JC, JC, and KC (By Her Litigation Guardian)* [2012] SASC104: Hepatitis B injections: In re H [2011] QSC 427). Children who are wards of the state/territory have issues relating to consent to medical treatment covered by relevant child welfare legislation in each state/territory.

There are a number of defences against an action in assault that are relevant to the provision of healthcare. The defence of necessity permits a health professional to carry out treatment without consent, provided the treatment is intended to avoid a greater risk of harm to the person. The defence operates in those circumstances when patients are unable to give consent and the treatment is necessary to preserve them from a serious danger to their life. An example would be a patient who has suffered head injuries in a car accident and is unconscious. It would be justified to perform whatever surgery is necessary to save the patient from death or a serious risk to their health.

Legislation may authorise particular acts without consent. For example, mental health legislation provides the rules for non-consensual treatment of mentally ill patients. With respect to consent provisions for mental health patients generally, nurses should consult their relevant mental health legislation in their State/Territory.

Finally, the defence of self-defence is applicable in the event that a patient or others assault a healthcare worker in anger, or vice versa. People who are assaulted are legally entitled to defend themselves, but the force used must not exceed what reasonably appears to be necessary to repel the attack.

Patient freedom of movement

During the course of clinical practice, a nurse will encounter patients who wish to leave a healthcare institution against medical advice. Unless there is some law that allows for the detention of patients without consent, then patients do have the right to leave.

The tort of false imprisonment compensates a person who has been subjected to an intentional and total restraint of movement without lawful justification. Restraint is either by total confinement or by preventing the person from lawfully leaving the place in which he or she is. The tort can be committed where a patient is too ill to move, or is unaware of the fact that he or she was imprisoned by reason that he or she is in a state of drunkenness, while asleep or while they were a lunatic (see *Meering* vs *Grahame-White Aviation Co Ltd* (1920) 122 LT 44. See also *Hart* vs *Herron* (1996) Aust Torts Reports 81; [1996] NSWSC 176). Mr Hart was detained and treated with ECT and deep sleep therapy at a private psychiatric hospital without proof of his consent. He successfully sued the psychiatrist for assault and false imprisonment.

The plaintiff must prove the confinement was total. If the person can leave by some reasonable alternative exit, there is no false imprisonment. Locking a patient in a room with no reasonable avenue of escape, or barring a patient from lawfully leaving a healthcare institution, could amount to false imprisonment in the absence of lawful justification.

Using bed rails, manacles and chemical restraints can also be regarded as false imprisonment if they are used without lawful justification and totally confine the patient. Removing a disabled person's wheelchair which they need to move about is another example. It can also amount to false imprisonment if a patient reasonably believes that any attempt to leave a healthcare institution will be prevented by a nurse, even if there are no physical restraints (psychological restraint). This could occur if a nurse gave the patient the impression that they would be prevented from leaving if they tried to do so; for example, telling the patient they could not leave until they saw a doctor and signed a release form. However, the patient would have to prove the submission to the nurse was complete and it was a reasonable response.

Hospitals develop policies requesting patients to see a doctor and to sign a release form in the event that a patient wishes to leave hospital against medical advice. There is no problem if a patient voluntarily agrees to the request. Some doubt exists as to whether hospital staff could detain a patient without consent in order to fulfil the hospital requirements. In the event that a patient leaves without advising staff, or refuses to stay to sign a release form and see a doctor, the patient should not be prevented from leaving and the events should be clearly documented in the hospital notes.

The fact that a patient wishes to leave hospital against medical advice does not relieve the staff from advising the patient of any deleterious effects a premature departure from hospital could entail, if the patient will remain to accept such advice. Wherever possible, staff should ensure that the patient fully appreciates the risks involved in leaving against medical advice.

Defences that can be raised against an allegation of false imprisonment include the common law defence of necessity, which permits the restraint of persons who are a danger to themselves or others. However, restraint is not justified if it is merely for the convenience of staff; there must be a real necessity to protect the patient or others. The restraint of a patient attempting to jump off the roof of a hospital, or threatening staff and other patients with violence, would be justified on this basis.

A second defence exists where legislation authorises the detention of persons (e.g. mental and public health Acts). A third lawful means of detaining patients is where a court authorises the detention of a person for treatment. Such orders are usually reserved for the detention of children when parents wish to remove a child in need of care from a healthcare institution. Finally, detention without consent is permissible to affect a lawful arrest when a person has committed a crime.

Patients' property

During the course of clinical practice, nurses will be faced with the prospect of taking charge of a patient's valuables, particularly when the patient is to be temporarily away from the ward to undergo surgery. When a patient's valuables are handed to a hospital for safekeeping, the law of bailment governs the relationship. The law of bailment is a contract and applies when one person (the bailor) delivers goods to another (the bailee) so that they may be used or stored until they are to be delivered back to the bailor.

Bailment may be for reward or gratuitous (free). When bailment is for reward, the bailee will be held liable to compensate for the loss of the goods according to the ordinary rules of negligence, whereas the bailee is only liable if gross negligence is shown in cases of gratuitous bailment. With respect to patients' valuables handed over to a hospital for safekeeping, the hospital is legally regarded as a bailee for reward and therefore has an obligation to exercise reasonable care in securing the safety of the valuables.

A hospital can become an involuntary bailee for patients' property. A hospital in New Zealand was held liable to compensate the estate of a deceased woman for a ring that disappeared from a woman's hand at the time of her death (*Southland Hospital Board vs Perkins Estate* [1986] 1 NZLR 373). The woman's personal control over her property ended with her death, and the hospital was held to be an involuntary bailee for the ring.

When a patient dies in hospital, any valuable property should be removed and kept in safekeeping to be handed over to the deceased patient's legal personal representative. Non-valuable items such as clothing and toiletries can be sent home with a relative or friend. Police usually deal with the property of a person who is brought in deceased on arrival.

Healthcare institutions draw up policies and procedures in order to fulfil the duty of care to protect a patient's valuables and nursing staff should follow these. The valuables should be recorded in a document that is signed by the patient. When the patient is unable to sign, the valuables should be recorded by one nurse and witnessed by another.

The valuables must then be stored in a safe place. For short-term care the valuables may be stored in a locked cupboard at ward level (not the dangerous drugs cupboard). If the valuables are to be cared for on a long-term basis, they should be stored in a hospital safe. Patients are generally required to sign for the goods upon return to them. In the case of a deceased patient, the person legally entitled to deal with the patient's property after death would sign for receipt of the valuables.

In the event that the goods are lost, the patient has the onus of proving negligence and the value of the property. Nurses are not trained in evaluating the quality of valuable goods such as jewellery, and should not attempt to describe such goods as being of any particular kind and value. For example, a sapphire and diamond ring in a gold setting should be described as a ring with blue and clear stones set in a yellow coloured band, even if the patient states that the stones are a sapphire and diamonds, and the metal is gold.

Where theft of valuables is suspected, the police should be notified. The police can undertake an investigation and lay criminal charges where they reasonably suspect a member of the nursing staff or other person is responsible.

CRIMINAL LAW

During the course of practice, a nurse may assault or cause serious bodily harm or death to patients. As well as providing facts that may be the subject of a civil action, such events may result in charges of criminal assault, criminal negligence, manslaughter or rarely murder. The prosecutor must prove both *mens rea* (guilty mind) as well as *actus reus* (an unlawful act). The *mens rea* element can be satisfied by proving that the accused committed an unlawful act, either with intent or could have foreseen that someone could suffer harm but nevertheless proceeded to commit the act.

Criminal assault

Assault can be the subject of a criminal charge as well as a tort. In addition to the elements required to prove civil assault, there must be proof of a forcible or hostile act of the accused, without the consent of the victim. If a patient is criminally assaulted (e.g. punched or kicked), the matter should be reported to administration and to the police, who can charge the responsible party with criminal assault. The same legal redress is available to nurses who are assaulted by others. When an assault takes place, which is intended to cause harm, it is referred to as an aggravated assault. Touching a patient in the course of diagnosis or treatment without consent may give rise to an action to recover compensation at civil law but is unlikely to be regarded as a criminal assault where the intent is to benefit the patient.

An assault with consent may not be an assault as is the case with most contact sports (e.g. a lawful boxing match). However, if an act is unlawful, it cannot be made lawful because of consent of the victim. Thus sexual relations with a minor remain unlawful even if the minor is consenting. Deceit as to the identity of a person or the nature of the act will vitiate consent. The consent of a patient to a diagnostic or therapeutic treatment obtained by a person impersonating a nurse or other health professional is invalid in law. Should a nurse examine a patient extending the examination to breasts or sexual organs beyond what is required for a legitimate examination, the nurse can be found guilty of a sexual assault. A radiologist pleaded guilty to sexual intercourse by various means with a minor aged 13 years after administering injections which made her lose consciousness (see *Staats vs R* [1998] NTSC 13).

Two defences to a charge of assault are misadventure and self-defence. To constitute misadventure, an assault occurs by accident. For example, a nurse slips on a wet floor and accidentally strikes a patient. Self-defence involves the use of force by one person to repel an attack on him or her. A person may use reasonable force to repel attacks, but must not use more violence than is necessary to repel the attack. The right of self-defence only lasts as long as any danger exists. A nurse would be entitled to exercise the right of self-defence if attacked by a patient or other person provided the nurse used no more force than was necessary to repel the attack. The onus of proving the reasonableness of the self-defence lies with the person relying upon it.

Criminal negligence/homicide

Nurses can be charged with criminal negligence where an act causing serious bodily harm or death shows such a high disregard for the life and safety of another that it goes beyond a mere matter of compensation at civil law. The death of a patient resulting from treatment by a nurse would amount to manslaughter where the nurse's practice was grossly negligent and the nurse did something no reasonably skilled person would have done. Charges of criminal negligence against healthcare workers are rare and are difficult to prove to the requisite standard required in criminal law (i.e. 'beyond a reasonable doubt').

A charge of murder could be laid where the nurse intended the patient to die or was grossly reckless as to whether the patient died. A nurse who assists or counsels another to suicide can be charged with aiding and abetting a suicide or attempted suicide. Criminal charges may result from a referral by a coroner to the relevant Crown law authorities following a coronial inquiry into the death of a patient.

A further issue is causation. The prosecutor must prove that the act led to the serious injury or death of the victim—a 'but for' test. This is not always easy to do. For example, if a person suffers brain damage as a result of an act (e.g. negligently given an overdose of a drug) and is placed on a life support system, then it cannot be said that the act has caused the death of the person. If the life support system is disconnected because the victim is brain dead, the question arises as to whether the defendant caused the death of the victim. When the initial act was the operative factor in causing the brain damage, then turning off the life support system does not break the chain of causation and a conviction for murder or manslaughter can stand. For example, a victim is brought to hospital as a result of a bashing causing brain damage. They are put on life support which is appropriately removed. It is the act causing the brain damage that causes the death, not the removal of the life support. But if the patient dies as a result of some other event, unrelated to the brain damage, then it cannot be said that the act causing brain damage was the cause of the death. In the latter case a charge of murder or manslaughter could not be made out. A charge of criminal negligence may still be made out.

VICARIOUS LIABILITY

When a nurse's act or omission has caused harm to a patient and the patient has successfully sued to recover compensation for that harm from the practitioner's employer, the question arises as to who is responsible for providing the compensation. Under the law of vicarious liability, an employer can be held responsible for the acts of its employees carried out in the course of their employment.

An employer's responsibility is limited to an employee's acts performed during the 'course of employment'. However, this term is fairly broad and encompasses all acts, authorised or not, which are reasonably within the scope of the employee's duties. Thus a healthcare employer can be held legally responsible to compensate an injured patient whose injuries resulted from an employee's negligence. It is only when a nurse's actions are so far removed from anything that can reasonably be held to be part of a nurse's role that an employer will escape responsibility. A nurse's failure to follow guidelines in a procedure manual would not be enough to excuse the employer unless there was a gross departure from standards.

Vicarious liability merely means that the healthcare employer will generally be the party that will be held responsible for compensating a successful plaintiff and does not negate the nurse's personal liability. The nurse may be joined as a co-defendant. Responsibility under vicarious liability applies with respect to civil wrongs, but normally does not apply to criminal acts. Thus a hospital may be found vicariously liable for a nurse who commits a civil assault by giving an injection without consent, but not if the nurse angrily punched a patient.

An independent nurse practitioner is solely liable for harm caused by that practitioner's practice. An independent practitioner in turn becomes vicariously liable for harm caused by a person employed by the practitioner to assist in the practice. It is essential that healthcare institutions and practitioners secure insurance cover in the event of successful litigation by a patient. This cover should be sufficient to pay the highest amount that could be awarded from time to time.

Even when an employer cannot be found to be vicariously liable because a person committing a wrong is not an employee, the courts have been prepared to find that an institution such as a hospital has a personal duty of care towards patients and others which is non-delegable. A hospital can be found negligent for harm caused to a patient by reason of its personal liability, when the act or omission of a visiting medical officer caused the alleged harm. When a hospital's policies and procedures could expose a patient to an unreasonable risk of harm, a duty arises to avoid that harm.

PATIENT RECORDS

Patient records are legal documents; therefore, it is important to keep accurate and complete records of all treatment and care administered to patients. The documents record the progress of patients admitted to healthcare facilities for the period of time that they are in care. Accurate and complete documentation can provide a good defence for a nurse who is faced with an action by a patient when the patient's record discloses that adequate and reasonable nursing care was delivered.

Even when adequate treatment may have been administered, failure to keep adequate patient records can lead to a finding of liability on the part of a nurse. Failure to record treatment may be accepted as evidence that such treatment was not in fact given. Overall failure to keep complete and adequate records can be regarded as a negligent omission, since a reasonable nurse would be expected to keep all patient record notes in order and up to date. It is reasonably foreseeable that a patient may suffer harm from failure to record a treatment given (e.g. a patient may be given two doses of a drug because a first dose was not recorded).

Although it is important that a patient's records be complete and up to date, a nurse should not write more than is necessary since this can lead to excessive questioning in evidence. In circumstances where a nurse offers treatment or advice, and a patient refuses, it would be prudent to include a notation to this effect in the patient record.

Patient records should be objectively written, and those responsible for writing records should avoid making value judgements. 'Patient has a headache' is a subjective statement and should be recorded as 'patient complaining of headache'. A description of the nature of the headache, the nursing action taken and the outcome of that action should follow this statement.

Records should be as near as possible contemporaneous with the event if they are to be accepted as reliable evidence in a court action. Delays in recording make the record less reliable as a true description of an event. In fact, a record made days after an event can be made to look as though it was an afterthought. Interlineations and notes made in margins should also be avoided, as they can suggest that information has been added to a record at a later date. It is for this reason that nurses are advised not to leave lines between individual reports.

Errors in recording should not be completely erased since this can appear suspicious in the event that a patient is suing on the basis of delivery of healthcare. Mistakes should be ruled through in a manner that enables others to be able to read what was initially written. A notation that the recording was made in error, signed by the person making the error, should be added to the record.

Nurses should be cognisant of the fact that personal information given by patients in the course of administering care is to be kept confidential. Patients are entitled to expect that nurses will maintain a high degree of confidentiality. Should a nurse breach a patient's confidentiality, the patient may be able to sue in defamation for unlawful disclosure if their reputation has been harmed, in negligence if they suffer foreseeable nervous shock, or in breach of contract. Commonwealth and state privacy Acts provide for investigation of complaints of breaches of privacy.

Access to a record can be granted to third parties with the consent of the patient. For all other purposes, access should be denied to all others except other health professionals treating the patient on a 'need to know' basis (i.e. those who have a genuine need to access the information in order to provide adequate care). Confidentiality may be legally breached by virtue of legal process (discovery and subpoenas), statutory authority, necessity and the criminal law.

Legislation generally provides that patients have a right of access to their medical records. The Commonwealth government and various state governments have enacted freedom of information legislation that gives people a right to have access to various documents, including personal documents held by public authorities. These Acts also provide for requesting that the documents be amended if there is any material that is false or misleading. In 2002, the New South Wales Government introduced the Health Records and Information Privacy Act, which gives patients the right to access their healthcare records held by private practitioners. Exceptions to disclosure can be found embodied in the various Acts.

As a general policy, patients should be given access to their records as freely as possible. A healthcare practitioner should be available when a patient is accessing their record in order to ensure that the patient understands the nature of what has been written and why it was written.

The Commonwealth Government has enacted the Personally Controlled Electronic Records Act 2012 to set up a National e-Health Records system. The Act provides for healthcare providers (section 42) and consumers (patients) to register (section 39). It is a voluntary process referred to as an 'opt-in' system. It is a condition of registration of a healthcare provider organisation that the organisation does not refuse to provide healthcare to a consumer or otherwise discriminate against a consumer in relation to the provision of healthcare because the consumer is not registered (section 46).

Those patients who register will be able to easily access information about their medical history, including test results and medications on-line. The system also enables patients to attend for treatment anywhere within Australia and to consent to health professionals accessing their relevant history. They will not have to remember every detail of their health history each time they consult a different practitioner or go to a healthcare facility. Patients will also be able to control which health professionals can view their records or add to their files and what is stored on them.

Although patient information is protected and there are privacy protection principles in place, the Act provides that there is mandatory disclosure for Coroners' matters. Disclosure to other courts or tribunals is with the consumers' consent. For the purposes of law enforcement, disclosure is when it is reasonably necessary.

REGULATION OF DRUGS

Each state and territory has specific legislation that regulates the supply and use of drugs and poisons within its jurisdiction (e.g. the Poisons and Therapeutic Goods Act 1966 (NSW)). The rules and regulations in relation to the drugs that nurses routinely administer to patients can be found within each relevant state or territory Act and any Regulations to the Act. While an Act may specify in broad terms the rules regarding the control of drugs and poisons, regulations formulated under the power of the Act set out in greater detail the specifics of the obligations of individuals under the Act.

Drugs and poisons are usually classified in Schedules according to the manner in which they may be supplied (e.g. Schedule 4 and Schedule 8 drugs are pertinent to nurses working in NSW). Changes in the Schedules take place when new drugs come into use or there are changes in the manner in which a particular drug may be supplied. For example, a drug that formerly required a doctor's prescription may be moved to a Schedule that permits the drug to be purchased over the counter from a chemist.

All nurses should become familiar with the relevant Act and any Regulations operating in the state or territory in which they work.

REGULATION OF NURSING PRACTICE

Prior to the introduction of the Health Practitioner Regulation National Law Act 2009 (The National Law) being adopted by each state and territory government, individual legislation in each state/territory governed the registration and discipline of nurses within its jurisdiction. As from July 2010 there is now a national system of primary and ongoing registration for nurses and other specified registered health professions and students, and for review of their conduct. The objects of the national registration is for the protection of the public by ensuring only suitably trained and qualified health practitioners can be registered to practise and to facilitate workforce mobility across Australia, the provision of high-quality education and training of health practitioners, rigorous and responsive assessment of overseas-trained practitioners, access to services provided by health practitioners in accordance with the public interest and to enable the continuous development of a flexible, responsive and sustainable Australian health workforce and innovation in the education of, and service delivery by, health practitioners (section 3).

The Australian Health Profession Regulatory Authority (AHPRA) is the national body responsible for the regulation, national registration and accreditation of health practitioners and the registration of students. AHPRA supports ten national health practitioners boards that are responsible for regulating each profession. A National Board can establish a State or Territory Board to enable it to exercise its functions more effectively. The primary role of the Boards is the protection of the public and to set standards and policies for the professions. With respect to nurses this is the Nursing and Midwifery Board of Australia (NMBA).

National Boards must develop registration standards for the health professions. These include standards for professional indemnity insurance, criminal history checks, continuing professional development, English language skills and recency of practice (section 46).

AHPRA, on behalf of the Boards, manages investigations into the professional conduct, performance or health of registered health practitioners in conjunction with relevant health complaints entities in the states and territories. The NSW government elected to implement a co-regulatory model by adopting parts of The National Law which deals with national registration and accreditation whilst retaining legislative control over handling complaints.

Under the National Law categories of registration are general, specialist, provisional, limited, non-practising or student. AHPRA is responsible for maintaining and publishing registers of practitioners and important information regarding each practitioner's registration; for example, conditions on registration. Conditions may be public or private. Public conditions are those which relate directly to the workplace and are made available to the public on the AHPRA website. Health-related conditions are not made available to the public. A registered health practitioner who has conditions on registration who knowingly or recklessly claims, or holds himself/herself to be registered without conditions, may become the subject of a health, conduct or performance action (section 120).

It is an offence, punishable by a fine, for a person to take or use a prescribed title that could reasonably be expected to induce a belief the person is registered under the National Law in the profession unless the person is so registered (section 113). Nor can a person who is not a registered health professional knowingly or recklessly take or use protected titles (sections 114 to 119).

In order to be eligible for general registration in a health profession, an applicant must be qualified for general registration in the health profession and have successfully completed a period of supervised practice or examination or assessment required by an approved registration standard for the health profession to assess their ability to competently and safely practise the profession, and they are a suitable person to hold general registration (section 52). The qualifications required for general registration are that the applicant must hold an approved qualification for the health profession or one that is substantially equivalent, or gained under a corresponding prior Act (section 53). Legal requirements for other categories of registration are prescribed in separate detail (sections 57 to 76). A National Board has the power to check an applicant's proof of identity (section 78) and to check their criminal history (section 79). The Board must give written notice to an applicant if it is proposing to refuse registration or to register an applicant subject to a condition to allow the applicant to make written or verbal submissions (section 81).

In NSW a person is competent to practise a health profession only if they have sufficient physical and mental capacity, knowledge and skills to practise the profession, and they have sufficient communication skills for the practice of the profession including an adequate command of the English language (section 139).

The relevant National Board maintains a register of students who are undertaking an approved program of study, or part of an approved program (section 89). The Board may ask education providers for a list of persons undertaking an approved program of study (section 88). Education providers must provide lists of persons who are not enrolled in an approved program of study who are undertaking clinical training in a health profession (section 91).

A National Board may endorse the registration of a registered health practitioner to administer, obtain, possess, prescribe, sell, supply or use a class of scheduled medicines (section 94). Also it can endorse nurse practitioners (section 95) and midwife practitioners (section 96). Other endorsements which may be granted are acupuncture (section 97) or approved areas of practice (section 98).

Registered health practitioners must apply annually for renewal of registration or endorsement if they wish to continue to practise. The application must be made no later than one month after the practitioner's period of registration ends (section 107). In addition to re-applying for registration annually and paying a fee, all practising registered practitioners are now obliged to undertake continuing professional development (CPD) for each profession they wish to remain registered for (section 128) and be able to demonstrate recency of practice. They must also declare inter alia that they do not have an impairment and that they have not practised the health profession during the preceding year without appropriate indemnity insurance (section 109). Other requirements include the disclosure of criminal charges and convictions, or disciplinary actions taken with respect to their profession in another jurisdiction (section 130). Applicants for renewal can make submissions regarding a Board's proposal to refuse the application for renewal of registration (section 111). Registered practitioners can surrender their registration by written notice to the National Board (section 137).

For each nursing profession, nurses must be able to demonstrate that they have undertaken at least 20 hours CPD annually. This must be documented and verifiable should the nurse be audited. The requirement for recency of practice is that the nurse has practised their profession for a period equivalent to a minimum of three months full time within the past five years. Practising includes clinical and non-clinical roles relevant to the delivery of nursing and midwifery services. Examples of non-clinical roles are management, regulatory, education, research and industrial (NMBA Fact Sheets). Nurses who elect to have non-practising registration are not required to undertake CPD. They cannot, however, practise nursing (section 75).

New South Wales elected to introduce a co-regularity model. Registration of health practitioners was transferred to the National body whereas conduct, competence and professional performance of nurses in New South Wales remains a State matter. The Health Practitioner Regulation National Law (NSW) No 86a amends the National Law to provide for a Health Professionals Council Authority (HPCA) to deal with complaints about registered health practitioners. There are individual Councils for each of the health professions in New South Wales. The Nursing and Midwifery Council of New South Wales (NMCNSW) is responsible for handling complaints regarding the conduct, competence and professional performance of nurses employed in NSW. Matters relating to a nurse's registration are handled by the Nursing and Midwifery Board of Australia (NMBA). The NMBA is the body to review conditions should a nurse with conditions on registration change his/her principal place of residence or predominant place of practice from NSW to another State or Territory. A review of conditions and undertakings may be made to the National Board (section 125) and in NSW to the Nursing and Midwifery Council (section 150C). The Council consults with the Health Care Complaints Commission (HCCC) regarding taking action with respect to complaints.

The legislation provides for a review or right of appeal against a decision of a Board, Council or disciplinary body to an appropriate judicial body. The above discussion provides an overview of some of the provisions of the National Law. It is not definitive and nurses should obtain a copy of the Act in the jurisdiction in which they practise in order to become fully cognisant of its provisions.

In addition to gaining knowledge of the legislative provisions governing nursing practice, all nurses should acquaint themselves with the various nationally agreed codes of practice, standards, frameworks and guidelines for professional practice governing the practice of nursing. For example, National Competency Standards, Codes of Professional Conduct, and Codes of Ethics for Registered Nurses, Midwives, Enrolled Nurses and Nurse practitioners in Australia.

The Nursing Council of New Zealand is set up under the Nurses Act 1977 and is the regulatory body for nursing and midwifery in New Zealand. The Council's primary role is the protection of the public. The Council is responsible for the registration and maintenance of standards for nurses and midwives in New Zealand. They are also responsible for investigating complaints regarding nurses and midwives and to impose sanctions such as conditions on registration. The Trans-Tasman Mutual Recognition Act 1997 mutually recognises the registration of professionals registered in New Zealand and Australia. The Act also permits the exchange of information regarding disciplinary action taken with respect to a nurse or conditions which have been placed on a practitioner's registration.

COMPLAINTS

During the course of their nursing practice, nurses may observe behaviour, professional or unethical, which they believe to be inappropriate or wrong. A nurse may feel obliged to report another professional for their actions. Reporting issues of unsatisfactory professional conduct or unethical behaviour through the proper channels is important in maintaining public confidence in the profession and maintenance of standards.

The National Law now requires mandatory notification of notifiable conduct by registered health practitioners and by employers. Notifiable conduct includes intoxication by alcohol or drugs whilst practising the profession, sexual misconduct in connection with their profession, an impairment which places the public at substantial risk of harm and significant departures from accepted professional standards which places the public at risk of harm (section 140). Impairment is defined as when a person has a physical or mental impairment, disability, condition or disorder (including substance abuse or dependence) that detrimentally affects or is likely to detrimentally affect a health practitioner's capacity to practise their profession, or a student's capacity to undertake clinical training (section 5). Registered health practitioners, in the course of practising their profession, must report other health practitioners whom they reasonably believe have behaved in a way that constitutes notifiable conduct, or students who have an impairment which may place the public at substantial risk of harm whilst undertaking clinical training (section 141). An employer of a registered health practitioner must notify the National Agency when they reasonably believe that the health practitioner has behaved in a way that constitutes notifiable conduct (section 142). The National Agency can report failures of employers to report notifiable conduct to the Minister. Education providers must notify the National Agency if a student has an impairment which may place the public at risk whilst undertaking clinical training (section 143).

Any person may make a complaint to AHPRA regarding a healthcare practitioner or institution. This includes members of the public, patients, former patients and their relatives. In NSW a complaint may be lodged with the HCPA or NSW Health Care Complaints Commission (HCCC) who can investigate the matter. The HCCC is required to consult with the relevant HCPA, which is the Nursing and Midwifery Council of New South Wales when the complaint is in respect of nursing, to consider the appropriate procedure for handling the complaint. Likewise the HCPA consults with the HCCC.

Health practitioners, employers and education providers make mandatory notifications on an approved form and forward to AHPRA. Complaints should be in writing containing particulars of the allegation. Each complaint must be dealt with expeditiously. Where complaints are made in good faith, the legislation provides that complainants are protected from civil, criminal and administrative liability; the complaint is not a breach of professional etiquette or ethics; nor does it constitute a departure from accepted standards of professional conduct; and no liability for defamation is incurred (section 237).

Grounds for complaints which may be made against a registered health practitioner include a criminal conviction or criminal finding, unsatisfactory professional conduct or professional misconduct, lack of competence, impairment and/or that the practitioner is not a suitable person (section 144). The fact that a matter complained of has occurred in the personal life of the nurse does not exclude it from giving rise to disciplinary proceedings to determine whether the behaviour is such that the nurse is not a fit and proper person to practise nursing. For example, information that a registered nurse has been convicted of downloading child pornography will be referred to AHPRA and this can lead to a disciplinary hearing with the prospect that disciplinary action will be taken and that the nurse's name may be removed from the register.

One issue that can face a nurse and which can give rise to a complaint is when a nurse enters into a financial, personal and/or sexual relationship with a patient or former patient. The fact that the nurse–patient relationship has ceased does not legitimise the relationship if the circumstances were such that the profession regards the relationship as unethical. This is particularly so when the nurse has become privy to a great deal of sensitive personal information regarding the patient's past and present life and health issues. Such matters are regarded as 'crossing the boundaries'. Whether or not such a relationship falls within prohibited behaviour will be decided on its facts. Nurses are well advised to seek advice regarding such actual or potential relationships, as it could lead to deregistration.

Similarly, nurses should not accept valuable gifts from patients. The nurse/patient relationship is such that a court may determine that there was 'undue influence' which brought about the giving of the gift. In matters involving health practitioners and patients, as in other dependent relationships, the courts consider that there is an imbalance of power. As such there is a presumption that 'undue influence' is an operative factor in the giving of a valuable gift. In such cases the recipient of the gift has the onus of proving to the court (rebutting the presumption) that the gift did not flow from undue influence. Even if such an issue is not raised in a court of law, the receipt of a valuable gift from a patient may find the nurse facing disciplinary proceedings.

Should a nurse choose to make a complaint to the administration of the institution in which they work, they must do so confidentially and restrict their complaint or report to senior authorities. In such cases, nurses should not take it upon themselves to discuss the issue with colleagues as this may lead them to being sued for defamation. Reports must be made in good faith.

Defamation Acts in the various states are now uniform and the same provisions apply across all states. The person complaining of being defamed must prove that what was said or written was capable of being defamatory of them, and that their reputation has been harmed. There are a number of defences available to a defendant in defamation proceedings, including 'qualified privilege'. This defence applies where the recipient has an interest or apparent interest in having information on some subject, the matter is published to them in the course of giving them information on that subject, and the defendant's conduct in publishing that information is reasonable. The information must be substantially true. Thus it could be argued that a nurse who passes on potentially defamatory material to the authorities in adherence to the above specifications would be able to avail themselves of this defence. It should be noted that the defence of qualified privilege is defeated if actuated by malice.

Nurses who feel that their complaints are not being handled appropriately may take it upon themselves to go outside the usual channels available to them thus becoming what is known as 'whistleblowers'. Legislation protecting whistleblowers is unsatisfactory in its scope and the way in which it protects whistleblowers. Legislation has been introduced largely to protect employees who disclose information about corrupt behaviour in the public sector. Nevertheless, employees who disclose such information may face the risk of being considered as breaching their duty of confidentiality to their employer, and suffer general censure or legal consequences from that employer.

The ways in which a whistleblower may report would also seem to be restricted. The Department of Parliamentary Services (2005) published a research note on whistleblowing, which commented that: 'Most Australian state jurisdictions provide that, for whistleblowers to be protected, the information is to be disclosed internally or to a "proper" or "investigating" authority.' Thus it is appropriate, and in some cases mandatory, for nurses to make a complaint through AHPRA, or the Council or the HCCC in NSW.

Certainly, it is accepted that reporting corrupt or risky behaviour of another health practitioner through the proper channels is a matter of public interest. Nurses who consider taking this path would need to take reasonable steps to satisfy themselves that what they are wishing to report is substantially true and a matter of public interest, and that they adhere to appropriate steps when doing so to protect themselves and to ensure that no unjustifiable complaints are made.

CONCLUSION

Knowledge of the law and its application to nursing practice has become a necessary component of a nurse's knowledge base. Nurses must be aware of and respect the legal rights of patients and the corresponding obligations of nurses in nursing care. Through an interest and knowledge of the law, a nurse can most effectively act as an advocate of patients by being involved in committees charged with the responsibility of formulating policies for the delivery of healthcare.

Failure to appreciate the legal rights of patients can lead a nurse to face a legal action mounted by a patient or some disciplinary action taken by a nursing board. Acknowledgment of, and adherence to, the legal rights of patients also goes a long way in maintaining the quality of nursing care delivered and the respect to be accorded to the profession. It is a professional obligation of all nurses to acquaint themselves with current legal issues touching upon the profession, and to do so by remaining up to date with their legal knowledge.

The discussion of the law and legal issues in this chapter is necessarily brief. This basic introduction does not purport to give legal advice. Should a nurse require legal assistance they should seek advice from a legal practitioner at the time that an adverse event arises.

REFLECTIVE QUESTIONS

1 To what extent do you believe that the common law adequately provides for the resolution of complaints by patients allegedly harmed by healthcare?

2 What resources could you draw on in preparing to face court proceedings in relation to your professional practice?

3 How can you ensure that you remain up to date with the legal issues associated with the practice of nursing?

RECOMMENDED READINGS

Chiarella M 2002 The legal and professional status of nursing. Churchill Livingstone, London

Forrester K, Griffiths D 2010 Essentials of law for the health professions, 3rd edn. Elsevier, Sydney

Johnstone M-J 1994 Nursing and the injustices of the law. WB Saunders, Sydney

Kerridge I, Lowe M, Stewart C 2009 Ethics and law for the health professions, 3rd edn. The Federation Press, Sydney

McIlwraith J, Madden B 2010 Health care and the law, 5th edn. Lawbook Company, Sydney

Staunton P, Chiarella M 2007 Law for nurses, 5th edn. Elsevier Science, Melbourne

ONLINE RESOURCES

Australian Health Practitioner Regulation Agency: www.ahpra.gov.au

Health Care Complaints Commission: www.hccc.gov.au

Law and Justice Foundation: www.lawfoundation.net.au

Nurses and Midwives Professional Standards Committee of New South Wales: www.austlii.edu.au

Nurses and Midwives Tribunal of New South Wales: www.austlii.edu.au

REFERENCE

Department of Parliamentary Services 2005 Whistleblowing in Australia: transparency, accountability … but above all, the truth. Research Note, Parliament of Australia, 14 February 2005, No 31

CHAPTER 12

The gendered culture of nursing: a historical review

Sandra Speedy

LEARNING OBJECTIVES

On completion of this chapter, readers will have:

- understood and appreciated the historical development of feminist thinking on concepts such as nursing work and science
- examined the role that gender plays in defining the world of nursing work
- developed greater insight into how the healthcare system and health professionals are impacted upon by the issue of gender
- briefly explored the influence that feminisms have had on the discipline of nursing
- understood how feminist theory has influenced nursing research
- considered the debate about the relative advantages and disadvantages that gender provides for nurses.

KEY WORDS

Gender, nursing work, feminism, patriarchy, power, organisational culture

INTRODUCTION

In order to consider a range of gender issues—which are of interest and relevance to nurses all over the world—this chapter will consider the gendered nature of nursing work. This will involve a review of understandings of feminism as they have evolved over time, given that gender and feminism are intricately linked. It is necessary to examine the nature of women who provide more than 90% of the nursing workforce (Maher et al 2008). It will also require some analysis of the nature of nursing work, as it is performed by women and men. Inherent in this discussion will be consideration of the role of society and science in determining views of the concept of 'woman', as well as the work women undertake. The chapter also considers briefly the influence of the feminisms on nursing, and the influence of nurses and nursing on feminism. Finally, the chapter examines the increasing role played by men in nursing, a gender issue of utmost importance for the future of nursing. It should be noted that there has been an extensive exploration of substantial volumes of literature that reflect classical thinking and debate over almost 20 years, most of which remains relevant to the concepts presented here.

CHANGING VIEWS OF THE NATURE OF FEMINISM

An important event highlighted some of the changing views of feminism. It was the 8th European Feminist Research Conference held in May 2012 in Budapest, Hungary. The prime motivator for this conference was recognition that there were serious concerns at regional, national and international levels, which forced feminist scholars to re-assess their 'theoretical and political toolbox' (www.8thfeministconference.org). These concerns related to social, political, economic, cultural and environmental matters, that resulted in 'increasingly racist politics and nationalist discourses across Europe, huge cutbacks in social services and education' (www.8thfeministconference.org), all of which resulted in a strengthening of conservative gender discourses towards women. It was not only Europe where these developments were initiated: one presenter from Morocco stated that 'gender issues in North Africa are largely determined by the socio-cultural sources of power and authority in the region' (Sadiqi 2012). She cited 'space-patriarchy' that associates the public space with men and the private space with women, suggesting that women are claiming status, functionality and dignity in the public sphere, while retaining their cultural role in the private sphere. Sadiqi questioned whether these attempts would be successful, or hijacked by conservative forces, or simply benefit a lucky elite. Milojevic (2008) supported the concept of embracing other perspectives. She noted that many African, Chinese and women from former socialist countries prefer to be involved in 'feminology' rather than 'feminism', which was perceived as Western feminism.

Hemmings (2012) suggested that gender equality has either been 'mainstreamed to the point of de-politicisation' or been sidelined by the urgent demands of the global financial crisis. She suggests that feminism, to be a significant force, must move beyond itself and ask questions that are more relevant to the political problem of gender in the current social, economic and financial climate. There are other forces that require us to take note of the impact of feminism, including generational differences, which will be considered later in this chapter.

THE GENDERED NATURE OF NURSING WORK

A consideration of the gendered nature of nursing work must examine the concept of woman, since the majority of nurses are women. Whatever societal views are held regarding women will influence perception of women's work—in this case, nursing work. Historically, perspectives on women were influenced by 'scientific' views about the nature of women, although it was also argued that perspectives on women influenced beliefs about the nature of science.

There is a considerable volume of literature that demonstrates a range of approaches and various viewpoints on woman as object and subject. Women have been examined from sociological, psychological, biological, philosophical or political perspectives—and other viewpoints as well. Many of these viewpoints featured devaluation of women, as any examination of the concepts of essentialism, biologism, naturalism or universalism demonstrate. In an insightful and historically important work, Grosz (1990) suggested that all of these terms, which argue the nature of women (and men, incidentally), fixed and defined the limits, because they 'are commonly used in patriarchal discourses to justify women's social subordination and their secondary positions relative to men in patriarchal society' (Grosz 1990:333). In their work, both David (2000) and Gherardi (1994:591) argued the similar point that 'masculinity and femininity are symbolic universes of meaning socially and historically constructed'. Today there are few, if any, scholars who would argue against these views.

Gherardi also suggested that the way we 'do gender' in our work 'helps to diminish or increase the inequality of the sexes: we use ceremonial work to recognize the difference of gender, and remedial work socially to construct the "fairness" of gender relationships' (Gherardi 1994:592). Ceci (2004) asserted that genders were identified by specific traits, virtues and behaviours that place us as either feminine or masculine—that is, identifiable and named as such. There is no question that in nursing each gender experiences 'cross-over', necessitating the management of dual presence in what are essentially separate symbolic contexts.

There are problems with constructing a 'universal feminism', since allowance must be made for difference and diversity between women, just as there is between women and men. This prompted some debate about whether men can be feminists (Wadsworth 2001). The question was raised: is feminism just a logical consequence of humanism? If so, there was no reason why men could not be feminists. Nevertheless, there are contrary views that humanism often ignores women and 'simply meant man-ism'. This is a digression for the interested reader to pursue.

However, what is also worthy of exploration are some of the views about women and nurses within a medical and health professions context, because these views were influenced by the concepts mentioned above. The issue of how women were constructed by science is also relevant here (Kane & Thomas 2000). Feminist literature argues that the masculinity of science is an image that has been perpetuated for centuries. This image creation was affected by textbook representations, curriculum organisation, classroom behaviour and stereotypical beliefs and attitudes. It distorts science, yet scientific method had not been successful in filtering out patriarchal bias in the scientific construction of women. In the early 1990s, Lather wrote with insight and clarity regarding this. She says:

> The claim of positivistic researchers that their method is sufficient protection against ideological incursion is debunked by feminist critiques of the conceptual and methodological orientations that reflect and reinforce sex-based inequality. Hence the construction of women brings into question that which has passed for knowledge in the human sciences.
> (Lather 1991:17)

The masculinity of science is only an illusion (albeit a powerful one), not an intrinsic part of its nature. Science is a social construct, and 'its development is inextricably linked with social relations, not least the relations between men and women' (Kelly 1985:76). This leads, of course, to using male as the norm and female as the referent, a strategy that has been exposed and rejected in a wide range of disciplines, including psychology, sociology, psychiatry, medicine, education and biology. As long ago as the 1970s, it was pointed out that 'male' medicine misunderstood the female body, and these debates have now extended to cover all aspects of women's health, not just those of childbirth and reproduction.

In nursing and medicine, the presence of increasing numbers of women at all levels of authority indicates a modicum of success in producing women-friendly services and conditions. This has come about only because women have been forced to reclaim their healing role, which was given a boost by the knowledge and insights in the classic treatise written by Ehrenreich and English (1979), documenting the exclusion of women-as-healers from professionalised, modern medicine. There has long been 'increasing institutional awareness of the deficiencies and sexism of specific institutional practices' (Evans 1997:42). This had both positive and negative effects. For the latter, it resulted in some feminists 'beating up' on nurses, thus earning the title of 'anti-nurse'. This was:

> ... predicated on the belief that nurses willingly capitulate to male (and/or medical) dominance, thereby making it difficult for 'real feminists' to achieve their goals. This ... 'complicity hypothesis' ... sees nurses as compliant with patriarchal demands to remain oppressed.
> (Buchanan 1997:82)

Using this argument, nurses were viewed as either the embodiment of the 'ideal' or 'good woman' (David 2000, Fealy 2004:653), conforming to masculine desires, or as the 'bad mother', 'thwarting women in their endeavours and assisting the medical profession in torturing women patients' (Buchanan 1997:82). In some ways this analysis, awareness and critique could and was viewed as hostile criticism; however, it provided us with a historical perspective of the alternative views and insights that can be growth enhancing for women and nurses, should these perspectives be objectively and critically considered.

Published studies over the last three decades indicate that we did not need feminists to 'beat up' on nurses—nurses do that very well to each other, whether they are feminists or not (Briles 1994, Center for American Nurses 2008, Curtis et al 2007, David 2000, Norris 2010). Horizontal violence has long been recognised by a range of authors, who suggested that nurses' self-hate and dislike of other nurses (which is very common in oppressed groups) was demonstrated by the lack of cohesion in nursing groups, as well as the phenomenon of 'eating our young' (Bent 1993, Kitson 2004, Roberts 2000). This concept arose out of the original work of Freire (2007) in his now classical work *Pedagogy of the Oppressed* (first published in 1968), which highlighted the relationship between the coloniser and the colonised, its power and its powerlessness. From these insights, we could conjecture that the systematic oppression of women would assist nurses to recognise the oppressive structures in which they practise. This:

> ... includes recognising that nurses are placed in a culture that does not value their attributes, rather than 'blaming' them for ranking lower on self-esteem and higher in

submissiveness in job-trait studies than do people in other occupations. Nurses must no longer assume that they are inherently inferior to the systems that surround them. (Bent 1993:298)

Awareness of the social construction of women and nursing and its oppressive nature must change the way nurses relate to each other, and refrain from 'horizontal violence'. There are many disadvantages resulting from such relationships, including medication and nursing errors that have no place in nursing care (Stanley 2010). It is clear that workplace bullying, a major form of violence, can have severe psychological and physical effects (Hutchinson et al 2006, Rodwell & Demir 2012), including clinical depression, attempted suicide and post-traumatic stress disorder (Branch et al 2012).

As David makes clear:

Nurses will never be able to expunge gender politics without first developing an understanding of how many use self-deception and how that action perpetuates nursing's professional mediocrity, limits freedom of thought and action, and preserves nurses' borderline status.
(David 2000:85)

This brings us to the work of nursing.

THE WORK OF NURSING

The role and function of nursing cannot be separated from those who undertake this activity. Literature published in the past two decades indicates that there are particular views held about women and nursing that create the definitions of women's work and nursing work, and, by implication, men's work (David 2000, Fealy 2004, McDonald 2012, Meadus 2000). Cheek and Rudge point out that:

... the low status of nursing and the way in which the work of nurses is devalued, especially when compared to other health professionals, can at least in part be explained by its gendered nature.
(Cheek & Rudge 1995:312)

Labelling nursing as 'women's work' creates a deterrent that 'inhibits recruitment of men into the profession and aids promotion of the sex imbalance in the nursing workforce' (Meadus 2000:9). Similar views were expressed by Anthony (2006) and Cude and Winfrey (2007). Nursing was thus viewed as a natural extension of the female role, valuing nurturance, caring, support, care and concern (Bent 1993, Brykczynska 1997, Evans 1997, McDonald 2012). These characteristics have been described as encompassing a 'tyranny of niceness' (Street 1995). Nevertheless, researchers have, over the decades, found that these characteristics were selectively eliminated during the educational and socialisation process (Doering 1992). For example, Treacy noted that current 'nurse training' endorses 'compliance, passivity and ladylike behaviour, but it negatively sanctioned other female traits such as intuition, empathy, and emotional expression' (Treacy 1989:88). These characteristics are still found in the literature, but are deemed as positive and essential traits nurses should possess (Winter 2009).

It should be noted that there are cultural differences, as Varaei et al (2012) and Creina and Meadus (2008) point out in a wide-ranging review of various countries' perceptions of nursing image. The descriptors 'compliance, passivity and ladylike behaviour' are words which were argued as suggestive of 'powerlessness', and 'intuitiveness, empathy and emotional expression' were often viewed as unscientific and hence unacceptable in the world of science. The social construction of women as emotional beings was also used to undermine their credibility as nurses (Ceci 2004). As David (2000:86) also pointed out: 'the gender dialectic is still so fundamental to gender politics that it permeates the traditions of nursing, such as the belief that nursing is woman's work'.

A powerful, grass-roots and sometimes painful description of the traits every nurse should have can be found on a blog commenced by Winter (2009) (accessed online at http://blog/soliant.com/). This blog is not reading for the faint-hearted.

Because of these stereotypes and beliefs, it was argued that women and nurses gravitate towards nursing as a career, while men are relatively inhibited from entering the nursing profession (Tugung & Villafana-Reynoso 2008). According to Evans (2004:321), the 'ideological designation of nursing as women's work has excluded, limited, and conversely, advanced the careers of men in nursing'. The issue of male advantage and/or disadvantage will be addressed later in this chapter.

Recent research has, however, taken a different approach to viewing gender and feminised occupations. McDonald (2012:16) found for nursing students, that 'performing gender successfully entails performances of femininity and masculinity for both women and men, requiring all nurses to do and undo dominant gender norms'. Thus it is just as important to 'examine the gender identity negotiation of women in female-dominated occupations as it is to examine the experiences of men'. Similar research targeting current practising nurses, and how they do and undo gender, could be illuminating.

In 1997 Evans noted that nineteenth-century science and rationality perceived the 'feminine' as an abstraction, which assisted in marginalising women within institutional practices. Women, as the literature informs us, were constructed as hysterical and intellectually inferior, while men were expected to conform to the stereotype of masculine behaviour. Thus, 'the "soft" feminine and the "hard" masculine then received institutional recognition and confirmation in particular practices' (Evans 1997:39). Feminists have sought to demonstrate the disjunction between supposed institutional objectivity and actual institutional practice. Specifically, the institution of medicine, for example, defined its values as non-gendered, while in practice they were deeply gendered (Evans 1997). This was exposed in many areas—for example, in the management of childbirth and women's sexuality (Erturk 2004).

Because the values that dominate our health system were so pervasive and reflected the values of society at large, 'it is a struggle for nurses to remain aligned to the person rather than the institution' (Huntington 1996:170). This created difficulties in nursing work, as the dominant discourses that shaped health, illness and perceptions of what it is to be a woman (and a man, incidentally) disadvantaged the individual. As Huntington (1996:170) pointed out: 'we have been left with only male language to explain the fundamentally female practice of healing bodies'. The only solution to this problem was to develop an alternative discourse to that constructed and dominated by orthodox scientific discourse characteristics of the medical world.

Clearly too, the feminist literature challenged the cultural code of organisations, designed around masculinity and femininity, which suggested that 'gender is deeply embedded in the design and functioning of organisations' (Davies 1995:44). These workplaces were (and continue to be) socially constructed, as is the position of 'nurse' (David 2000), neither of which are gender-neutral, and operate on masculine values for their legitimation and affirmation (Gherardi 1994). Nurses therefore found it difficult to function within such gendered organisations, and frequently resorted to 'blaming the victims', who were usually other nurses struggling with their day-to-day functioning within a hostile environment (Center for American Nurses 2008). Alternatively, they adopted a victim mentality, rather than recognising the dysfunctionality of their workplaces (Kitson 2004). Thus:

> [W]omen, in a very important sense, cannot be 'at home' in the public world—it is constructed in such a way that assumes home is somewhere else, somewhere far away and different.
> (Davies 1995:62)

More recently, however, Sadiqi (2012) noted that, in Morocco, feminists are attempting to gain greater access to public space, whilst retaining their existing private space. She states: '… women are now engaged in short, medium and long term actions that are not only transforming the region but also women and men's mentalities'. They are engaging in social programs, targeting citizenship rights, promoting religious and textbook reforms and engaging in political decision making in their local communities. This does not negate the fact that nursing historically provided a haven for women who sought to control their lives within a professional context (and still does for some), but there were significant limits to what could be achieved (Kane & Thomas 2000). In fact, David (2000) suggested that this was delusion, because power does not belong to women in a male-dominated system (see also Paliadelis 2005, 2008, Paliadelis et al 2007).

As we continue our searching of pertinent literature, we find a range of other historical scholarly work that demonstrates the further weakening of nursing's value. Historically, Gamarnikow (1978) linked nursing to domesticity; Treacy (1989) suggested that the invisibility of nurses' contribution to care reflected the invisibility of much of the work contribution of women in society. Other scholars have pointed out that the sexual division of labour in the home disadvantages women in the workplace, which creates enormous stress for working women and, in this case, nurses. This taps into the work of feminist scientists who have 'identified "women's work" the "caring professions", "unpaid domestic labour", "the double shift" and other manifestations of the apparently "natural" social division of labour' (Evans 1997:59).

It was pointed out by many scholars that caring itself is a gendered construct, since notions of professional caring were derived from traditional concepts of caring as a feminine obligation (Caffrey & Caffrey 1994, Ekstrom 1999, Falk Rafael 1996, Paliadelis et al 2007, Wuest 1997). Caring in nursing was constructed as an inherently feminine pastime, and traditionally received little social or economic recognition; it was perceived as women's work, as unintellectual, unskilled and emotional, and thus likely to perpetuate gender exploitation (Bubeck 1995, Ceci 2004, Henderson 2001). It was long believed that the work nurses undertake in order to provide care does not require any particular skill or knowledge; it was considered to be a quality that women possess 'naturally' (Falk Rafael 1998, Henderson 2001, Zebroski 2001).

However, this view was also challenged. For example, Meadus (2000) cited research demonstrating that men enter nursing because of their desire to care for others, thus challenging the stereotype that only women nurses care. He also noted that such men run the risk of being perceived as 'gay' because of this role violation. This viewpoint was challenged by Bubeck (1995:114), when she noted that 'part of the practice of care is to focus on the needs of the other, to become attentive, to be selfless'. The construction of masculinity makes caring very difficult for men; they also escaped from the care burden through the 'public/private' split in responsibilities of women and men (Tronto 1999).

Nursing's detractors long promoted the idea that nurses were 'doers' rather than 'thinkers'; that is, nurses did not need to 'think' to do nursing, as long as they could 'do' certain tasks. This resulted in an anti-intellectual bias, which created the perception that the 'intelligent nurse was not a good practical nurse' (Fealy 2004:652), a myth that threatened the academic preparation of nurses (Liaschenko & Peter 2004). This, in no small measure, led to a significant devaluation of nursing, assisted by the unequal power relations that characterised the position of nursing vis-a-vis medicine (David 2000). For many years, this view was used to justify the low-level education provided to nurses prior to their entry into the higher education system.

That caring was assumed not to require knowledge was not without practical consequence. The replacement of registered nurses with less skilled personnel could be considered less of a reflection of economic rationalism than a reflection of the idea that caring was unskilled activity intrinsic to domesticity and womanhood. To engender nurse caring as feminine, therefore positioning it as innately instinctive to women, was to deny the advanced knowledge and skills that lay within the therapeutic caring acts of nurses. Despite the fact that 'emotional labour' was a vital and necessary part of the nursing labour process, it 'tends to be marginalized as a skill that a predominantly female nursing workforce would naturally possess' (Bolton 2000:580).

The concept of emotional labour was derived from the insightful work of Hothschild (1983) who suggested that stress occurs to those involved, as they needed to repeatedly suppress their felt emotions while they expressed contradictory feelings. This dissonance created emotional deadening and distancing from authentic feeling. Emotional labour was conceived as a 'gift in the form of authentic caring behaviour' (Bolton 2000:586), which truly reflected the state of 'being a nurse' or acting out the social construction of the 'ideal nurse' (Mazhindu 2003:249). The fact that it was under-theorised and not appreciated was of serious concern (Henderson 2001).

Emotion work was hard labour, because it required containment of emotions and/or denial of feelings. Relief measures were sought to cope with this continuous labouring. Relief was found in 'backstage regions', such as the nurses' station, where profound irritation with patients or emotional anguish could be expressed, where nurses could 'drop their public mask' and express their true feelings (Weir & Waddington 2008). As Fineman (1993:21) indicated, 'off-stage settings are not emotion-free ports'. Here, implicit feeling rules came into play; colleagues could then express emotion to a degree that would be cathartic for them, but would also maintain organisational order.

Despite the fact that it is now acknowledged that emotional labour does occur in organisations, and that employers have expectations about what sort of emotion employees should feel in particular contexts, emotion work tends to be privatised and moved out of the realm of organisational responsibility (Boyle 2002a, 2002b, Martinez-Indigo et al 2007). The organisation that does not support staff for emotional labour work is faced with significant staff dissatisfaction levels that impact negatively (Chou et al 2012). Emotional labour work involves remaining continually vigilant and sensitive to the environment, constantly noting and responding to others' emotional states, alleviating resultant distress, and assisting those who are 'inappropriately emotional' to regain their stability (Lupton 1998). The fact that this creates workplace stress for nurses was rarely acknowledged (McVicar 2003, Mann & Cowburn 2005).

Given that emotional labour work is emotionally and physically demanding (requiring high levels of interpersonal and intrapersonal skills and competencies) (McQueen 2004, Myerson 2000, Nicolson 1996), it must be acknowledged. There are three reasons for this. First, emotion work remains largely invisible. Second, it requires the development of awareness and of a vocabulary to describe this work as a competency. Third, this work is predominantly done by women, it is 'women's work' and therefore 'natural' (Huynh et al 2008). Women tend to be more involved in the caring and service professions (as in nursing) than are men, and also perform much of the 'backstage' or behind-the-scenes work (Goffman 1959). While this work has in the past been perceived as trivial, it is usually of a supportive nature, enhancing the intellectual capability or productivity of organisations (Lupton 1998), reducing burnout and retaining staff (Bartram et al 2012). This is not to say that men do not 'do' emotional labour; some do. However, management is still predominantly done by men, and their power to demand emotional labour from both women and men is maintained by management, although it is 'often constructed as (non)emotions' (Hearn 1993:161). On the other hand, Boyle's (2002a) research on emotional labour and masculinities places men in a lose–lose predicament, given that males are not viewed to have a primary 'caring' role.

It is important not to forget the value of relationships that nurses develop with their patients, with relatives and carers. This requires using the self in caring mode which can be critical to recovery, and which can be very demanding. Sandelowski makes the point that those who engender nursing as female:

> ... inadvertently minimise or deny nursing its record of expertise and innovation within technology, the primary roles nurses have played in the deployment of technology and the power and remuneration that comes with technological knowledge and skills in a high-technology culture.
> (Sandelowski 1997:172)

For readers who seek to further explore the relationship of nurses to technology, it is recommended that they read Chapter 16 of this book.

Historical and traditional expectations that surround caring as a feminine and nursing activity involve subjugation of the self and selfless devotion to duty (Caffrey & Caffrey 1994). In some circumstances nurses experience feelings of powerlessness and eventually burn out, as a result of suppression of their own feelings and needs (Demerouti et al 2000). Others suggest that emotional labour is an integral part of caring in nursing (Henderson 2001, Weir & Waddington 2008). For an excellent and comprehensive analysis of caring in nursing, refer to Chapter 5 of this text.

THE INFLUENCE OF FEMINISMS ON THE DISCIPLINE OF NURSING

'The feminisms' refers to the variety of theoretical approaches to the advocacy of equal rights for women, accompanied by a commitment to improving the position of women in society. They were informed by a range of theoretical propositions, which include liberal feminism, socialist feminism, radical feminism, postmodern feminism, postcolonial feminism (Rancine 2003), feminist ethics (Peter et al 2004), third wave feminism, ecofeminism and black feminism (Rockler-Gladen 2008).

This chapter has developed the argument, derived from decades of literature, that women and nurses are devalued in general, notwithstanding that gains have been made in recent years. Feminist nurses, and others, have provided feminist analyses of their clinical practice, their educational understandings and their research. It is most notable that the feminisms have been promoted more by nursing scholars than practitioners, which has led to some uneasiness between the two groups. This may have arisen because the feminisms have an 'image' problem due to stereotypical views of what constitutes a feminist.

In reality, the feminisms are political perspectives, which seek to balance societal power, to gain equalities and autonomies for women of all races, classes, ethnicities, ages, disabilities, sexualities and professional status (Peter et al 2004). These feminisms offer the opportunity for nurses to recognise and analyse the unequal power relations that have been discussed earlier in this chapter, and to develop a raised consciousness about gender issues (Dendaas 2004, Meadus 2000, Valentine 2001). Feminist analyses have been extended to clinical practice to examine nursing and healthcare contexts, particularly 'managed care' from the 'feminist philosophical assumption that "the personal is political"' (Georges & McGuire 2004:11).

It is noteworthy that the feminisms have been eschewed by a large number of women, particularly younger women (Baumgardner & Richards 2003). This may be partly attributed to (mis)understandings of the meaning of feminism. Those who seek to denigrate feminism and what it can offer suggest that feminists are 'man-haters' and therefore separatists; a number of other jaundiced and inaccurate epithets are hurled at them.

Nevertheless, the literature also suggests that Generation Y women may believe that feminism is passé 'because it worked' (Wynter 2006). The argument runs that the successes of feminism must sow the seeds of its failure to be seen as relevant for adults of the present generation. Jayatilaka (2001) likens feminism to fluoride, suggesting that 'feminism is like fluoride—we scarcely notice we have it—it is simply in the water'. And the new generation of women can take advantage of the gains of their fore-mothers, but 'do' their feminism in different ways, as well as perceiving the importance of feminism from different perspectives (Hemmings 2012).

In reality, one can espouse feminist philosophy or be driven from a feminist perspective while celebrating womanhood, whatever individualistic form it takes. Thus, women can enjoy male company, be interested in fashion and enjoy their youth and femininity. The key point is that feminism can be individually practised, which includes making choices about life. This can range, for example, from career choice and relationship definition, to shaving whatever parts of our body we wish, wearing nail polish and make-up and even enjoying relationships with males. Feminism is thus about taking control of one's life, respecting one's womanhood as well as men; feminists can (and do) enjoy male company. The radical left of the 1970s' view was that all men were rapists and perpetrators of violence. The reality is that some were, but the majority were not. So adopting a feminist perspective did not mean rejecting relationships with men; there could be (and often is) a natural and harmonious co-existence between women and men.

Generational differences are a vital component of this historical review (Milojevic et al 2008). It has been suggested that these groups can be divided into the 'Greatest Generation (born 1925–1945), Baby Boomers (born 1946–1964), Generation X (born 1965–1977) and Generation Y (born 1978–2000)' (Lavoie-Tremblay et al 2010).

There is a strong view that women of Generation X and Y, in failing to identify with feminism, are rejecting the radical feminist notion of what it means to be a feminist (Wynter 2006). As Jayatilaka (2001) notes, such women might be identified as feminist if they were recognised as doing it in their own way. Rockler-Gladen (2007) suggested that this is 'third wave feminism', developed in the 1990s, which 'focuses more on the individual empowerment of women and less on activism' in economic, political, social and personal areas. Essentially, this means that there is greater emphasis on using personal empowerment as a way to begin social change. It is this approach that is criticised by other feminists who believe that personal empowerment is unlikely to foster social change. Third wave feminism has also been identified as 'postfeminism'—a concept explored in a study by Aronson (2003). She found that, while younger women were more ambivalent about supporting feminism, they were supporters, and might, under the right conditions, become the drivers for the next wave of the feminist movement.

So while it is true that the feminisms have not been adopted wholeheartedly by nurses, they certainly have had an impact. Some feminists have been hypercritical of nursing and nurses because of the latter's inability to embrace feminist theories: they believe that nursing as a women's field needs 'rescuing'—that it is a victim of patriarchy and needs help in recognising this. As previously noted, some feminists place the blame for the continuance of nursing oppression at the feet of nurses who collude with their oppressors to prevent change in the system (David 2000). In this way, nurses are viewed as weak and compliant with the dominant forces that seek to retain the status quo, or as deceiving themselves. This may be a deliberate act, but it is more likely that insight and awareness have not been developed, thus disadvantaging nurses and nursing (Giddings 2005).

Nursing, however, provided fertile ground for the development of feminist theories, as these provided useful perspectives for nurses who worked with disempowered and marginalised groups in their practice. Many nurses recognised that they are also disempowered, marginalised and disadvantaged within the healthcare system (Ceci 2004), and were developing understandings of these processes in order to action change. But while this is an ongoing movement, it is certainly no easy task.

While feminist theories have focused on nursing and the development of nursing research, there is a significant 'halo effect' that works against the valuing of nursing research. In accepting the premise that women and nurses are devalued in general, by 'scientific' researchers in particular, nursing research itself is devalued, because it is done by women and nurses. The qualities that define a 'good nurse' are quite distinct from those defining a 'good researcher'. Hicks (1999, 1997) argued that 'research has fundamentally masculine connotations and nursing is quintessentially feminine' (Hicks 1999:130), which in itself contributed to the relative paucity of nursing research output. At this time, it seemed that two cultures were in collision: nursing and research (Neuman 1999, Valentine 2001). This is not necessarily the case today, as will be discussed shortly.

There is a long history of males who, in the past, were the academics and intellectual and political gatekeepers of Western thought. They constructed and reproduced knowledge. But with the deconstruction and reconstruction of knowledge by feminists who have challenged the 'received view', nurses can take advantage of the liberalising approach inherent in the scholarly work published since the 1970s and 1980s in academic feminism and nursing. Since this time, feminist critics of science have exposed the history and assumptions of science and identified its masculinist practices.

Evans (1997:54) argued that 'women then had to fight and argue their way back into science—and a scientific epistemology and community that they had had little or no part in constructing'. Not only were they literally absent from science, there was also a wider absence of the 'feminine' and an absence from the findings and conclusions of science. This was not surprising because 'the questions that science identified as important were determined by the construction of the social world in which men occupied the public, and women the private, space' (Evans 1997:54).

According to Huntington (1996), this created an opportunity for scientific knowledge to maintain the control of women (primarily through their bodies), as men constructed a knowledge base that was able to be extrapolated to women. She continued: 'nurses ... have not addressed the issue of the place of science in nursing nor the impact this has had on nursing generally, and the nursing of women in particular' (Huntington 1996:168). This, of course, had implications for nursing work and nursing research, as it suggested that nurses were instrumental in maintaining a medical ideology for women patients, calculated to be negative and oppressive (Buchanan 1997).

Part of the rejection of masculinist science was fostered by scholars, intellectuals and researchers who adopted the 'emancipatory science' perspective promulgated by the Frankfurt School of Sociology and Philosophy. The inaugural address given by Habermas in 1965, entitled 'Knowledge and interest', defined emancipatory science as 'one which reveals the relationship of knowledge and interests which the objectivist attitude conceals' (Hagell 1989:227). This included a rejection of logical positivism as the only or most appropriate approach to research; interpretive and other qualitative forms were deemed by many to be superior for a range of disciplines, including nursing.

In the 1960s, the nursing discipline was given opportunities for development by a nursing science that was driven by an empiricist or logical positivist philosophy. Edwards (1999) suggested that nursing was driven to claim its science base for reasons of prestige and status, as well as a need to be perceived as a 'successful' profession. He concluded that nursing did not qualify as a legitimate science, since it had to be empirical (and was not). Nurse researchers and scholars acknowledged the inappropriateness for *all* nursing research to be undertaken using the empiricist model, because many of the questions framed were not valid for nursing knowledge development (Whittemore 1999). Winters and Ballou (2004:533) argued that 'legitimate science includes both empirical and non-empirical scientific methods'.

However, if we return to the argument that has been developed, given society's attitudes to women, and hence nurses, there is more value in conforming to the dominant culture (i.e. 'scientific research' that is acceptable to masculinist science). This is not appropriate, however, because it will not answer many of the questions nursing asks. Thus, Winters and Ballou (2004:533) proposed that nursing should work towards integrating 'all applicable modes of scientific inquiry into the discipline'.

An alternative approach for the development of nursing knowledge underpinned by feminist principles provided nurses with understandings of what it was they knew, and what it was they experienced, which involved reclaiming and renaming nursing's experiences and knowledge of the social world lived in and daily constructed. Rancine (2003:91) contended that there were other promising and more appropriate ways of developing knowledge that supported social activism, including that deriving from nursing research. These included the use of critical and feminist approaches to explore 'health issues related to race, gender, and social classes'. This built on the work of Doering (1992:25), who suggested that feminism and post-structuralism were particularly relevant to nursing because they incorporated the concepts of the female experience and of power. These concepts reflected the historical, social and political dynamics in which the discipline of nursing operated. They encompassed a theme central to nursing—that of powerlessness, characterised by oppression, submission and male domination.

It is important to note that feminist research 'permits the recognition and exploration of socio-cultural factors that transcend gender' (Jackson 1997:87), which signalled that, while the concept of oppression was central to feminism, it was clearly shared with other groups (Evans 1997). Thus:

> Accepting that experiences around oppression and struggle are not exclusive to women permits recognition that institutionalised patriarchy and androcentricity are oppressive to all but those of the dominant class, race and gender.
> (Jackson 1997:87)

This insight attempted to deal with the charge by Allen et al (1991) that feminist research marginalised men. These authors raised the question of whether research involving only women simply 'supports a conceptual scheme that reinforces the material subjugation of women' and thus 'perpetuates problematic social categories' (Allen et al 1991:50). They concluded, somewhat controversially, that 'a better strategy is to deconstruct the dichotomy itself and to expand awareness of the diverse contemporary and historical forms of gendered existence' (Allen et al 1991:56), which subsequently occurred.

It was thus reasonable to support the view that the value of feminist research was that it 'empowers women and addresses issues that can make a difference to the quality of life for all humankind' (Parker & McFarland 1991:66). There were those who believed that nursing research should be approached from a much broader perspective and incorporated a range of paradigms (Brayton 1997, accessed online 2012, and Milojevic 2008, accessed online 2012, who also recommended there be a 'futures lens' applied). The method used is defined by the questions being asked. Unfortunately, too, the method may be driven by other motives, such as economic rationalism and the need to obtain research funding, regardless of the ethical and moral imperatives that would normally guide research behaviour. But it was clear that the research approach took into account the context in which it was to be conducted, and for nursing this had political and power implications. There was no question that gender was a critical and all-encompassing variable to be acknowledged. And it was feminist theory that has largely been responsible for raising nursing's consciousness in this domain.

MEN IN NURSING: THE DEBATE CONTINUES

It has long been noted that men are a minority in nursing, despite the fact that their numbers have increased over the decades. In 2005, the nursing workforce in the United States consisted of 5.9% men (Donley 2005, Janiszewski Goodin 2003), increasing to 6.6% (American Association of Colleges of Nursing 2011), while in 1998 they comprised 4.4% of the Canadian workforce (Meadus 2000). Note that this had improved to 5.1% by 2008 (see Table 12.1), and is now suggested to be between 5 and 10% (McDonald 2012).

Table 12.1
Registered nurses gender breakdown

	Female	Percentage	Male	Percentage
Australia[1]	169,800	92.8%	13,244	7.2%
Canada	219,161	94.9%	11,796	5.1%
Denmark	50,817	96.5%	1,850	3.5%
Germany	10,003	94.5%	582	5.5%
Iceland (2003)	3,112	98.7%	40	1.3%
Ireland[2]	35,990	92%	3,129	8%
New Zealand	29,782	93.5%	2,056	6.5%
Norway (2003)	50,691	92.5%	2,056	7.5%
Sweden	107,382	90%	11,983	10%
United Kingdom	580,000	89.9%	65,000	10.1%
United States[3]	N/A	95%	N/A	5%

[1] Labour Force, Australian, Detailed, Quarterly: www.abs.gov.au/ausstats/abs@nsf/mf/6291.0.55.003.
[2] Loughrey M 2008 Just how male are male nurses? Journal of Clinical Nursing 17:1327–1334. This article suggests that the ratio of female to male general nurses is approximately 20:1.
[3] Donley Sr R 2005 Challenges for nursing in the 21st century. Nursing Economic$ 23(6):312.
Source: International Council of Nurses Nursing Workforce Profile 2004. Online. Available: www.icn.ch/Flash/SewDatasheet04.swf 8 Aug 2008.

This compares to statistics from Britain, where male nurses constitute 10.1% of the qualified nursing workforce (Marsh 2012), while in Australia it is approximately 9.6% (Australian Institute of Health and Welfare 2012). In Germany, male nurses comprise 18% of the nursing workforce (McDonald 2012). The International Council of Nurses Nursing Profile (2004) provides an international snapshot of the gender breakdown of nurses in a range of countries (see Table 12.1).

In the United States, male students comprised 8.6% in baccalaureate programs, 9.6% in masters' programs and 6.7% in doctoral programs (American Association of Colleges of Nursing 2002). In the United Kingdom, 14% of nursing students are male. The proportion of male nursing undergraduate students in Australia increased from 11.9% in 1987–90 to 15.9% in 1995 (Brown 1998). It is unfortunate that updated Australian statistics are unable to be located.

A very early Australian study by Sharman et al (1996) concluded that women were supporting men in the workforce and the home, often at the expense of their own career advancement. More recently, Brown and Jones (2004) found that taking a career break, or working less than full time, significantly reduced women's chances of occupying senior positions. This was based on any significant interruption of full-time work, rather than seniority.

What is historically interesting is that this finding was previously highlighted in other traditionally female occupations, such as teaching, physiotherapy, occupational therapy, librarianship and social work (Williams 1992). What it demonstrated was that males tended to move into powerful positions over the largest occupational group in the health workforce, nursing, an occupational group that was traditionally 'managed, taught, disciplined and organised almost entirely by women' (MacGuire, cited in Sharman et al 1996). There was little doubt that 'the ideological climate, socialisation processes and women's family and domestic responsibilities underlie a glass ceiling for women and a glass elevator for men in non-traditional occupations' (Sharman 1998:56).

Nevertheless, males continued to be viewed as increasingly disadvantaged and reduced to 'lifting machines' (Shakespeare 2003:53). Loughrey's research (2008) indicated that male nurses viewed themselves as a source of strength and valued for their ability to deal with aggressive patients. The negative side of this was, however, that male nurses accounted for up to 60% of nurses who were deregistered, when accused of physical abuse.

While men in some numbers were relative newcomers to nursing, they were increasingly being promoted to higher levels than women, despite their disproportionate numbers; furthermore, they seemed to have less experience and fewer qualifications (Evans 2004). This appears to have been due to a recruitment campaign, which attacked the negative stereotype of men in nursing, and highlighted the fact that management positions were 'made ripe for male capture', thus positioning men with 'poor formal educational qualifications' (Evans 2004:326) for leadership positions. As indicated earlier in this chapter, male nurses appear to be promoted to management positions regardless of their qualifications, which has long been recognised in the cited literature.

Some years ago, Brown's study (1998) found that men were overrepresented in senior nursing administrative positions. Although men comprised only 8% of the registered nurse workforce, they held 22% of senior nursing positions. Poliafico (1998) indicated that this comparative figure was only 6% in the United States, and suggested that there was a common misconception that men held a disproportionate number of administrative positions. Brown (1998:21) considered a range of explanations as to why this was happening in Australia. One of the most compelling was that women were seen to be invading the workplace, since workplaces were constructed by men. So it was that even in 'women's occupations', such as nursing, where it may be expected that men would be perceived as not fitting in, the overriding culture of the workplace turned this disjunction into a benefit for men.

Thus men who entered nursing were seen to be 'lowering themselves, losing status by undertaking "women's work"' (Brown 1998:21), yet were expected to be better workers than female nurses. They retained the benefits of their ascribed gender role: they were seen to be the 'breadwinner', to have leadership qualities, to be worth mentoring (since they were more likely to be serious about their career) and they were more likely to be assisted in accessing 'power networks' in nursing. Hicks (1999) argued that if men in these top positions behaved consistently with the findings of research studies, then they were most likely to reproduce themselves at these top-level positions. This would then serve to widen the gender/power divisions in nursing.

Further evidence that men were being promoted to the highest levels of service in nursing, despite their numerical minority, was provided by Boughn (2001:23) who noted that 'men who go into nursing rise like cream in milk' because they expected practical rewards and set up their lives to achieve and retain these, whereas women failed to recognise their economic and political power. More recently, it has been suggested that males gravitate towards administrative and more highly paid nursing jobs to reduce role strain and discomforting dissonance (Stott 2004). This led to some interesting scholarly work that interrogates masculinities and gender (Anthony 2006, Brown 2009, McDonald 2012).

A study which examined senior nursing administrative positions in the United Kingdom found that, in 1987, 8.6% of registered nurses were men, but 50.3% held chief nurse/advisor posts, and 57.8% were directors of nursing education (Gaze 1987). There has been a disproportionate increase of males in senior nursing positions in the United Kingdom (Ford et al 2010; Vere-Jones 2008), which also occurred in the United States. It should be noted, however, that there was a concerted effort in the United Kingdom to 'defeminise' management within nursing, enabling men to be more easily promoted into these positions (Carpenter 1977). McDonald (2012:2) does point out that there can be disadvantages of being 'kicked upstairs' to administrative and management positions: for example, they may be excluded from performing certain tasks, such as maternity and newborn nursing duties.

Jenkins (1989) noted that Florence Nightingale had a vision that nursing would always be under the control of women; she saw no place in nursing for men, just as there was no place for men in controlling nursing. Mackintosh (1997) and Meadus (2000) believed that the contribution of men to nursing was not recognised and that it was time for affirmative action in favour of men for nursing to survive the twenty-first century. This means 'that the Nightingale image must be counter-balanced by the entry and acceptance of larger numbers of men into the profession' (Meadus 2000:10, also see Chung 2001).

This view was rejected by other researchers who suggested that nursing, rather than increasing male numbers, should introduce feminist strategies to enhance the power of women nurses, since their lower disproportionate voice in academic writing and actual power in practice requires improvement (Ryan & Porter 1993:43, Shields et al 2011). Other research that focused on the experience of male nurses suggested that attrition was a major issue, due to the treatment given to males (Kelly et al 1996, Morin 1999).

To counteract the inequities experienced by men in nursing, the American Assembly for Men in Nursing was formed in 1971 (Evans 2004). Its aims were 'to recruit more men into the profession, to provide support to those men who already are nurses, and to increase the visibility of men in nursing' (Poliafico 1998:43). Evans (2004) documented how nursing associations acted as gatekeepers of change, limiting men's participation in nursing, including the refusal of approval to employ male nurse educators, on the grounds that it was inappropriate for men to teach women how to nurse. Gendered attitudes, which were 'reinforced and perpetuated by patriarchal societal institutions and processes' (Evans 1997:231), continue. The solution lay in challenging stereotypes of femininity and masculinity and, in the latter case, of assisting male nurses to critically examine their 'gender curio status' (Loughrey 2008). For McDonald (2012) it is also an issue of female nurses critically examining their gender norms and values. The matter of addressing structural relations is also an obvious requirement for change.

CONCLUSION

The aim of this chapter was to bring into sharp focus the gendered culture of nursing. Quite clearly there are inequities at work that can be documented with respect to control, management and leadership in nursing. Additionally, there are more subtle ways that gender impacts on nursing. This chapter has argued that historically, nursing work in all its forms (including clinical practice, education and research), mostly undertaken by women, has been affected severely by gender because of its construction and the context in which nursing is carried out (Valentine 2001). Becoming aware of such systematic oppressions is the first step in changing paternalistic structures and systems that operate to disadvantage nurses, their patients and the overall healthcare system (Giddings 2005).

Over a decade ago, David (2000:90) suggested that nurses 'must reframe the sociopolitical reality and give it back'; otherwise they will continue to be 'shackled in servitude, denied freedom to acknowledge the full benefit of their health and healing practices'. This remains true today. Failure to challenge the stereotypes rife in nursing effectively results in collusion 'with nursing's power brokers in maintaining for the nurse the status of "trained worker" as opposed to that of "learned professional"' (Fealy 2004:654). And such challenges are part of that which the feminisms sought to contribute to the nursing profession, and continue to do, in many but subtle ways.

REFLECTIVE QUESTIONS

1 What do you think the feminisms have to offer to the various generations of nurses, from 'baby boomer' to 'generation Y', and to the discipline of nursing, including its academic and clinical aspects?

2 Do you believe that the role and function of nursing cannot be separated from nurses who undertake it? If so, why is this? If you disagree, outline your arguments to support your position.

3 What do you think of the fact that men in nursing, despite their numerical minority, have the majority of leadership positions? Why do you think this is? What implications does this have for nursing as a profession?

RECOMMENDED READINGS

Barrett M, Phillips A (eds) 1992 Destabilizing theory: contemporary feminist debates. Polity Press, Cambridge

Caro J, Fox C 2008 The F word: how we learned to swear by feminism. University of New South Wales Press, Sydney

Davies C 1995 Gender and the professional predicament in nursing. Open University Press, Buckingham

Donley R 2005 Challenges for nursing in the 21st century. Nursing Economic$ 23(6):312–318

Dux M, Simic Z 2008 The great feminist denial. Melbourne University Press, Melbourne

Jayatilaka G 2001 Rebranding feminism? Geethika Jayatilaka's talk. Online. Available: www.thefword.org.uk/features/2001/12/rebranding_feminism_geethika_jayatilakas_talk 6 Aug 2008

REFERENCES

Allen D G, Allman K K M, Powers P 1991 Feminist nursing research without gender. Advances in Nursing Science 13(3):49–58

American Association of Colleges of Nursing 2002 Annual state of the schools. Online. Available: www.aacn.nche.edu/media/annual report02.pdf 14 Feb 2003

American Association of Colleges of Nursing 2011 New AACN data show an enrolment surge in baccalaureate and graduate programs amid calls for more highly educated nurses. Online. Available: http://www.aacn.ncha.edu/news/articles/2012/enrollment-data 24 August 2012

Anthony A S 2006 Tear down the barriers of gender bias. Men in Nursing Journal August:43–49. Online: www.meninnursingjournal.com

Aronson P 2003 Feminists or postfeminists? Young women's attitudes toward feminism and gender relations. Gender and Society 17(6):903–922

Australian Institute of Health and Welfare 2012 Nursing and midwifery workforce. Online. Available: http://www.aihw.gov.au/nursing-midwifery-workforce/ 24 August 2012

Bartram T, Casimir G, Djurkovic N, Leggat S G, Stanton P 2012 Do perceived high performance work systems influence the relationship between emotional labour, burnout and intention to leave? A study of Australian nurses. Journal of Advanced Nursing 68(7):1567–1578

Baumgardner J, Richards A 2003 The number one question about feminism. Feminist Studies 29(2):448–454

Bent K N 1993 Perspectives on critical and feminist theory in developing nursing praxis. Journal of Professional Nursing 9(5):296–303

Bolton S C 2000 Who cares? Offering emotion work as a 'gift' in the nursing labour process. Journal of Advanced Nursing 32(3):580–586

Boughn S 2001 Why women and men choose nursing. Nursing and Health Care Perspectives 22(1):14–24

Boyle M V 2002a Sailing twixt Scylla and Charybdis. Women in Management Review 17(3/4):131–141

Boyle M V 2002b You wait until you get home: emotional regions, emotional process work and the role of off-stage support. Paper presented at the 'Third emotions in organisational life conference', Bond University, Gold Coast

Branch S, Ramsay S, Barker M 2012 Workplace bullying, mobbing and general harassment: a review. International Journal of Management Reviews Online, 6 June

Brayton J 1997 What makes feminist research feminist? The structures of feminist research within the social sciences. Online. Available: www.unb.ca./PAR-L/win/feminmethod.htm August 2012

Briles J 1994 The Briles report on women in healthcare: changing conflict to collaboration in a toxic workplace. Jossey-Bass, San Francisco

Brown B 2009 Men in nursing: re-evaluating masculinities, re-evaluating gender. Contemporary Nurse 33(2):120–129

Brown C R 1998 Gender segmentation in the paid work force: the case of nursing. Unpublished PhD thesis. Griffith University, Brisbane

Brown C, Jones L 2004 The gender structure of the nursing hierarchy: the role of human capital. Gender, Work and Organization 11(1):1–25

Brykczynska G (ed) 1997 Caring: the compassion and wisdom of nursing. Arnold, London

Bubeck P E 1995 Care, gender and justice. Clarendon Press, Oxford

Buchanan T 1997 Nursing our narratives: towards a dynamic understanding of nurses in literary texts. Nursing Inquiry 4(2):80–87

Caffrey R, Caffrey P 1994 Nursing: caring or codependent? Nursing Forum 29(1): 12–17

Carpenter M 1977 The new managerialism and professionalism in nursing. In: Stacey N, Reid M, Heath C, Dingwall R (eds) Health and the division of labour. Croom Helm, London, pp 165–191

Ceci C 2004 Gender, power, nursing: a case analysis. Nursing Inquiry 11(2):72–81

Center for American Nurses 2008 Lateral violence and bullying in the workplace. February:1–12

Cheek J, Rudge T 1995 Only connect … feminism and nursing. In: Gray G, Pratt R (eds) Scholarship in the discipline of nursing. Churchill Livingstone, Melbourne

Chou H Y, Hecker R, Martin A 2012 Predicting nurses' well-being from job demands and resources: a cross-sectional study of emotional labour. Journal of Nursing Management 20:502–511

Chung V 2001 Men in nursing. Minority Nurse. Online. Available: http://www.minoritynurse.com/men-nursing/ 14 August 2012

Creina J, Meadus R J (2008) Despite the barriers men nurses are satisfied with career choices. Canadian Journal of Career Development 7(1):30–34

Cude G, Winfrey K 2007 The hidden barrier: gender bias: fact or fiction. Association of Women's Health, Obstetric and Neonatal Nurses (AWHONN) 11(3):255–265

Curtis J, Bowen I, Reid A 2007 You have no credibility: nursing students' experiences of horizontal violence. Nurse Education Prac 7(3):156–163

David B A 2000 Nursing's gender politics: reformulating the footnotes. Advances in Nursing Science 23(1):83–94

Davies C 1995 Gender and the professional predicament in nursing. Open University Press, Buckingham

Demerouti E, Bakker A B, Nachreiner F, Schaufeli W B 2000 A model of burnout and life satisfaction amongst nurses. Journal of Advanced Nursing 32(2):454–464

Dendaas N 2004 The scholarship related to nursing work environments: where do we go from here? Advances in Nursing Science 27(1):12–21

Doering L 1992 Power and knowledge in nursing: a feminist poststructuralist view. Advances in Nursing Science 14(4):24–33

Donley R 2005 Challenges for nursing in the 21st century. Nursing Economic$ 23(6):312–318

Edwards S D 1999 The idea of nursing science. Journal of Advanced Nursing 29(3):563–569

Ehrenreich B, English D 1979 For her own good: 150 years of experts' advice to women. Pluto, London

Ekstrom D N 1999 Gender and perceived nurse caring in nurse–patient dyads. Journal of Advanced Nursing 29(6):1393–1401

Erturk Y 2004 Considering the role of men in gender agenda setting: conceptual and policy issues. Feminist Review 78(1):3–21

Evans J 2004 Men nurses: a historical and feminist perspective. Journal of Advanced Nursing 47(3):321–332

Evans M 1997 Introducing contemporary feminist thought. Blackwell, Oxford

Falk Rafael A 1996 Power and caring: a dialectic in nursing. Advances in Nursing Science 19(1):3–17

Falk Rafael A 1998 Nurses who run with the wolves: the power and caring dialectic revisited. Advances in Nursing Science 21(1):29–42

Fealy G M 2004 'The good nurse': visions and value in images of the nurse. Journal of Advanced Nursing 46(6):649–656

Fineman S 1993 (ed) Emotion in organizations. Sage, London

Ford S, Santry C, Gainsbury S 2010 Top hospitals show bias for male nurse directors. Nursing Times.net Online. Available: http://www.nursingtimes.net/whats-new-in nursing 24 August 2012

Freire P 2007 Pedagogy of the oppressed. Continuum, New York

Gamarnikow E 1978 Sexual division of labour: the case of nursing. In: Kuhn A, Wolpe A M (eds) Feminism and materialism. Routledge & Kegan Paul, London

Gaze H 1987 Man appeal. Nursing Times 83(20):24–27

Georges J M, McGuire S 2004 Deconstructing clinical pathways: mapping the landscape of health care. Advances in Nursing Science 27(1):2–12

Gherardi S 1994 The gender we think, the gender we do in our everyday organizational lives. Human Relations 47(6):591–601

Giddings L S 2005 Health disparities, social injustice and the culture of nursing. Nursing Research 54(5):304–312

Goffman I 1959 Presentation of the self in everyday life. Overlook Press, New York

Grosz E 1990 Conclusion: a note on essentialism and difference. In: Gunew S (ed) Feminist knowledge: critique and construct. Routledge, London

Hagell E I 1989 Nursing knowledge: women's knowledge. A sociological perspective. Journal of Advanced Nursing 14:226–233

Hearn J 1993 Emotive subjects: organizational men, organizational masculinities and the (de)construction of 'emotions'. In: Fineman S (ed) Emotion in organizations. Sage, London

Hemmings C 2012 A genealogy of ambivalence: Emma Goldman, postfeminists and feminist politics for our times. The Politics of Location Revisited: Gender@2012. 8th European Feminist Research Conference, May, Budapest, Hungary

Henderson A 2001 Emotional labour and nursing: an under-appreciated aspect of caring work. Nursing Inquiry 8(2):130–138

Hicks C 1997 The research–practice gap: individual responsibility or corporate culture? Nursing Times 93(39):38–39

Hicks C 1999 Incompatible skills and ideologies: the impediment of gender attributions on nursing research. Journal of Advanced Nursing 30(1):129–139

Hothschild A R 1983 The managed heart: the commercialisation of human feeling. University of California Press, Berkeley

Huntington A 1996 Nursing research reframed by the inescapable reality of practice: a personal encounter. Nursing Inquiry 3(3):167–171

Hutchinson M, Vickers M, Jackson D, Wilkes L 2006 Workplace bullying in nursing: towards a more critical organisational perspective. Nursing Inquiry 13(2): 118–126

Huynh T, Alderson M, Thompson M 2008 Emotional labour underlying caring: an evolutionary concept analysis. Journal of Advanced Nursing 64(2):195–208

International Council of Nurses Nursing Profile 2004 Online. Available: www.icn. ch/Flash/SewDatasheet04.swf 8 Aug 2008

Jackson D 1997 Feminism: a path to clinical knowledge development. Contemporary Nurse 6(2):85–91

Janiszewski Goodin H 2003 The nursing shortage in the United States of America: an integrative review of the literature. Journal of Advanced Nursing 43(4):335–350

Jayatilaka G 2001 Rebranding feminism? Geethika Jayatilaka's talk. Online. Available: www.thefword.org.uk/features/2001/12/rebranding_feminism_geethika_jayatilakas_talk 6 Aug 2008

Jenkins E 1989 Nurses' control over nursing. In: Gray G, Pratt R (eds) Issues in Australian nursing 2. Churchill Livingstone, Melbourne

Kane D, Thomas B 2000 Nursing and the 'f' word. Nursing Forum 35(2):17–25

Kelly A 1985 The construction of masculine science. British Journal of Sociology of Education 6:33–154

Kelly N R, Shoemaker M, Steele T 1996 The experience of being a male student nurse. Journal of Nursing Education 35(4):170–174

Kitson A 2004 Drawing out leadership. Journal of Advanced Nursing 48(3):211

Lather P 1991 Feminist research in education: within/against. Deakin University Press, Geelong

Lavoie-Tremblay M, Leclerc E, Marchionni C, Drevniok U 2010 The needs and expectations of Generation Y nurses in the workplace. Journal for Nurses in Staff Development 26(1):2–8

Liaschenko J, Peter E 2004 Nursing ethics and conceptualizations of nursing: profession, practice and work. Journal of Advanced Nursing 46(5):488–495

Loughrey M 2008 Just how male are male nurses ...? Journal of Clinical Nursing 17(10):1327–1334

Lupton D 1998 The emotional self. Sage, London

McDonald J 2012 Conforming to and resisting dominant gender norms: how male and female nursing students do and undo gender. Gender, Work and Organisation 19(1):508–527

Mackintosh C 1997 A historical study of men in nursing. Journal of Advanced Nursing 26:232–236

McQueen A C H 2004 Emotional intelligence in nursing work. Journal of Advanced Nursing 47(1):101–108

McVicar A 2003 Workplace stress in nursing: a literature review. Journal of Advanced Nursing 44(6):633–642

Maher J M, Lindsay J, Bardoel A, Advocat J 2008 Flexibility and more? Nurses working and caring. School of Political and Social Inquiry and the Australian Centre for Research in Employment and Work, Monash University, Melbourne

Mann S, Cowburn J 2005 Emotional labour and stress within mental health nursing. Journal of Psychiatric and Mental Health Nursing 12:154–162

Marsh B 2012 More men than ever work as hospital nurses. Online. Available: http://www.dailymail.co.uk/health/article-145183/ 24 August 2012

Martinez-Indigo D, Totterdell P, Alcover C M, Holman D 2007 Emotional labour and emotional exhaustion: interpersonal and intrapersonal mechanisms. Work and Stress 21(1):30–47

Mazhindu D 2003 Ideal nurses: the social construction of emotional labour. European Journal of Psychotherapy Counselling and Health 6(3):243–262

Meadus R J 2000 Men in nursing: barriers to recruitment. Nursing Forum 35(3): 515

Milojevic I 2008 Feminism, future studies and the futures of feminist research. Journal of Policy, Planning and Future Studies 40(4):313–318

Milojevic I, Hurley K, Jenkins A 2008 Introduction: futures of feminism. Futures 40:313–318

Morin K H 1999 Mothers: responses to care given by male nursing students during and after birth. Image: Journal of Nursing Scholarship 31(1):83–87

Myerson D E 2000 If emotions were honoured: a cultural analysis. In: Fineman S Emotion in organizations, 2nd edn. Sage, London

Neuman C E 1999 Taking charge: nursing, suffrage and feminism in America, 1873–1920 (review). Journal of Women's History 10(4):228–235

Nicolson P 1996 Gender, power and organisation: a psychological perspective. Routledge, London

Norris T L 2010 Lateral violence: is nursing at risk? Tennessee Nurse 73(2):1

Paliadelis P 2005 Rural nursing unit managers: education and support for the role. The International Electronic Journal of Rural and Remote Health Research, Education Practice and Policy 5(1):325. Online. Available: http://rrh.deakin.edu.au

Paliadelis P 2008 The working world of nursing unit managers: responsibility without power. Australian Health Review 32(2):256–264

Paliadelis P, Cruickshank M, Sheridan A 2007 Caring for each other: how nurse managers 'manage' their role. Journal of Nursing Management 15(8):830–837

Parker B, McFarland J 1991 Feminist theory and nursing: an empowerment model for research. Advances in Nursing Science 13(3):59–67

Peter E, Lunardi V L, Macfarlane A 2004 Nursing resistance as an ethical action: literature review. Journal of Advanced Nursing 46(4):403–416

Poliafico J K 1998 Nursing's gender gap. Registered Nurse 61(10):39–43

Rancine L 2003 Implementing a postcolonial feminist perspective in nursing research related to non-Western populations. Nursing Inquiry 10(2):91–102

Roberts S J 2000 Development of a positive professional identity: liberating oneself from the oppressor within. Advances in Nursing Science 22(4):71–83

Rockler-Gladen N 2008 Third wave feminism: personal empowerment dominates this feminist philosophy. Online. Available: http:feminism.suite101.com/article. cfm/third_wave_feminism 6 August

Rodwell J, Demir D 2012 Psychological consequences of bullying for hospital and aged care nurses. International Nursing Review 59(4):539–546

Ryan S, Porter S 1993 Men in nursing: a cautionary critique. Nursing Outlook 41(6):262–267

Sadiqi F 2012 The shifting gender roles in North Africa: the crisis of patriarchy in the digital age. The Politics of Location Revisited: Gender@2012. 8th European Feminist Research Conference, May, Budapest, Hungary

Sandelowski M 1997 (Ir)reconcilable differences? The debate concerning nursing and technology. Image: Journal of Nursing Scholarship 29(2):169–174

Shakespeare P 2003 Nurses' bodywork: is there a body of work? Nursing Inquiry 10(1):47–56

Sharman E 1998 The glass elevator: how men overtake women in the nursing higher education workforce in Australia. Unpublished PhD thesis, University of New South Wales, Sydney

Sharman E, Short S, Black D 1996 Why so many? The masculine mystique and men in the nursing higher education workforce in Australia. Conference proceedings of the 'Changing society for women's health conference', Australian National University, Canberra

Shields L, Hall J, Namum A A 2011 The 'gender gap' in authorship in nursing literature. Journal of the Royal Society of Medicine 104(11):457–464

Stanley K M 2010 The high cost of lateral violence in nursing. Sigma Theta Tau International Leadership Summit, Atlanta Georgia (24 April)

Stott A 2004 Issues in the socialisation process of the male student nurse: implications for retention in undergraduate nursing courses. Nurse Education Today 24:91–97

Street A 1995 Nursing replay: researching nursing culture together. Churchill Livingstone, Melbourne

Treacy M P 1989 Gender prescription in nurse training: its effects on health provision. In: Hardy L K, Randell J (eds) Recent advances in nursing: issues in women's health. Churchill Livingstone, Edinburgh

Tronto J C 1999 Caring: gender-sensitive ethics. Hypatia 14(1):112–120

Tugung K, Villafana-Reynoso A 2008 Men in nursing: a look at the minority in the nursing field. March 3. Online. Available: http://malesinnursing.blogspot.com.au 28 August 2012

Valentine P E B 2001 A gender perspective on conflict management strategies of nurses. Journal of Nursing Scholarship 33(1):69–79

Varaei S, Vasimoradi M, Jasper M, Faghihzadeh S 2012 Iranian nurses self-perception – factors influencing nursing image. Journal of Nursing Management 20:551–560

Wadsworth Y 2001 What is feminist research? Paper presented at Bridging the Gap: Feminisms and Participatory Action Research Conference, Boston, June

Weir H, Waddington K 2008 Continuities of caring? Emotion work in a NHS direct call centre. Nursing Inquiry 15(1):67–77

Vere-Jones E 2008 Why are there so few men in nursing? Nursing Times.net Online. Available: http://www.nursingtimes.net/why-are-there-so-few-men-in-nursing/849269.article 24 August 2012

Whittemore R 1999 Natural science and nursing science: where do the horizons fuse? Journal of Advanced Nursing 30(5):1027–1033

Williams C 1992 The glass escalator: hidden advantages for men in the 'female' professions. Social Problems 39(3):253–267

Winter R 2009 Top 10 traits every nurse should have. Online. Available: http://blog.soliant.com August 2012

Winters J, Ballou K A 2004 The idea of nursing science. Journal of Advanced Nursing 45(5):533–535

Wuest J 1997 Illuminating environmental influences on women's caring. Journal of Advanced Nursing 26(1):49–58

Wynter V 2006 Feminism is passé because it worked. Online. Available: www.onlineopinion.com.au/view.asp?article=4781 6 Aug 2008

Zebroski S A 2001 The gender lens: caring and gender. Journal of Comparative Family Studies 32(2):322–323

CHAPTER 13

Power and politics in the practice of nursing

Jean Gilmour and Annette Huntington

LEARNING OBJECTIVES

After completing this chapter, the reader will:

- understand the nature of power and politics
- have an awareness of different theoretical conceptions of power
- understand the way in which nurses possess power individually and collectively
- understand the advocacy role and how it relates to power
- appreciate the complexities of whistleblowing and its consequences.

KEY WORDS

Power, politics, agency, influence, advocacy, whistleblowing

NURSING AND POLITICS

Nursing is a political activity. Politics, in the broadest sense of the word, is part of all nurses' lives, especially in the large institutions within which many of us work. It is therefore important to think about power and politics. At the very least, we need to understand that the health sector is a highly politicised environment at both micro and macro levels, and that it is not an apolitical or neutral site. As nurses, we have considerable power in this highly political arena.

Health is fundamental to life, and nurses are intimately involved in caring for the sick and supporting the healthy, either directly or indirectly, wherever they are working. Nurses are in a privileged position in that millions of people every day put their trust in nurses and assume that nurses will always work on the public's behalf. When you become a nurse, you accept the obligations and expectations that go with being in that highly responsible and highly respected (particularly by the general public) role. With registration comes the commitment and accountability to work within a code of ethics, at the centre of which is the safety and wellbeing of those for whom you provide care. Key to the delivery of safe care is using the power that you have wisely, and being aware of the moral and ethical obligations you have because of this position of trust.

Every nurse has a degree of power. Even as a newly registered nurse you immediately have power over patients/clients, who are nearly always in a less powerful position due to your knowledge of both health and illness, and the healthcare system. Knowledge is power, and just the ability to impart or withhold information puts nurses in a privileged position in relation to the people and/or communities with whom they work. Henderson's (2003) research in Western Australia exploring the power imbalance between nurses and patients clearly highlighted this, as the nurses in the study showed a reluctance to share any meaningful power with the patients. As the author says: 'This imbalance of power was most evident in information-giving and during nurse–patient interactions, where nurses used their power to maintain control' (Henderson 2003:504).

More recent Australian research around vital information provision for Yolngu from North West Arnhem Land who have chronic illness (Lowell et al 2012) and family caregivers of people with dementia (Bauer et al 2011) also reports disempowering gaps in health professionals' communication. In contrast, patients involved directly in information exchanges at bedside handovers as nurses changed shifts in a Queensland hospital ward study commented that they felt acknowledged as partners and that there was recognition that they had a 'legitimate right to information on their condition' (McMurray et al 2011:22).

In addition to an individual nurse's power in the patient/client relationship, nurses as a collective also have considerable potential power. In many countries, nurses are the largest occupational group in the healthcare sector. In New Zealand, there are 48,563 practising registered nurses (Nursing Council of New Zealand 2012a) and in Australia 260,121 registered nurses (Australian Institute of Health and Welfare 2011). Many of the reforms and restructuring that have taken place in Western health systems in recent years are focused on controlling and managing this considerable workforce—often due to the perceived cost of providing nurses' services in the health sector. However, these same numbers give nurses power—power that can be used to influence the health system and improve it for both nurses and the public. McKenna (2010:397) argues: 'If nurses began to speak with one voice, the power emanating from such a unified workforce would move political mountains'. To be active in such a way, nurses require an understanding of power and its effects, and the way that they can use their power to enhance the health and wellbeing of people.

Power is often considered a negative and oppressive attribute. However, more recent definitions of the nature of power discussed in this chapter incorporate the notion of power as constructive and constitutive, as well as having the potential to be destructive and oppressive. These definitions also provide nurses with a new way of considering power, where we can view nurses as being powerless in certain situations but very powerful in other circumstances. This representation frees us from the idea of inherent powerlessness and/or being victims, simply through being nurses. Rethinking and reshaping of nurses' positioning in terms of agency is important in this era of intense governmental scrutiny and concerns about controlling health sector costs which impact on the resourcing of nursing care and workforce retention (Huntington et al 2011).

In this chapter the concept of power is explored with its multiple meanings and understandings. Nurses' political power is then examined followed by a discussion of power in practice, including issues of advocacy and whistleblowing.

UNDERSTANDING POWER

Power is a concept that has many meanings and definitions; different perceptions of power will influence people's actions and the outcomes of these actions. Simple definitions consider power to involve something one person has over another (Poggi 2001), and the potential to be influential; that is, make your ideas known to others and gain their support (Sullivan 2004). Harrison and Dye (2008) suggest influence is a form of power where particular effects are produced through a system of reward and punishment. They also argue that power is based on access to intertwined resources such as wealth, education, political influence and economics. Resources are not evenly distributed through society, and those with power control resources through rewards or the threat of deprivation of resources.

A nursing example of the nexus between power and control is the organisation of nurses' work life and conditions through shift rosters. Rotating shift work has negative effects on nurses' health and wellbeing (Chan 2008, Huntington et al 2011, Samaha et al 2007). Enabling nurses to have shift choices and shift stability would be a sound managerial approach. However, rostering practices are enacted in a range of ways, from an autocratic top-down directive with no space for personal preferences, to a participatory style of management where the nurses in a ward or unit manage their own roster and the allocation of patient care. Ultimately, the manager or clinical leader has control over shift allocation processes.

Michel Foucault (1980), a French philosopher, has another viewpoint on power. He conceptualises power as being exercised, productive and as emulating from below. This view means that people traditionally constructed as powerless and oppressed can be represented as having agency—defined as the capacity to act and exert power, and therefore effecting the way it is enacted. Power circulates, rather than being localised 'never in anybody's hands, never appropriated as a commodity or piece of wealth' (Foucault 1980:98). People are simultaneously affected by power relationships and participate in those relationships.

Foucault's definition highlights the flow of power in everyday practices and relationships, and the inherent potential for the exercise of power as a productive force in social relationships. He also differentiates power relations from relations of force or violence where there are no choices. The significant factor for nurses in this representation of power is that power relationships involve the possibility of resistance—the person over whom power is exercised has the capacity to react and respond in a range of ways (Foucault 1983). Using the example of shift rosters discussed earlier, a study of Australian, New Zealand and United Kingdom nurses (Huntington et al 2011) found nurses reduced their hours of work or changed practice settings in response to unsatisfactory shift allocation and workload.

POLITICS AND POWER

Politics permeates all aspects of life. Chaffee et al (2012:5) define politics as 'the process of influencing the allocation of scarce resources'. As to who is influential, Lasswell (1958) describes them as those who get the most of what there is to get. If success in politics is judged by control over resources, nurses historically have been unsuccessful in the political arena when judged by factors such as pay parity with equivalent professional groups or satisfactory working environments. Sullivan (2004) argues that historical factors still impact on nurses' degree of influence in contemporary healthcare, with values such as personal discipline, a focus on service and obedience being seen by some as fundamental characteristics of nurses.

While many nurses have effectively engaged in politics at all levels, stereotypical views of nursing (discussed in Chapter 1), along with the issues around the gendered nature of nursing (discussed in Chapter 12), have limited the full realisation of nurses' and nursing's potential for political action, influence and advocacy. Takase et al (2001) also argue that nurses have been historically disadvantaged by their close relationship with medical colleagues. This has positioned the practice of nursing as subservient to the practice of medicine, and impacts negatively on nurses' perception of themselves. This perception can inhibit nurses from seeing the power that their increasing professionalisation confers.

Politics at state and national level is often thought of as only involving government. Governments are critical bodies for regulating behaviour in that 'government lays down the "rules of the game" in conflict and competition between individuals, organizations, and institutions within society' (Harrison & Dye 2008:198–9). But politics, seen as the exercise of power in the form of influence, is also part of everyday life. Engaging in political action—learning to be more influential in relation to matters that count—is therefore a possibility for all nurses. Sullivan (2004) suggests that influence exists through relationships and is more significant than authority. It is gained through position or respect for knowledge and skills. She also suggests that influence is earned through effort and that the skills of influence can be learnt, the most crucial factor being the personal decision to become influential.

Nurses tend to think that because they are good people doing a good job they should be valued and fairly rewarded and, if that does not happen, they blame themselves or the profession (Sullivan 2004). However, nurses may in fact be unrewarded due to not effectively engaging in the underlying political game, which requires adherence to a particular set of rules that they may not even know exists. Critically, we as nurses must therefore recognise the existence and reality of politics, the legitimacy and necessity of being involved in politics and learn skills to gain greater influence if personal and professional goals are to be achieved. Sullivan (2004) identifies some possible workplace strategies for developing influence, including:

- reciprocity with other workers (i.e. exchanging favours)
- having a good understanding of the informal information that circulates within the organisation
- avoiding confrontation
- compromising when necessary to achieve a more important goal
- networking
- accepting responsibility for individual actions, both positive and negative, and
- finding a mentor.

The idea of playing workplace politics may not initially resonate with the cherished nursing ideal of teamwork, but having influence and developing assertive and satisfying interdisciplinary relationships are essential factors in nurses being active in ensuring the provision of high-quality nursing care.

NURSES' COLLECTIVE POLITICAL POWER

All people have political power as individuals, but nurses also have great potential as a collective body to exercise their power. Australian and New Zealand nurses are well educated at graduate level and have an evidence-based body of knowledge to support nursing practice. Nurses also work in wide-ranging roles in healthcare, spanning clinical, management, research, teaching and health policy domains that provide multiple opportunities to exert influence.

A key element of realising collective power is having formal ways to organise groups of people with a common cause that is well articulated and appeals to broad segments of the population. In nursing, the protection, support and influence derived from the power of the collective is realised through professional organisations. This power is shown clearly in situations such as the guaranteed nurse–patient ratios negotiated in Victoria in 2001 and more recently in New South Wales after a concerted campaign in 2010, initiatives which have had a major impact on the working environment for nurses. Another example of collective bargaining power is the Multi Employer Collective Agreements negotiated by the New Zealand Nurses Organisation. These agreements would be impossible to negotiate at an individual level.

One of the most important choices you will make as a registered nurse, therefore, is the decision to join a professional body. There are many organisations that primarily serve to advance the interests of the nursing workforce. As nurses, there is the opportunity to be involved and shape the political activity of these organisations through contribution as a member or at governance level. While nurses are often considered a homogeneous group, it is important to accept that nurses are enormously diverse. As a result, while the overall goal of nursing may be shared by everyone in the profession, individual nurses will not always share worldviews at either the macro or micro level. Therefore, using the power nurses have means being highly skilled at working not only with diverse population groups, but also with diverse nurses and nursing groups. Nurses have widely differing philosophical and political positions, and one strategy for managing this diversity is through the focus that professional organisations can bring. This means that individual difference can be accepted, but organisational power can focus on collective professional issues.

The particular structure and focus of nursing groups varies considerably, but the broad areas of interest are industrial or employment concerns and what are loosely called 'professional issues'. The choice of which professional body to join should be given careful thought considering their role, focus and achievements and what they can provide. An overview of Australian and New Zealand organisations is provided at www.nurses.info/organizations_australia_newzealand.htm.

An example of nurses successfully using their collective political power to advance practice through the legislative process is the gaining of prescribing authority. Australian and New Zealand nurses have advocated for changes in legislation and governmental processes to enable nurses (usually advanced practitioners) to prescribe in their scope of practice. In New Zealand, extending prescribing rights to nurse practitioners has been contentious, with some members of the medical profession, such as general practitioners, concerned about potential competition for funding (Mackay 2003). After a drawn-out and contested political process, the Medicines (Designated Prescribers: Nurse Practitioners) Regulations 2005 provided a framework for nurse practitioner prescribing. This initial legislative platform is a starting point in expanding the prescribing role of registered nurses in order to more effectively meet the treatment needs of specific population groups. Developments since include the regulation Medicines (Designated Prescriber—Registered Nurses Practising in Diabetes Health) Regulations 2011 which enables authorised diabetes nurses to prescribe a range of medications. Further developments to allow clinical nurse specialists limited prescribing rights are also currently being progressed in New Zealand.

Jones' (2004) description of the approach taken by the Royal College of Nursing (RCN) in the United Kingdom points out the political skills required to advance the nursing agenda. He notes that the implementation of nurse prescribing required 'political machination, the need to construct an effective case, and deft manoeuvring within the corridors of power' (Jones 2004:266). Initial elements of the strategy to increase political influence included focusing on a clear objective, taking advantage of an existing opportunity (which in the United Kingdom was the review of community nursing), developing alliances with the British Medical Association and pharmacists and ensuring a unified professional position by managing internal concerns raised by groups such as practice nurses.

Table 13.1 lists some ways of developing influence through knowledge, communication skills and action.

POWER IN PRACTICE

Knowledge carries with it power and authority, but not all forms of knowledge are created equal. In the preceding section on nurses' political power, we discussed the power that nurses have as a collective. However, there is ample evidence to suggest that nurses have been conspicuously silent, or have been silenced, at times when it has been vital that patients have had vocal, assertive and knowledgeable advocates. Chiarella (2000) argues that, within the legal system, nurses are seen as a separate but subordinate group to medicine, which impacts on the authority of nurses' testimony and their opportunities to speak:

> Today or tomorrow or the next day, a nurse may or may not intervene to stop a doctor from making a mistake, which might harm the patient. It will not depend on the law. It will depend on how brave they are. They operate inside (or outside) a legal framework, which insufficiently recognises their work and their presence.
> (Chiarella 2000:198)

Table 13.1
Developing influence through knowledge, communication skills and action

Knowledge	Communication skills	Action
Nursing knowledge base		
Evidence-based clinical practice knowledge Patient and family knowledge/agendas/issues Policy/legislation knowledge at government, discipline and organisational levels	Articulate and assertive verbal communication Clear and appropriate written communication meeting academic/media/political/popular conventions, depending on context	Respond in a timely and coherent manner Document using appropriate channels Take opportunities to be involved in shaping policy through submissions and committee work Use information technology competently for communication and information retrieval
Understanding power		
Relationship of knowledge with power Power as a circulating force The capacity for resistance Differentiation of power relations and force relations	Professional introductions Title parity Adhere to professional code of dress Prepare accounts demonstrating importance of nursing work	Take leadership opportunities—formal and informal Accept responsibility Use knowledge to inform patients and families Act as an advocate
Understanding the rules of the game		
Nursing Healthcare teams Organisations Communities	Network within and outside the profession Develop and use relationships with media and politicians	Develop respectful and communicative relationships within and outside nursing Be tenacious Enlist support from broader communities of interest in issues of concern to nursing

One instance of the devaluation of nurses' knowledge and authority by the medical profession, with lethal results, involved 12 children who died during or shortly after undergoing cardiac surgery in a Canadian hospital in 1994. Nurses involved in the cardiac surgery service had made sustained attempts to voice their concerns through the appropriate hospital channels during the preceding year, but these had not been taken seriously (Ceci 2004). Medical peers of the surgeon dismissed the validity of claims by several nurses that there were competency issues on the grounds that nurses did not have medical expertise. In a similar Australian example, the repeated complaints of Queensland nurses about the actions of an incompetent surgeon, who was eventually implicated in at least 13 patient deaths, were not acted upon by the hospital Director of Medical Services (Davies 2005).

When nurses themselves feel powerless, however, they may choose not to act, and this can also have dire consequences. One example of this was revealed during New Zealand's Cartwright Inquiry into cervical cancer, which revealed unethical medical research practices and the lack of informed consent about treatment options. The approach to treatment, carried out from 1966 until the early 1980s, studied the progression of cervical cancer in situ in a group of women, without offering medical intervention, until progression to invasive cancer (Coney 1988). Nurses throughout this period working at this particular hospital did not openly voice their concerns or ensure the women had been provided with the information necessary to make an informed choice about participation. Judge Silvia Cartwright stated that:

> ... nurses who most appropriately should be advocates for the patient, feel sufficiently intimidated by the medical staff (who do not hire or fire them) that even today they fail or refuse to confront openly the issues arising from the 1966 trial.
> (Committee of Inquiry into Allegations Concerning the Treatment of Cervical Cancer at National Women's Hospital and into Other Related Matters 1988:172)

Although by speaking out the nurses at that time may not have been able to stop particular medical practices, their complicity through silence is something that nurses in New Zealand have had to acknowledge. Constructing ourselves as powerless and lacking in agency can lead to nurses behaving unethically and not putting patients' best interests at the centre of our professional obligations.

Buresh and Gordon have offered a powerful critique of nurses' lack of visibility and voice in the public arena, and suggest many strategies for 'creating a voice of agency' (Buresh & Gordon 2006:25). Expressing agency is built upon the realisation of the importance of nurses' work and the confidence of nurses themselves. To make this agency explicit requires change at the fundamental level of day-to-day practice. Every encounter with patients, families and other staff members is an opportunity to communicate, verbally and non-verbally, messages about the competency and the knowledge base underpinning our decisions and practices.

Expressing agency begins right at the first introduction to patients and colleagues. For example, status can be reinforced through the use of both first and last names rather than just first name, along with title and role, a professional standard of dress and non-deferential body language. Buresh and Gordon (2006) have written extensively on the necessity for nurses to take every opportunity to educate people they meet about what they do and why they do it:

> To convey the content of nursing, nurses must describe the complexity of care they give and the clinical judgments they use. They must be careful not to depict themselves as extensions of the doctor's agency in their discussions with patients and families, the broader public, the media, and political representatives.
> (Buresh & Gordon 2006:67)

As nurses, we are highly educated practitioners with both formal education in, and considerable informal knowledge of, the culture and processes of the health system within which our clients and patients find themselves. This has important implications for power relationships between ourselves and the people for whom we care.

An example of our everyday exercise of power is the categorisation of people through the practice of assessment and the ensuing allocation of resources to them. Assessment requires recording a range of information and judging whether a person meets certain predetermined criteria for normality and/or abnormality. The distribution of a wide range of resources, including the time and expertise of nurses and other health professionals, medical equipment, pharmaceuticals and access to the care setting, can be determined by nursing assessment. From a Foucauldian perspective, the assessment process therefore needs to incorporate opportunities for patients and their families to exercise some control. This can be achieved by providing information about the purpose, scope and implications of the assessment in clear language, obtaining informed consent and validating the documented information with the person concerned.

Power can also be used by nurses to improve practice and the experiences of the people and groups with whom we are working. We have chosen to highlight two particular situations or practices where power can be used by the individual nurse. The first of these is the advocacy role that for many nurses is an integral part of day-to-day practice, and the second is what is commonly called 'whistleblowing'.

Advocacy

Advocacy consists of taking action on behalf of a person, or supporting an individual or group to gain what they need from the system. This role is now considered a fundamental element of practice at all levels (Priest 2012). The *Code of Ethics for Nurses in Australia* states from the outset that nurses must take action when the standard of care is considered unacceptable; 'this includes a responsibility to question and report what they consider to be unethical behaviour and treatment' (Australian Nursing and Midwifery Council, Royal College of Nursing, Australia and the Australian Nursing Federation 2008:4). The increasingly overstretched and changing world of service delivery means that, more than ever before, nurses need to understand and enact this advocacy role at the micro and macro level.

Nurses may work on behalf of a person or group to advocate for resources or appropriate treatment and care. However, this approach could be seen as limiting the empowerment of individuals or groups—as in many instances it may be more appropriate to support a person or community to advocate for themselves (MacDonald 2006). It is important to recognise that acting as an advocate does not involve taking over the situation. This can result in a nurse acting out what he or she feels is best for the person, rather than acting to ensure that the person achieves what they want (Henderson 2003). Supporting individuals or groups to take action still involves the nurse in an act of advocacy, but one that reflects a more Foucauldian approach to power, in which everyone has power but may need support and information to enact that power. If a nurse is not able to act in this way, then the appropriate action is to ensure that the person or group has access to another source of advocacy.

To be able to act effectively as an advocate, nurses need the following:

- understanding of the politics, culture and systems of health sector institutions and health service delivery
- respect for the client or community and their rights
- understanding of relevant clinical issues

- understanding of ethical issues
- commitment to the client and/or group, and
- understanding of the need for evidence and the way it can be used to support decisions.

Advocacy can be used at all levels in the health system. It can be part of day-to-day practice in relationships with patients and clients, or it can involve influencing service delivery to enhance services for a client group or community as a whole. Advocacy at service delivery level aims to address health outcome disparities between different groups of the population. For instance, in New Zealand there are well-documented health disparities between Māori and non-Māori (Robson & Harris 2007). The Treaty of Waitangi negotiated in 1840 created a Crown obligation to preserve certain Māori rights and protections that can be applied to health service access and care (Kingi 2007). Consequently a key objective of *The New Zealand Health Strategy* (Minister of Health 2000:viii) is to 'ensure accessible and appropriate services for Māori'. Nurses are well placed to detect access and treatment issues and advocate for services that provide equitable healthcare.

Many nurses are also key players in special interest groups working with people with particular health issues. Patient and family representative groups are effective lobbyists often accorded a voice in health policy development. Joint initiatives with these groups offer productive alliances to further nurses', and health consumers', agendas focused on improving healthcare services (Davies 2004). For example, the Health and Disability Commissioner in New Zealand has established the New Zealand *Code of Health and Disability Services Consumers' Rights* (1996), which aims to protect consumers' rights, works in conjunction with a consumer advocate and has established a complaints system (see www.hdc.org.nz). Similarly a Queensland Ministerial Consumer Advisory Committee has been set up to support consumer involvement and advocacy in the health sector (Health Consumers Queensland 2011). It is important that nurses understand that there are limits to their advocacy skills, and that in some areas people may prefer external or non-health professional advocates. External advocates can be provided by special interest sector groups, or be paid independent advocates. Part of our advocacy role is to be aware of the form of advocacy that is preferred by the clients or patients concerned, and to be able to discuss this in an informed manner.

Whistleblowing

Whistleblowing requires assertive action in voicing concerns in the interests of the public about patient safety or serious misuse of resources. The Australian Nursing and Midwifery Council (2008:10) defines whistleblowing as employee information disclosure 'about misconduct, illegal, unethical or illegitimate practices that are within the control of their employers; to a person or an organisation that has the authority or power to take action'. There may be disclosure to authorities external to the organisational reporting processes.

Whistleblowing is an extremely serious action. There are major implications that must be considered by a nurse when he or she decides to take this step as nurses involved in whistleblowing situations, as whistleblowers and as those complained about, report significant negative emotional responses. A qualitative study of fourteen nurses who experienced a whistleblowing event reported that the nurses suffered a range of adverse emotional consequences (Peters et al 2011). The participants talked about various responses including sadness, depression, anxiety and panic attacks. Prolonged periods of time were spent reflecting on the experience. Disrupted family relationships have also been reported (Wilkes et al 2011). Nurses who take such action are courageous and need the support of colleagues, friends and family. Too often, those who choose to take a stand can feel isolated and are at risk of reprisal such as harassment and loss of employment (Brown 2006, Jackson et al 2010).

Jackson and Raftos (1997) found in their research with registered nurses that whistleblowing was an extremely difficult decision, and one that left the nurses feeling exposed and unsupported. However, this study also highlights the way in which these particular nurses put their moral obligation to the residents above the possible harm they may experience themselves. The concept of 'personal resilience' is considered important in terms of being able to positively cope with adverse situations, and practise in difficult workplaces. It involves developing strategies such as productive professional networks and focusing on personal development in areas such as the maintenance of a positive attitude, work–life balance and emotional insight (Jackson et al 2007).

The public media has been used by some whistleblowers to draw attention to health issues. The media can serve a useful purpose in promoting accountability but also creates intense public scrutiny and critique, confidentiality concerns and may present an unbalanced picture (Firtko & Jackson 2005). Professional nursing guidelines are now available to inform decision making about when a situation is serious enough to warrant adopting a whistleblowing stance, guide how action should be taken and who to approach external to the organisation. The United Kingdom Nursing and Midwifery Council (2010) has developed a guideline, Raising and Escalating Concerns, which was produced in response to inquiry findings of systemic healthcare failure and patient neglect over many years (Francis 2010). All nurses received a copy of the guidelines. The United Kingdom guidelines stipulate that nurses and midwives must report public safety concerns (Nursing and Midwifery Council 2010) as does the Code of Professional Conduct for Nurses in Australia which states:

> Where nurses make a report of unlawful or otherwise unacceptable conduct to their employers, and that report has failed to produce an appropriate response from the employers, nurses are entitled and obliged to take the matter to an appropriate external authority.
> (Australian Nursing and Midwifery Council 2008:3)

Guidelines for taking action in reporting and escalating serious concerns include (i) acting immediately if people are put at risk because of another's action, (ii) using usual internal reporting procedures and informing the appropriate authority, (iii) providing written documentation, (iv) respecting patient confidentiality and (v) escalating the concern to an appropriate external healthcare or professional authority only after internal avenues are exhausted and after seeking expert advice (Greene & Latting 2004, Nursing and Midwifery Council 2010). The whistleblowing actions of Toni Hoffman, the Nurse Unit Manager of an Intensive Care Unit at a Queensland hospital, which were taken in response to concerns about the competence of a surgeon, follow these steps. She persistently communicated her concerns about specific cases that demonstrated issues with surgical clinical competence to the appropriate authorities, verbally and in writing. Her evidence was supported by written statements from

227

other nurses. As a last resort she approached the local Member of Parliament and her documentation was eventually tabled in the Queensland Parliament; processes were then initiated to address major and systemic health service issues (Davies 2005).

The need to legally protect people in whistleblowing situations is recognised with specific legislation aiming to ensure disclosures are investigated and to protect whistleblowers from retaliation. In New Zealand there exists the Protected Disclosures Act 2000 while Australian examples include the South Australian Whistleblowers Protection Act 1993, the Queensland Whistleblowers Protection Act 1994, the New South Wales Protected Disclosures Act 1994 and The Western Australia Public Interest Disclosure Act 2003. The legislation is variable across jurisdictions in terms of who is eligible for protection and the type of public sector wrongdoing covered (Brown 2006) and so it is essential to investigate what the applicable legislation provides in terms of protection.

The serious lapses in safe and humane healthcare noted in this chapter are rooted in systemic organisational inadequacies; as individuals nurses have been driven to bravely act against prevailing practices or alternatively have been part of the invisible forces enabling injustices to be perpetuated. Recent government and professional responses have been to clearly articulate to health services the criteria to be used as a basis in monitoring and improving the quality and safety of healthcare along with health professional accountability to act effectively when patient safety is at jeopardy (Australian Commission on Safety and Quality in Health Care 2010, Australian Nursing and Midwifery Council 2008, Nursing Council of New Zealand 2012b).

CONCLUSION

Nursing services are pivotal in the provision of healthcare. Nurses are mediators between healthcare institutions, with their associated mysterious practices, language and technologies, and the person—translating and making the health system understandable for the individual or community. Nurses are a powerful group, expert in terms of their knowledge base, their practice and their understanding of the impact of health on people and communities. This knowledge and experience places the nurse in a very powerful position in terms of being able to influence people they are working with to make particular decisions regarding their health and wellbeing. Understanding and being consciously political at both the collective and the individual levels is central to working with patients and clients to improve their experience of healthcare and their health outcomes.

REFLECTIVE QUESTIONS

1 Do you think you are influential as a nurse? If so, how have you become influential? If not how could you be more influential?

2 How can power imbalances between you and your patients be minimised in everyday practice?

3 What do you think patients and families need to know to be effective advocates for themselves and others?

4 What do you think are the most important steps to take when raising concerns about healthcare issues?

RECOMMENDED READINGS

Buresh B, Gordon S 2006 From silence to voice: what nurses know and must communicate to the public, 2nd edn. ILR Press, Ithaca

Stanley D 2011 Power, politics and leadership. In: Stanley D Clinical leadership: Innovation into action. Palgrave Macmillan, South Yarra, pp 290–310

Sullivan E J 2004 Becoming influential: a guide for nurses. Pearson/Prentice Hall, New Jersey

REFERENCES

Australian Commission on Safety and Quality in Health Care 2010 Australian Safety and Quality Framework for health care. Putting the framework into action: getting started. Guide for the health care team. Online. Available: http://www.safetyandquality.gov.au/wpcontent/uploads/2011/01/ASQFHC-Guide-Healthcare-team.pdf 11 July 2012

Australian Institute of Health and Welfare (AIHW) 2011. Nursing and midwifery labour force 2009. Bulletin no. 90. Cat. no. AUS 139. AIHW, Canberra. Online. Available: www.aihw.gov.au/publicationdetail/?id=10737419682 11 July 2012

Australian Nursing and Midwifery Council, Royal College of Nursing, Australia and the Australian Nursing Federation 2008 Code of ethics for nurses in Australia. Online. Available: www.nrgpn.org.au/index.php?element=anmc+code+of+ethics 11 July 2012

Australian Nursing and Midwifery Council 2008 Code of professional conduct for nurses in Australia. Online. Available: www.nrgpn.org.au/index. php?element=anmc+code+of+ethics 11 July 2012

Bauer M, Fitzgerald L, Koch S, King S 2011 How family carers view hospital discharge planning for the older person with a dementia. Dementia 10(3):317–323

Brown A 2006 Public interest disclosure legislation in Australia: Towards the next generation. Commonwealth Ombudsman, NSW Ombudsman, Queensland Ombudsman, Australia

Buresh B, Gordon S 2006 From silence to voice: what nurses know and must communicate to the public, 2nd edn. ILR Press, Ithaca

Ceci C 2004 Nursing, knowledge and power: a case analysis. Social Science and Medicine 59:1879–1889

Chaffee M, Mason D, Leavitt J 2012 A framework for action in policy and politics. In: Mason D, Leavitt J, Chaffee M (eds) Policy and politics in nursing and health care, 6th edn. Saunders, St Louis, pp 1–18

Chan M (2008) Factors associated with perceived sleep quality of nurses working on rotating shifts. Journal of Clinical Nursing 18:285–293

Chiarella M 2000 Silence in court: the devaluation of the stories of nurses in the narratives of health law. Nursing Inquiry 7(3):191–199

Committee of Inquiry into Allegations Concerning the Treatment of Cervical Cancer at National Women's Hospital and into Other Related Matters 1988 The report of the committee of inquiry into allegations concerning the treatment of cervical cancer at National Women's Hospital and into other related matters. The Committee, Auckland

Coney S 1988 The unfortunate experiment. Penguin Books, Auckland

Davies C 2004 Political leadership and the politics of nursing. Journal of Nursing Management 12:235–241

Davies G 2005 Queensland public hospitals commission of inquiry report. The State of Queensland. Online. Available: www.qphci.qld.gov.au/Final_Report.htm 11 July 2012

Firtko A, Jackson D 2004 Do the ends justify the means? Nursing and the dilemma of whistleblowing. Australian Journal of Advanced Nursing 23(1):51–56

Foucault M 1980 Two lectures. In: Gordon C (ed) Power/knowledge. Pantheon Books, New York, pp 78–108

Foucault M 1983 Afterword: the subject and power. In: Dreyfus H, Rabinow P Michel Foucault: beyond structuralism and hermeneutics, 2nd edn. University of Chicago Press, Chicago, pp 208–226

Francis R 2010 Report of the Independent Inquiry into care provided by Mid Staffordshire NHS Foundation Trust January 2005 – March 2009. The House of Commons, United Kingdom. Online. Available: www.midstaffs inquiry.com/assets/docs/Inquiry_Report-Vol1.pdf 11 July 2012

Greene A D, Latting J K 2004 Whistle-blowing as a form of advocacy: guidelines for the practitioner and organization. Social Work 49(2):1–13

Harrison B C, Dye T R 2008 Power and society: an introduction to the social sciences, 11th edn. Thomson Wadsworth, Belmont, California

Health Consumers Queensland 2011 Health advocacy framework. Strengthening health advocacy in Queensland. Online. Available: http://www.health.qld.gov.au/hcq/publications/hcq_framework_may11.pdf 11 July 2012

Henderson S 2003 Power imbalance between nurses and patients: a potential inhibitor of partnership in care. Journal of Clinical Nursing 12(4):501–508

Huntington A, Gilmour J, Tuckett A, Neville S, Wilson D, Turner C 2011 Is anybody listening? A qualitative study of nurses' reflections on practice. Journal of Clinical Nursing 20(9–10):1413–1422

Jackson D, Firtko A, Edenborough M 2007 Personal resilience as a strategy for surviving and thriving in the face of workplace adversity: a literature review. Journal of Advanced Nursing 60(1):1–9

Jackson D, Peters K, Andrew S, Edenborough M, Halcomb E, Luck L, Salamonson Y, Wilkes L 2010 Understanding whistleblowing: qualitative insights from nurse whistleblowers. Journal of Advanced Nursing 66(10):2194–2201

Jackson D, Raftos M 1997 In uncharted waters: confronting the culture of silence in a residential care institution. International Journal of Nursing Practice 3:34–39

Jones M 2004 Case report. Nurse prescribing: a case study in policy influence. Journal of Nursing Management 12:266–272

Kingi T R 2007 The Treaty of Waitangi: A framework for Māori health development. The New Zealand Journal of Occupational Therapy 54(1):4–10

Lasswell H 1958 Politics: who gets what, when, how. World Publishing Company, New York

Lowell A, Maypilama E, Yikaniwuy S, Rrapa E, Williams R, Dunn S 2012 'Hiding the story': indigenous consumer concerns about communication related to chronic disease in one remote region of Australia. International Journal of Speech – Language Pathology 14(3):200–208

MacDonald H 2006 Relational ethics and advocacy in nursing: literature review. Journal of Advanced Nursing 57(2):119–126

Mackay B 2003 General practitioners' perceptions of the nurse practitioner role: an exploratory study. The New Zealand Medical Journal 116(1170):356. Online. Available: www.nzma.org.nz/journal/116-1170/356 11 July 2012

McKenna H 2010 Nurses and politics—laurels for the hardy. International Journal of Nursing Studies 47(4):397–398

McMurray A, Chaboyer W, Wallis M, Johnson J, Gehrke T 2011 Patients' perspectives of bedside nursing handover. Collegian 18(1):19–26

Minister of Health 2000 The New Zealand health strategy. Ministry of Health, Wellington

Nursing and Midwifery Council 2010 Raising and escalating concerns: Guidance for nurses and midwives. United Kingdom. Online. Available: www.nmc-uk.org/Documents/Raising-and-Escalating-Concerns/Raising-and-escalating-concerns-guidance-A5.pdf 11 July 2012

Nursing Council of New Zealand 2012a The New Zealand nursing workforce: a profile of nurse practitioners, registered nurses, and enrolled nurses 2011. Wellington. Online. Available: http://www.nursingcouncil.org.nz/download/186/31march2011.pdf 23 July 2012

Nursing Council of New Zealand 2012b Code of conduct for nurses. Wellington. Online. Available: http://www.nursingcouncil.org.nz/download/283/coc-print.pdf 23 July 2012

Peters K, Luck L, Hutchinson M, Wilkes L, Andrew S, Jackson D 2011 The emotional sequelae of whistleblowing: findings from a qualitative study. Journal of Clinical Nursing 20(19–20):2907–2914

Poggi G 2001 Forms of power. Polity Press, Cambridge

Priest C 2012 Advocacy in nursing and health care. In: Mason D, Leavitt J, Chaffee M (eds) Policy and politics in nursing and health care, 6th edn. Saunders, St Louis, pp 31–38

Robson B, Harris R (eds) 2007 Hauora Māori standards of health IV. A study of the years 2000–2005. Te Rōpū Rangahau Hauora a Eru Pōmare, Wellington

Samaha E, Lal E, Samaha N, Wyndham J 2007 Psychological, lifestyle and coping contributors to chronic fatigue in shift-worker nurses. Journal of Advanced Nursing 59:221–232

Sullivan E J 2004 Becoming influential: a guide for nurses. Pearson Prentice Hall, New Jersey

Takase M, Kershaw E, Burt L 2001 Nurse–environment misfit and nursing practice. Journal of Advanced Nursing 35(6):819–826

Wilkes L M, Peters K, Weaver R, Jackson D 2011 Nurses involved in whistleblowing incidents: sequelae for their families. Collegian 18(3):101–106

CHAPTER 14

Becoming a nurse leader

Patricia M Davidson and Siriorn Sindhu

LEARNING OBJECTIVES

At the completion of this chapter, the reader will be able to:

- describe the social, economic and political trends influencing contemporary nursing practice globally
- identify the differences between the terms 'leadership' and 'management'
- recognise strategies for undergraduate nurses to develop to become nurse leaders
- appreciate the importance of evidence-based practice in facilitating optimal patient outcomes
- identify professional and organisational factors that facilitate effective leadership and strategic management.

KEY WORDS

Clinical leadership, clinical management, nurse practitioner, transformational leadership, evidence-based practice

INTRODUCTION

Nursing leadership is critical for implementing evidence-based, ethical practice and promoting optimal patient outcomes. Promoting competence in nursing care and ensuring safe and effective work environments are important in providing high-quality patient care. This chapter describes contemporary trends influencing clinical practice, models of nursing care delivery and aspects of leadership in the clinical setting (Zittel et al 2012). This chapter will also discuss the desirable attributes of leaders in the clinical workplace and the role of expert clinical practice in forging a professional identity for nursing.

The chapter also provides insights into the way expert practitioners, functioning as leaders in the clinical setting, can face challenges and successfully implement strategies to improve patient care and advance nursing practice.

As you read through this chapter, it is important as a beginning nurse to consider the attributes that you need to develop to become a nurse leader and how these manifest in modern healthcare environments (Scott & Miles 2013). It is never too early to focus on developing your leadership style or begin critiquing others' leadership styles.

Effective leaders cultivate a reflective and self-reflective self-appraisal of their strengths and weaknesses as part of a lifelong learning process. Nurse leaders also engage in activities to develop competencies and personal skills in their personal and professional life.

It is also important for you to consider that leadership is manifest and crucial at all levels of nursing practice—from novice to expert. You will also observe leadership styles that are positive and enabling as well as dominating and destructive. Unfortunately, you will probably experience each of these leadership styles in your career. Learning to work with a range of leadership and managerial styles is an important part of your personal and professional development.

As you observe the behaviours of your peers, you can probably see the emergent characteristics of future nursing leaders; for example, how your colleagues deal with challenges in both the classroom and the clinical setting. Increasingly we are aware that the level of nursing competence as well as the quality of working environments influence patient outcomes requiring effective leadership (Griffiths et al 2012).

Even in your early days of practice you can shape the future of patient care and the nursing profession through engaging in critical discussion, reflective practice and providing a voice for patients and their families (Hurley & Hutchinson 2012). This will require focusing on both personal and professional development.

Internationally, contemporary clinical, administrative and policy environments in healthcare provide challenges to both professionals and consumers. Increased demands for clinical services, rising healthcare costs and health workforce shortages are just some of the issues you will face as you begin your nursing career (Gantz et al 2012). In spite of these obstacles, the healthcare setting has never been so welcoming for dynamic nurse leaders and managers. This is because contemporary healthcare systems are no longer based upon hierarchical medical leadership but are more inclusive and interdisciplinary (Davidson et al 2006).

Increasingly, there is emerging evidence of the unique contribution of nurses to patient care. It is critical that nurses provide leadership and direction for models of care development and delivery in policy, practice and research.

At many levels of organisations you will see nurse leaders functioning in organisation, policy and nursing-specific leadership positions (McSherry et al 2012). The growth of nursing research and scholarship has demonstrated the unique and valuable contributions of nurses to health-related outcomes, particularly related to promoting care continuity and coordination of care (McLaughlin et al 2013). As a consequence, nurses are not only in leadership positions but also demonstrating the contribution of nursing care to patient outcomes (Aiken et al 2012).

Given the importance of skilled nurses in achieving optimal patient outcomes and global nursing workforce shortages, the Robert Wood Johnson Foundation (RWJF) and the Institute of Medicine (IOM) in the United States (US) launched a two-year initiative in response to managing the challenges of contemporary healthcare systems. Four key messages were identified as part of this process:

- Nurses should practise to the full extent of their education and training.

- Nurses should achieve higher levels of education and training through an improved education system that promotes seamless academic progression.

- Nurses should be full partners, with physicians and other healthcare professionals, in redesigning healthcare in the United States.

- Effective work force planning and policy making require better data collection and information infrastructure.

This exciting report underscores the importance of independent nursing practice and the relationship to patient outcomes. It also labels a clear path of the importance of interprofessional practice. Although this report focuses on the US it has resonance internationally for nursing development.

The mandate for advanced practice creates an exciting milieu for nurses to work in an interdisciplinary context. These new opportunities create increased responsibility to work with an evidence-based, ethical and collegial framework. Accountability, integrity, ethical and expert practice are core values of all professions (Snellman & Gedda 2012). For nursing this should be the essence of our work and manifest in our practice and interactions.

In order for nurses to function effectively in dynamic clinical environments and exert their influence to optimise patient care, they need to appreciate the multiple factors that impact upon nursing practice and healthcare delivery. These factors are as diverse as the nature of nursing practice itself. It is also important to consider that, regardless of the healthcare system in which you will work, healthcare delivery is provided in a political context that is strongly influenced by economic factors and prevailing cultural and social values (van Olmen et al 2012).

The crucial role of leadership has been recognised in many aspects of nursing practice and professional interactions (Scott & Miles 2013). In this chapter, we explore clinical leadership within a global context and discuss the implications for developing enabling knowledge, skills and attitudes to perform professionally and with credibility in policy, education, practice and research.

HEALTHCARE IN CONTEXT

Contemporary healthcare settings are often portrayed as systems in crisis as they battle increasing demands and diminishing resources (Williams & Maruthappu 2013). This is the same for both developed and developing countries (Basu et al 2012). Across the globe population ageing and the increasing burden of chronic conditions challenges healthcare delivery and professional practice (Beaglehole et al 2012, Zittel et al 2012).

Many healthcare systems are designed for acute procedural care where current epidemiological trends emphasise the importance of community-based care (Henderson & Rubin 2012). Emerging economies such as China and Thailand face unique challenges relating to the changing status of nursing and rapid epidemiological transitions (Sindhu et al 2010). Nurse leaders in these countries are leading systemic change in healthcare systems.

Currently, the worldwide nurse staffing shortage continues to attract government and public comment (Littlejohn et al 2012). Nurses, along with many other professional groups, are experiencing workforce shortages. However, in countries such as the Philippines there is a paradoxical surplus due to the burgeoning of nursing courses to meet a perceived global nursing shortage and the export of nursing skills (Littlejohn et al 2012). This emphasises the importance of considering nursing workforce issues within the context of global economies.

In healthcare systems commonly portrayed as being in a crisis state, pointing the finger at nurses and nursing models of education creates an all too easy scapegoat (Jackson & Daly 2008). Yet the challenges facing health are global and strongly mediated by factors such as epidemiological transitions, increased migration and globalisation of economic factors (Bisht et al 2012). Taking the time to consider these forces is critical in assessing current clinical situations and planning for your future and the nursing professions.

As you begin your nursing journey and struggle with acquiring skills and terminology, terms such as leadership and mentorship can appear distant, remote and have limited relevance. However, it is important to consider that you and your colleagues are the nurse leaders of the future and have a personal and professional responsibility to develop the necessary skills and competencies. Leadership is rarely an historical accident; rather, it is a set of knowledge, skills and attributes that is developed over time and enacted in particular situations (Scott & Miles 2013). Therefore, as you read over this chapter, consider the knowledge and skills that you will need to develop to prepare yourself for a leadership role.

As the skill mix of nursing diversifies in the clinical setting, particularly with growing numbers of enrolled nurses and assistant roles, the registered nurse role will increasingly take on a role of leadership and coordination. No matter how small or large your clinical team is, you will need to inspire and motivate and lead your team to achieve negotiated goals and deliver effective clinical care (Kumar 2013). Skills such as effective communication, reflection, listening and critical thinking are crucial in developing these roles. Take the time to develop these skills and to seek feedback from your peers.

OPPORTUNITIES FOR CLINICAL NURSING LEADERS

A commitment to equity and access are driving healthcare reforms in many countries, such as Australia, New Zealand, the United States, the United Kingdom, Thailand and Malaysia (Clements et al 2012, Heyland 2012). Nurses undertake a crucial role in these reforms from the primary to tertiary care sectors (Clements et al 2012). Technological innovation has improved clinical outcomes for many non-communicable diseases (NCDs). These NCDs (heart disease, stroke, cancer, diabetes and chronic respiratory diseases) will be a high burden on societies globally (Beaglehole et al 2011).

Healthcare professionals are increasingly challenged to deliver healthcare in an equitable and accessible manner while dealing with issues of quality and safety

(Zrelak et al 2012). Globalisation refers to the increasing patterns of interdependency throughout the world attributable to migration, knowledge exchange, communication and trade patterns. Globalisation and health are inextricably linked and increasingly we need to consider issues beyond our local environment in healthcare policy and delivery (Davidson et al 2003, London & Schneider 2012). The burden of tuberculosis and HIV AIDS are just some recent examples of clinical conditions that have resulted as a consequence of living in a globalised world (Limmahakhun et al 2012).

Frequent travel, migration and other social and political factors can impact on the health and wellbeing of individuals and communities through the spread of disease and political and social unrest (Riaz 2013). In many countries throughout the world, issues such as refugee health and migration challenge the health and social care systems and also polarise community opinion (Kalt et al 2013).

Within a climate of healthcare reform, nurses now also have increasing opportunities to influence healthcare policy and practice globally. This new position of power is evidenced by nurses holding influential positions and driving practice changes following credible scientific research and advocacy (Joel & Stallknecht 2000).

Significant barriers may exist to advancing nursing roles, such as opposition from powerful groups, including medical organisations (Jones 2005). However, these challenges are not insurmountable and stewardship by effective nurse leaders is necessary. Demonstrating outcomes that show the quality and safety of nursing and midwifery care is critical in gaining acceptance and endorsement.

There are examples across a range of nursing and midwifery practice where innovative models of care have improved patient outcomes by challenging traditional views and perspectives. Innovative models of midwifery care, such as early discharge care, have improved the experiences of mothers and their babies (Homer et al 2002).

Recognising that the greatest power base for nurses and midwives exists within the practice domain is important. The demonstration of clinical excellence and innovation is an important factor in overcoming scepticism surrounding innovative practice. For example, nurses in the management of chronic heart failure have demonstrated their ability to influence patient outcomes and policies through nurse-coordinated programs and advanced practice nursing roles (Stewart et al 2012).

As a consequence, clinical leadership in the practice setting is an important tool, and strategies to achieve this are discussed below. A clinical leader is a nurse who demonstrates the ability to influence and direct clinical practice (Nicol 2012). This clinical leader also has a vision for the direction of practice and healthcare delivery. Their vision is informed by expert knowledge and analysis of the social, political and economic trends influencing healthcare.

Contemporary nursing leaders need to be flexible and innovative in collaborative practice models. Pressures on the healthcare system—for example, financial pressures and increasing chronic disease burden—represent significant challenges for nurses. However, innovative models of care, increasing emphasis on independent nursing practice and institution of clinical governance structures will likely serve nurses in addressing these challenges.

POLICY FRAMEWORKS FOR NURSING PRACTICE

In order to engage an organisational system, direct change and assert leadership, it is important to appreciate what 'drives' this process. This observation is relevant at both a macro and a micro level of operation. Politics and organisational strategy can be just as intriguing and complex within a hospital ward or community health centre as at the bureaucratic or parliamentary levels. However, at all levels it is important to be aware of social, political and economic factors that influence healthcare delivery (Davidson et al 2006). Politics in nursing is discussed in more detail in Chapter 13 of this text.

The working environment of nurses is influenced by the social, economic and political systems of the healthcare system. Social, political and economic environments across the world influence practices and trends in healthcare delivery. In some instances, policy can be either a barrier to or a facilitator of clinical leadership. The emerging role of the nurse practitioner in Australia, Thailand and New Zealand is an example where significant policy and legislative reform has created a context to promote advanced nursing practice in spite of opposition and scepticism from some medical professional groups.

A shortage in numbers of medical practitioners has seen evolving roles in developing economies such as Thailand (Sumet et al 2012) and Africa (North & Hughes 2012). Policy initiatives in the United Kingdom have seen the embedded nature of practice nurses working in general practice whereas in Australia this is an emergent and evolving role (Halcomb et al 2010). Internationally, healthcare professionals strive to ensure the delivery of safe and effective evidence-based care. Frameworks to monitor the quality and safety of healthcare are important in monitoring the efficacy and effectiveness of nurse-led models of care.

Strategies for promoting the quality and safety of patient care are mechanisms through which healthcare organisations are held accountable for adhering to evidence-based practice standards, continuously improving the quality of their services and ensuring high standards of care (Aiken et al 2012). As you engage in your clinical placements and nursing studies, consider the factors in which nursing care can shape the outcomes of patients.

Falls prevention, mouth care and pressure care are examples of essential nursing care that influence patient outcomes (Berry & Davidson 2006). Increasingly considering the complex factors within healthcare systems can also influence nursing practice and patient outcomes. Measuring nurse-sensitive patient outcome indicators, that is nursing tasks that influence patient outcomes, is of increasing importance (Furukawa et al 2011).

CHANGING MODELS OF CARE DELIVERY

A variety of care delivery models are used in healthcare—some relate to nursing only and are historic, while others are interdisciplinary and responsive to emerging practice trends. The changing healthcare environment—characterised by increasing short-stay surgery, decreasing lengths of stay and numbers of acute beds, combined with increasing patient acuity related to co-morbidities—requires vastly different models of care delivery from even a decade ago. Novel models of care are commonly developed in response to actual or perceived deficits in existing care delivery.

A description of common nursing models is provided in Table 14.1. It is important to note that to date the majority of discussion and evaluation of nursing care models have been undertaken in the acute care setting. It is important that nurses review these models and their applicability and relevance to contemporary healthcare systems.

Ensuring a negotiated taxonomy and relevance to scope of practice in local contexts is likely to be of great importance for future models of nursing care.

Table 14.1
Common care delivery models

Care delivery model	Characteristics
Functional nursing	Ward-based care with allocation of specific clinical tasks, such as medication administration, to nursing staff
Team nursing	Ward-based care where a small team of nurses (perhaps with different educational preparation, skills and competencies) provides care to a designated number of patients
Patient allocation/total patient care	Ward-based care provided by a registered nurse on a shift-by-shift basis to a defined number of patients
Primary nursing	Ward-based care with a registered nurse assigned to patients for their entire admission period. Within this model a plan of care is developed, implemented and evaluated by the 'primary' nurse, with 'associate' nurses continuing the plan in the absence of the 'primary' nurse
Care management/clinical pathways	Ward or hospital-based multidisciplinary coordinated patient care for a specific case type (e.g. patients with total hip replacement). This model frequently incorporates a 'critical' or 'clinical path' tool to 'map' and document care, including the sequence and timing of interventions and variances from expected outcomes
Case management	Hospital, outreach and/or community-based multidisciplinary care that provides continuity of care for a specific case-type of patients (e.g. patients with heart failure and chronic obstructive pulmonary disease) across the entire episode of care from hospital to community

Source: Davidson P M, Hickman L 2012 Managing client care. In Crisp J, Taylor C (eds) Fundamentals of nursing, 4th edn. Elsevier, Sydney, p 129

Patients are admitted to acute care hospitals primarily for collaborative or independent nursing care, as many medical diagnostic and therapeutic procedures can now be conducted in ambulatory care settings, except in critical or emergent circumstances. However, efficient and effective care also requires continuity of patient management beyond the traditional hospital admission period to encompass the entire episode of care, particularly for those with continuing chronic disease.

Programs that promote nurse coordination of care are emerging across many diagnostic conditions, including cancer, diabetes, heart disease, arthritis and chronic obstructive pulmonary disease (Sindhu et al 2010). Similarly, there are programs in early childhood and midwifery care. As you consider your options for nursing in the future, it is important to remember that, in the future, a large proportion of nursing care will be provided in the community and primary care settings. Many countries around the world are adopting primary healthcare approaches to decrease health disparities and the lack of dependence on the acute care setting (Taylor et al 2013).

Increasing adoption of technology will see nursing interventions delivered by tele-health and web-based media. This is likely to require the development of a suite of skills and resources to work in this setting effectively. Performing effective interventions over the phone or internet are likely to be of increased importance (Car et al 2012). This will also have implications for the regulation of professional practice and the monitoring of health outcomes.

WHAT IS LEADERSHIP?

Leadership is an attribute of an individual to work with, inspire and motivate others to work towards a defined goal or mission (Daly, Speedy & Jackson 2003). The dynamic and changing healthcare systems place change as a focus in contemporary health environments. Unless nurses choose to be swept along by change, they need to actively engage the process on both a personal and a professional level.

An important attribute of a leader is to formulate an action plan and support their team in achieving negotiated goals. There is an increasing discourse and discussion of leadership within the nursing profession. The concepts that make nursing leadership unique are the requisites for evidence-based healthcare: responsibility for the care and safety of patients; and the need for evaluation of clinical practice.

Leadership has long been an important part of the function of any organisational structure. Leadership styles vary along a continuum from authoritative to participatory, although common characteristics for leaders include being a visionary and having a plan to take individuals and services into the future. O'Rourke and colleagues define a visionary leader as one who can simultaneously have a vigilant focus on promoting health, with the capacity to build teams, articulate and demonstrate what others cannot see and address immediate challenges, as well as leading their team into a future of often uncharted waters (O'Rourke 2006, O'Rourke & Davidson 2004). Leadership is influenced by the values of individuals and organisations, as well as society. Values are a set of beliefs and concepts derived from knowledge, experience and aspiration (Weis & Schank 2004).

Values can be: *personal*, such as the importance placed on honesty and integrity; *professional*, such as the emphasis placed on reflective practice, accountability and continuing professional development; and *organisational*, such as the emphasis placed on patient outcomes and adherence to policy. In order to function effectively and avoid role conflict, there needs to be a congruency between the values and beliefs of the individual and the organisation in which they work. Where there is a mismatch is often a recipe for discord, conflict and low work satisfaction.

As you choose your work setting, it is important that you take the time to understand the mission and values of the organisation and ensure that these are congruent with your own belief system. The confluence between personal, professional and organisational values and leadership styles can often determine not only successful leadership styles but also your 'fit' within an organisation. That is how committed you are personally to the direction of the organisation and how happy you are within the organisation.

Figure 14.1 illustrates desirable attributes of effective clinical leaders. This leadership is linked to the cultural values of the systems, resources and support available. A distinction of leadership characteristics is made between transactional, transformational, connective and renaissance leaders (Cook 2008). Transactional leadership focuses on transactions or exchanges between leaders and others, with self-interest the key motivator. In contrast, transformational leaders create a culture of leadership for all stakeholders, generating empowerment, open dialogue and inclusive decision making (Davidson et al 2006). An additional concept, 'breakthrough leadership', incorporates role modelling, clarification of own values and respect for others' views (Lett 2002). Role modelling, mentoring and succession planning are vital aspects in preparing current and future nursing leaders.

Jackson describes servant leadership as an important and emerging trend where the servant-leader does not work in isolation, but rather actively searches for opportunities to build connections to promote creativity and enabling and mutually beneficial relationships (Jackson 2008). Regardless of the leadership style it needs to be a good fit with broader organisational contexts to promote quality and safety of patient care and the work satisfaction and retention of nurses in the workplace (Cummings et al 2010).

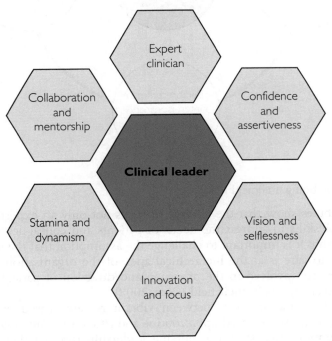

Figure 14.1
Attributes of a clinical leader

WHAT MAKES A CLINICAL LEADER?

In organisations such as hospitals and community health settings, there are different nursing leaders functioning at all levels. The individuals who readily come to mind are often those who are very visible in organisations, such as directors of nursing. However, it is important to differentiate between management and leadership. Management refers to the planning and organisation of services. The term 'leadership' infers that an individual is visionary and pivotal in directing and shaping clinical practice (Allan et al 2008). Implicit in functioning as a clinical leader is a significant mentoring role as shown in Figure 14.2.

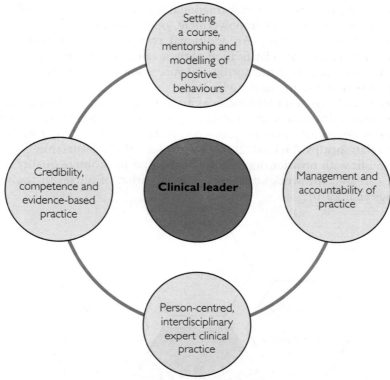

Figure 14.2
Framework for being a clinical leader

These attributes show that the clinical leader is not only an expert clinician but uses his or her skills to address the needs of patients and colleagues. In discussing clinical leadership it is important to challenge the assumption that the leader making the difference to care is at the hierarchical apex of the organisation (Cook 2008). Clinical leaders are involved in the provision and direction of patient care and are implicitly clinical experts in their field (Cook 2008).

Often a differentiating focus between vibrant research-based, evidence-based practice cultures and those based upon routine and ritual is the nursing leader (Cook 2008). Organisations that stimulate nursing leadership through their involvement in organisational decision making and promoting nursing research and innovative practice frequently have better patient outcomes (Wong & Cummings 2007).

Increasing numbers of individuals are living with chronic and complex conditions and require the professional services of different occupational groups. Nurses have demonstrated their ability to work as part of a team and be collaborative and participatory in their actions and decision making (for more on teamwork, see Chapter 15).

There are two critical factors in healthcare as clinicians face the complexities of current patient care: the need for specialised clinical experts; and the need for these professionals to collaborate. Interdisciplinary healthcare teams with members from many disciplines increasingly work together to optimise patient care (Reeves et al 2008). Examples of these teams are found in trauma, neonatal retrieval, geriatric assessment and drug and alcohol areas of clinical practice.

PROMOTING LEADERSHIP IN THE PRACTICE SETTING

Given the challenges facing contemporary health systems, focusing on clinical leadership development strategies is of crucial importance. Empowering nurses to have control and influence over their practice is of increasing importance. This leadership role has to be undertaken within the complexity of healthcare systems. It is important that nurses undertake this role with credibility, competence and capability and interact with their colleagues respectfully and collegially.

In order to address these factors, a number of strategies have been implemented across the globe. These include: clinical professoriate positions; clinical development units; practice development strategies; clinical leadership programs; and initiatives focusing on promoting evidence-based practice. The outcomes of these strategies are variable and commonly influenced more by local contextual and management factors rather than the value and the ethos of these programs. Regardless of the model undertaken the following factors are critical: (1) increasing the voice of nurses at the decision-making table; (2) encouraging nurses' control over their practice; (3) promoting science and scholarship in nursing practice; (4) fostering an emphasis on patient outcomes and nurse-sensitive measures; and (5) working more effectively and efficiently in interprofessional practice environments.

An example of successful leadership models are embedded in the 'Magnet' programs, which have been widely implemented in the United States and in several Australian sites (McHugh et al 2012). Magnet status is an award status administered by the American Nurses' Credentialing Center (ANCC), an affiliate of the American Nurses Association, to hospitals that satisfy a set of criteria designed to measure the strength and quality of their nursing. This ranges from a focus on specific nursing tasks to the quality of functional relationships within the organisation.

Many Magnet-accredited facilities have demonstrated optimal nursing outcomes in respect of nurse-sensitive patient outcome indicators, such as pressure areas and falls. These programs have a strong influence across all levels of the organisation from human resources to customer relations. Programs that employ such an approach are likely to have a greater chance of sustainable integration of strategies to promote clinical leadership. Strategies that foster clinical leaders within interdisciplinary care models espouse and profile the important role of nurses in improving health outcomes.

As you move through practice areas during your clinical placements, observe and critically evaluate strategies that you consider enabling for clinical leaders. Strategies that support a culture of collaborative clinical decision making, as well as an emphasis on education and reflective practice, are just some examples.

Box 14.1

Example of an innovative nurse-led model of practice

Nurse-led care is delivered using a comprehensive approach to patient care using the best available evidence. Advanced practice nurses work in collaboration with medical practitioners and offer a valuable contribution to the clinical care of acute and chronically ill patients. In the community there are many nurse-led models in chronic care, such as heart failure.

There has also been an increase in the nursing role in procedural techniques, such as gastroscopy and vascular access devices. Often dedicated positions can lead to higher procedural volume and technical expertise. Increasing numbers of patients are requiring insertion of central venous catheters and as a consequence the rate of catheter-related bloodstream infections has increased. A series of studies undertaken by nurse leaders has shown some compelling data in decreasing catheter-related infections and improved procedural and organisational outcomes through increased technical competence and a comprehensive approach to patient care. Nurse leaders in Australia are leading the establishment of the evidence base of nurse-led vascular access devices through technical competence, expertise and monitoring of patient outcomes (Alexandrou et al 2009, Yacopetti et al 2010). This is an exciting approach to improving the quality and safety of patient care through nursing leadership and advanced practice.

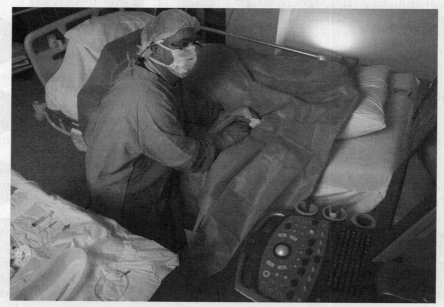

Evan Alexandrou—advanced practice nurse in vascular access

Professional societies and organisations to promote clinical leadership

Professional societies play an important role in terms of providing not only an environment of collegiality, but also leadership, mentorship and promotion of clinical excellence (Astley et al 2007). These aims are achieved through development of policy documents, publication of professional journals, conduct of scientific meetings and sponsorship of research and attendance at professional meetings. Some organisations serve the nursing profession broadly, focusing on an array of nursing issues, while others maintain a specialty focus. Examples of this in Australia are specialty groups such as the Australian College of Critical Care Nurses (ACCCN) and the Australasian

Cardiovascular Nursing College (ACNC) and more generic organisations such as the Australian College of Nursing and, internationally, Sigma Theta Tau International and the International Council of Nursing (ICN).

Sigma Theta Tau International is an international organisation promoting leadership globally through scholarship, knowledge and technology to improve the health of the world's people. There are chapters of Sigma Theta Tau throughout the world. The Sigma Theta Tau International Leadership Institute (ILI) focuses on the development and advancement of nurses as exceptional healthcare leaders. The ILI assists nurses internationally to develop leadership skills by creating and sharing knowledge.

Increasingly, professional nursing organisations are playing a role in terms of social advocacy and also mentoring and supporting nursing colleagues in developing countries. Particularly in situations of social disadvantage, nurses can play an important role in advocacy. What is increasingly apparent in a variety of settings is that a united voice can be a powerful force. For example, the International Council of Nursing has taken strategic stances on issues such as ethical recruitment and women's health.

Take the time to view the information and resources on the following professional nursing organisation websites presented in Box 14.2, particularly in respect of professional development and the ongoing evaluation and development of nursing practice. These sites can also provide an opportunity to reach out to other nursing colleagues globally.

Box 14.2

Examples of Professional Nursing and Midwifery Organisations

- the Australian College of Critical Care Nurses: www.acccn.com au
- the Australian College of Midwives: www.acmi.org.au
- the Australasian College of Cardiovascular Nurses: www.acnc.net.au
- the Australian Nurse Practitioner Association: www.nursepractitioners.org.au
- the Australian and New Zealand College of Mental Health Nurses: www.healthsci.utas.edu.au/nursing/college/index.html
- Australian College of Nursing: www.rcna.org.au
- Sigma Theta Tau International: www.nursingsociety.org
- the International Council of Nursing: www.icn.ch/

LEADERSHIP IN EVIDENCE-BASED PRACTICE

The assessment of the cost-effectiveness and efficacy of nursing interventions and the relationship to patient outcomes is becoming increasingly important. Patient outcomes are largely dependent on implementing the best available evidence. You will hear a lot of discussion about evidence-based practice. This term refers to the implementation of the best available evidence within the context of the patient's needs, knowledge and belief systems, and using the clinician's expertise (Sackett et al 1996).

As a consequence, nurse leaders have to be increasingly focused not only on assessing the needs of the patients and their families, but also on measuring outcomes (Chang et al 2011).

Outcome evaluation continues to be an important way in which nurses demonstrate their influence, not only to others but also to each other. This underscores that, to be an effective clinical leader beyond the charismatic attributes, nurses need to not only interpret and implement clinical evidence, but also evaluate the efficacy of nursing interventions. Clinical leaders recognise that strategies to support research and scholarship are important to develop the evidence base for supporting nursing practice.

Significance of expert clinical practice

Expert clinical practice remains the foundation of the nursing profession's standing in communities. Clinical practice, informed by nursing science, is what makes nursing exceptional and unique, and is the key to our autonomous, professional practice. This underscores the importance of emphasising expert nursing within models of professional practice, education and research. Nursing roles such as clinical nurse specialists, clinical nurse consultants and nurse practitioners are crucial in advocating for expert nursing care. Internationally and even nationally, the names for these roles may differ, but the fundamental attributes are similar.

Nurses who function as leaders in these roles carry not only the privilege but also the professional responsibility to direct healthcare practices to optimise the health of the populations they serve and also to foster the professional development of their colleagues. This is achieved through promoting evidence-based practice, nursing scholarship and developing and delivering care that is tailored to the needs of patients and their families.

Take the time to review the code of conduct of peak nursing organisations, such as the Australian Nursing and Midwifery Council in Australia, the Nursing Council of New Zealand in New Zealand, the Thai Nursing Council in Thailand and the Board of Nursing Philippines as well as the organisations in Box 14.2. The recommendations of these peak bodies should provide the blueprint for your professional actions and professional practice.

LOOKING TO THE FUTURE

In this chapter we have discussed the challenges, strategies and progress for clinical leadership. Contemporary health systems are facing considerable challenges because of the increasing burden of chronic conditions, population ageing and fiscal constraints. Yet never before has the importance of nursing care and the evidence to support nursing interventions been so strong.

It is an exciting time to be embarking on a nursing career and never before has leadership been so crucial. As you begin your nursing career, it is important to try to turn challenges into opportunities. You will be working in rapidly evolving settings, and the practice environments you enter in the next few years are likely to be radically different on the tenth anniversary of your graduation. Focusing on the needs of patients and their families is important in shaping care models for the future and also in setting your compass for the future.

The test remains to influence nursing practice through positive and enabling leadership strategies and to develop innovative approaches to dealing with challenges facing current clinical environments. In order to achieve this, a system of mentoring, career progression and succession planning in the clinical setting needs to be created and nurtured. Clinical and academic settings require a culture that develops innovation and fosters leadership potential (Donaldson & Fralic 2000).

CONCLUSION

It is important to realise that at every level of an organisation, and regardless of whether nurses work in clinical, education or management streams, they have the potential to influence and direct patient care by exemplary leadership and excellence in clinical practice. The potential for nursing practice to influence clinical outcomes is an empowering and motivating concept. As you embark upon your nursing career, seek enabling clinical environments and mentors who will guide you along your professional journey. Taking the time to develop your interpersonal, communication and leadership skills will be critical for you having a productive and satisfying nursing career.

REFLECTIVE QUESTIONS

1. How can leadership in the clinical setting influence the quality and safety of patient care? Please identify both positive and negative leadership behaviours and styles and formulate a model for what you consider an effective leader to be.

2. What are nurse-sensitive patient outcome indicators? Identify an indicator from one of your clinical practice settings and consider how nursing leadership can influence the capacity to achieve optimal outcomes.

3. Identify a professional nursing organisation, and review their activities relating to leadership. Why are professional organisations important in formulating a professional identity and advocating for quality and safety in healthcare environments?

4. Can you identify some of your personal characteristics that will enable you to undertake a leadership position? Once you have identified these factors, what are some strategies for fostering your leadership from what you have read in this chapter?

RECOMMENDED READINGS

Cummings G G, MacGregor T et al 2010 Leadership styles and outcome patterns for the nursing workforce and work environment: a systematic review. International Journal of Nursing Studies 47(3):363–385

Davidson P M, Elliott D, Daly J 2006 Clinical leadership in contemporary clinical practice: implications for nursing in Australia. Journal of Nursing Management 14(3):180–188

REFERENCES

Aiken L H, Sermeus W, Van den Heede K et al 2012 Patient safety, satisfaction, and quality of hospital care: cross sectional surveys of nurses and patients in 12 countries in Europe and the United States. BMJ: British Medical Journal 344:1717

Alexandrou E, Frost S, Spencer T et al 2009 Nurse led central venous catheter insertion: an integrative review. Australian Critical Care 22(1):61

Allan H T, Smith P A, Lorentzon M 2008 Leadership for learning: a literature study of leadership for learning in clinical practice. Journal of Nursing Management 16(5):545–555

Astley C M, Portelli L, Whalley G A, Davidson P M 2007 Coming of age: affiliate member profile and participation in the Annual Scientific Meeting of the Cardiac Society of Australia and New Zealand. Heart, Lung and Circulation 16(6):447–451

Basu S, Andrews J, Kishore S et al 2012 Comparative performance of private and public healthcare systems in low- and middle-income countries: a systematic review. PLoS medicine 9(6):e1001244

Beaglehole R, Bonita R, Alleyne G et al 2011 UN high-level meeting on non-communicable diseases: addressing four questions. The Lancet 378(9789):449–455

Beaglehole R, Bonita R, Horton R et al 2012 Measuring progress on NCDs: one goal and five targets. The Lancet 380(9850):1283–1285

Berry A M, Davidson P M 2006 Beyond comfort: oral hygiene as a critical nursing activity in the intensive care unit. Intensive and Critical Care Nursing 22(6):318–328

Bisht R, Pitchforth E, Murray S F 2012 Understanding India, globalisation and health care systems: a mapping of research in the social sciences. Globalization and Health 8(1):32

Car J, Huckvale K, Hermens H 2012 Telehealth for long term conditions. BMJ: British Medical Journal 344:e4201

Chang S, Gholizadeh L, Salamonson Y et al 2011 Health span or life span: The role of patient-reported outcomes in informing health policy. Health policy 100(1):96–104

Clements B, Coady D, Gupta S (eds) 2012 Health care reform in advanced and emerging economies. International Monetary Fund, Washington DC

Cook M 2008 The renaissance of clinical leadership. International Nursing Review 48(1):38–46

Cummings G G, MacGregor T, Davey M et al 2010 Leadership styles and outcome patterns for the nursing workforce and work environment: a systematic review. International Journal of Nursing Studies 47(3):363–385

Daly J, Speedy S, Jackson D 2003 Nursing leadership. Elsevier Australia

Davidson P M, Meleis A, Daly J, Douglas M M 2003 Globalization as we enter the 21st century: reflections and directions for nursing education, science, research and clinical practice. Contemporary Nurse 15(3):162–174

Davidson P M, Elliott D, Daly J 2006 Clinical leadership in contemporary clinical practice: implications for nursing in Australia. Journal of Nursing Management 14(3):180–187

Donaldson S K, Fralic M F 2000 Forging today's practice-academic link: a new era for nursing leadership. Nursing Administration Quarterly 25(1):95–101

Furukawa M F, Raghu T, Shao B B M 2011 Electronic medical records, nurse staffing, and nurse-sensitive patient outcomes: evidence from the National Database of Nursing Quality Indicators. Medical Care Research and Review 68(3):311–331

Gantz N R, Sherman R, Jasper M, Choo C G E K et al 2012 Global nurse leader perspectives on health systems and workforce challenges. Journal of Nursing Management 20(4):433–443

Griffiths P, Richardson A, Blackwell R 2012 Outcomes sensitive to nursing service quality in ambulatory cancer chemotherapy: systematic scoping review. European Journal of Oncology Nursing 16(3):238–246

Halcomb E J, Davidson P M, Brown N 2010 Uptake of Medicare chronic disease items in Australia by general practice nurses and Aboriginal health workers. Collegian: Journal of the Royal College of Nursing Australia 17(2):57–61

Henderson E J, Rubin G P 2012 Development of a community-based model for respiratory care services. BMC Health Services Research 12(1):193

Heyland D K 2012 Health care reform. Arch Intern Med 172(22)

Homer C S E, Davis G K, Cooke M, Barclay L M 2002 Women's experiences of continuity of midwifery care in a randomised controlled trial in Australia. Midwifery 18(2):102–112

Hurley J, Hutchinson M 2012 Setting a course: A critical review of the literature on nurse leadership in Australia. Contemporary Nurse:1908–1919

Jackson D 2008 Servant leadership in nursing: a framework for developing sustainable research capacity in nursing. Collegian: Journal of the Royal College of Nursing Australia 15(1):27–33

Jackson D, Daly J 2008 Nursing and pre-registration nursing education under the spotlight again. Collegian (Royal College of Nursing, Australia) 15(1):1

Joel L, Stallknecht H 2000 A global connection. AJN The American Journal of Nursing 100(10):109

Jones M L 2005 Role development and effective practice in specialist and advanced practice roles in acute hospital settings: systematic review and meta-synthesis. Journal of Advanced Nursing 49(2):191–209

Kalt A, Hossain M, Kiss L, Zimmerman C 2013 Asylum seekers, violence and health: a systematic review of research in high-income host countries. American Journal of Public Health doi 10.2105/AJPH.2012.301136:e1–e12

Kumar R D C 2013 Leadership in healthcare. Anaesthesia & Intensive Care Medicine 14(1):39–41

Lett M 2002 The concept of clinical leadership. Contemporary Nurse 12(1):16–21

Limmahakhun S, Chaiwarith R, Nuntachit N et al 2012 Treatment outcomes of patients co-infected with tuberculosis and HIV at Chiang Mai University Hospital, Thailand. International Journal of STD & AIDS 23(6):414–418

Littlejohn L, Campbell J, Collins-McNeil J 2012 Comparative analysis of nursing shortage. International Journal of Nursing 1(1):21–26

London L, Schneider H 2012 Globalisation and health inequalities: can a human rights paradigm create space for civil society action? Social Science & Medicine 74(1):6–13

McHugh M D, Kelly L A, Smith H L et al 2012 Lower mortality in magnet hospitals. Medical care doi: 10.1097/MLR.0b013e3182726cc5

McLaughlin M K, Speroni K G, Kelly P et al 2013 National survey of hospital nursing research, part 1: research requirements and outcomes. Journal of Nursing Administration 43(1):10–17

McSherry R, Pearce P, Grimwood K, McSherry W 2012 The pivotal role of nurse managers, leaders and educators in enabling excellence in nursing care. Journal of Nursing Management 20(1):7–19

Nicol E D 2012 Improving clinical leadership and management in the NHS. Journal of Healthcare Leadership 4:59–69

North N, Hughes F 2012 A systems perspective on nursing productivity. Journal of

Health Organization and Management 26(2):192–214

O'Rourke M W 2006 Beyond rhetoric to role accountability: a practical and professional model of practice. Nurse Leader 4(3):28–44

O'Rourke M, Davidson P M 2004 Governance of practice and leadership: implications for nursing practice. In: Daly J, Speedy S, Jackson D (eds) Nursing leadership. Elsevier Australia, pp 327–343

Reeves S, Zwarenstein M, Goldman J et al 2008 Interprofessional education: effects on professional practice and healthcare outcomes. Cochrane Database of systematic reviews 1

Riaz H 2013 Public health failings behind Pakistan's measles surge. The Lancet 381(9862):189

Sackett D L, Rosenberg W, Gray J et al 1996 Evidence based medicine: what it is and what it isn't. BMJ 312(7023):71–72

Scott E S, Miles J 2013 Advancing leadership capacity in nursing. Nursing Administration Quarterly 37(1):77–82

Sindhu S, Pholpet C, Puttapitukpol S 2010 Meeting the challenges of chronic illness: a nurse-led collaborative community care program in Thailand. Collegian: Journal of the Royal College of Nursing Australia 17(2):93–99

Snellman I, Gedda K M 2012 The value ground of nursing. Nursing Ethics 19(6): 714–726

Stewart S, Carrington M J, Marwick T et al 2012 Impact of home versus clinic based management of chronic heart failure: the WHICH?(Which Heart failure Intervention is most Cost-effective & consumer friendly in reducing Hospital care) multicenter, randomized trial. Journal of the American College of Cardiology 60(14):1239–1248

Sumet S, Suwannapong N, Howteerakul N, Thammarat C 2012 Knowledge management model for quality improvement in the hemodialysis unit of a non-profit private hospital, Bangkok, Thailand. Leadership in Health Services 25(4):306–317

Taylor E F, Machta R M, Meyers D S et al 2013 Enhancing the primary care team to provide redesigned care: the roles of practice facilitators and care managers. Annals of Family Medicine 11(1):80–83

van Olmen J, Marchal B, Van Damme W et al 2012 Health systems frameworks in their political context: framing divergent agendas. BMC Public Health 12(774): 1–13

Weis D, Schank M J 2004 An instrument to measure professional nursing values. Journal of Nursing Scholarship 32(2):201–204

Williams C, Maruthappu M 2013 'Healthconomic Crises': Public Health and Neoliberal Economic Crises. American Journal of Public Health 103(1):7–9

Wong C A, Cummings G G 2007 The relationship between nursing leadership and patient outcomes: a systematic review. Journal of Nursing Management 15(5):508–521

Yacopetti N, Alexandrou E, Spencer T R et al 2010 Central venous catheter insertion by a clinical nurse consultant or anaesthetic medical staff: a single-centre observational study. Critical Care and Resuscitation 12(2):90–95

Zittel B, Ezzeddine S, Makatjane M et al 2012 Divergence and convergence in nursing and health care among six countries participating in ICN's 2010 Global Nursing Leadership Institute. International nursing review 59(1):48–54

Zrelak P A, Utter G H, Sadeghi B et al 2012 Using the agency for healthcare research and quality patient safety indicators for targeting nursing quality improvement. Journal of Nursing Care Quality 27(2):99–108

CHAPTER 15

Becoming part of a multidisciplinary healthcare team

Anne Hofmeyer and Greta G. Cummings

LEARNING OBJECTIVES

After reading this chapter, students should be able to:

- explain the relationship between social capital and multidisciplinary teamwork
- explain how these factors influence nursing and the provision of safe quality healthcare
- provide an overview of issues related to leading and influencing others in teams
- appreciate working with different generations
- identify strategies for new graduates to build resilience in teamwork
- understand the importance of self-reflection, awareness, resilience and developing ties with trusted mentors.

KEY WORDS

Multidisciplinary teams, teamwork, social capital, networks, communication, leading, influencing, quality, resilience, nursing

INTRODUCTION

The aim of this chapter is to examine the basic concepts, benefits and challenges of multidisciplinary teamwork in healthcare using a social capital framework. Social capital is defined as the norms and networks that enable people to act collectively to achieve desired outcomes (Woolcock & Narayan 2000). Our re-framing of the concept of teamwork using a social capital framework to achieve desired outcomes offers new insights that may contribute to your ongoing development as an engaged and resilient team member in your career.

The position of governments, professional organisations, policy makers and funders worldwide is that health system renewal is dependent on the health professions working collectively and cohesively in teams to promote organisational success and provide integrated and quality healthcare services (D'Amour & Oandasan 2004, Gaboury et al 2009, Kohn et al 1999, O'Neill et al 1998, WHO 1999). There is widespread evidence that effective teamwork and communication is critical to safety in many areas of society such as healthcare and aviation (Boyce et al 2009, Hamman 2004, Leonard et al 2004). Medical errors, adverse events and patient harm are associated with poor teamwork and ineffective or insufficient communication (Leonard et al 2004, Murphy 2012). Indeed, the Institute of Medicine suggested that lessons about safety teamwork practices in aviation could be applied in healthcare (IOM 2001). Safety errors in healthcare and aviation have been directly associated with poor communication and poor teamwork, so team training skills should have equal importance with theoretical and technical training in curricula for successful outcomes (Hamman 2004).

In what follows, we use arguments and evidence from the social sciences, quality and safety, leadership and professional practice to re-frame a broader discussion about multidisciplinary teamwork in nursing. We contend that all individuals have the capacity to influence team norms. At best, these influencing and leading actions contribute to the desired outcomes for patients in general, and nurses' career aspirations in particular. We call for greater attention to relational issues when considering the meaning of teamwork for the individual nurse, with other nurses, and with other disciplines. To this end, we describe how an individual's enduring set of beliefs, norms, attributes and values shapes their resilience and interactions with others that, in turn, builds social capital in multidisciplinary teams to deliver desired outcomes.

WHAT IS A MULTIDISCIPLINARY TEAM?

Multidisciplinary teams are dynamic entities because healthcare professionals can move in and out of a group in response to changing circumstances. Some teams exist for a specific purpose and then are disbanded. Most teams have sub-groups because people naturally flock together, but the key requirement for cohesive functioning is that all people commit to the team effort. Murphy (2012:91) reminds us that, 'teamwork is not an automatic consequence of placing people together'. Xyrichis and Ream (2007) define teamwork as a:

> dynamic process involving two or more health professionals with complementary backgrounds and skills, sharing common goals, and exercising concerted physical and mental effort in assessing, planning, or evaluating patient care. This is accomplished through interdependent collaboration, open communication and shared decision-making. This in turn generates value-added patient, organisational and staff outcomes. (2007:238)

Studies investigating teamwork have been most prevalent in human resource management (Sewell 2005), organisational behaviour (Wilson et al 2005) and industries such as commercial aviation (Hamman 2004). Teamwork in healthcare is linked to desired outcomes for providers in terms of enhanced job satisfaction (Brunetto & Farr-Wharton 2006, Rafferty et al 2001), for patients in terms of increased satisfaction with safe, high-quality patient-centred care (Finn et al 2010, Kohn et al 1999, Leonard et al 2004), and for healthcare organisations in terms of reform (Finn et al 2010), increased productivity and cost-effective healthcare delivery (Brunetto & Farr-Wharton 2006, Kalisch & Lee 2010, Leonard et al 2004) and workforce retention (Xyrichis & Ream 2007). Newcomers and less experienced staff are able to access a broader range of support when they are members of highly functioning teams (Carter & West 1999).

To set the scene about working in multidisciplinary teams, imagine yourself as the nurse in the following narrative and then consider your response:

The coordinator says she is looking for nurses to work a shift tomorrow in two medical units (A and B) each with the same number and types of patients, lifting equipment and staffing. However, you have worked in both units previously and consider there were critical differences between the units in terms of team relationships and work practices. In your experience, nurses working in Unit A have social and professional norms that create a team environment where:

- you feel valued, respected and trusted, and new staff fit in easily;
- those in leadership roles value staff and consider their ideas in decision making;
- you are able to hold an opinion that is different from those in positions of authority, ask challenging questions and remain on good terms;
- feedback about performance is constructive and problems are resolved promptly, effectively and respectfully;
- a culture of constant improvement and evidence-based practice exists;
- it is safe to ask for help, advice and information;
- everyone is willing to share their knowledge and skills and help each other out to get the work done (reciprocity); and
- sick leave and workplace injuries are low (Hofmeyer 2003).

On the other hand, in your experience, the nurses working in Unit B have social and professional norms that create an environment where:

- new nurses or strangers have to prove themselves as trustworthy before being trusted and included;
- formal leaders have a command and control style and allow unethical fragmented team practices to continue unchecked;
- diverse views lead to conflict and those holding such views are scapegoated, excluded or marginalised;
- it is safer to remain silent and maintain the status quo;
- feedback is callous, punitive and blaming;
- problems are ignored and eventually erupt into conflict;

- calls to adopt new work practices are resisted;
- some nurses only help friends (tit for tat) but are unwilling to help others in the team;
- nurses who ask for help are judged as inadequate or incompetent; and
- sick leave is high; and a plethora of policies and rules exist (Hofmeyer 2003).

The descriptors in the narrative about Unit B illustrate levels of mistrust, self-interest and fragmented team cohesion. When you worked in Unit B, you remember the nurses were unsupportive and provided you with incomplete information that hampered your ability to provide quality care for your patients. They scoffed when you described a new wound care product that could potentially improve the care of a patient in the unit. During the shift, they helped each other out to get their work done, but then sat in the office while you finished your patient care alone (Hofmeyer & Scott 2007).

These vignettes about team relationships illustrate why you prefer to relieve in Unit A. Such insights about both units may explain why some multidisciplinary teams work more cohesively and effectively than others, and why nurses prefer to work in some teams and not in others. Inadequate staffing and resources have traditionally been considered a key causative factor in fragmented work environments. But we suggest a major contributing factor is the extent to which nurses perceive that other team members collaborate with them. Put simply, the quality, diversity and ethics of your relationships will help or hinder you to do your job. The extent to which your ties with others are respectful, cooperative and trusting will influence your ability to access the resources (e.g. evidence, knowledge, information, advice and support) that you need to provide quality and safe healthcare. This is why you as a new graduate nurse will need a range of networks with nurses who have different expertise, knowledge and skills and who are willing to support your ongoing professional development and practice.

What sorts of people fulfil these criteria and why do you listen to them and not others? Whose advice do you seek? What are their personal attributes, expertise and qualities? What is it about that person that gives you confidence to ask questions? We suggest that it is their enduring set of norms, beliefs and values that influences the manner in which they interact and communicate with you. Norms socialise people into expected behaviours in a given context, such as in families, sporting teams, tipping in a restaurant or not littering. These social expectations promote social conformity, reward people who conform and penalise those who do not meet the expectations. However, a problem can arise if individuals are not aware of the implicit expectations and violate the expected norms of group behaviour. So if we think about social norms in the context of multidisciplinary teams, what would be some examples of expected norms? Most likely the social norms about communicating and collaborating together as a cohesive team in Unit A would be examples of your expectations. You might value a person who was cooperative and helped anyone (e.g. reciprocity) not just their friends. So you would have confidence that you could depend on others in the team to support you in your learning and delivering desired outcomes.

Current debates about multidisciplinary teamwork stress the importance of communication and collaborative practice to improve the safety, quality and cost-effectiveness of healthcare services (ACSQHC 2011). In response, professional organisations in

Australia and beyond have developed standards and teamwork and communication competencies to guide the professional practice of registered nurses and midwives (ANMC 2006). Quality and safety in healthcare is informed by current evidence that is dependent on effective teamwork and communication between healthcare providers (ACSQHC 2011, IOM 2001, Kalisch & Lee 2010, Leonard et al 2004, Salas et al 2009). The Institute of Medicine in the US analysed over 100 definitions of quality of care in healthcare services and developed a definition in 1990 that remains relevant today:

> The degree to which health services for individuals and populations increase the likelihood of desired health outcomes and are consistent with current professional knowledge.
> (IOM 1990:21)

Implicit in this definition is the expectation that healthcare professionals must be using 'current professional knowledge' and research evidence in their decision making. The ongoing problem of the haphazard use of current evidence in healthcare decision making was highlighted by Grol and Grimshaw (2003) who reported that 30%–40% of patients did not receive care based on current evidence, and 20%–25% of care provided was not needed or potentially harmful.

On the face of it, arguments about improving teamwork are commendable, but the practicalities and challenges of learning to work together are poorly understood. Idealising the notion of multidisciplinary teams and teamwork fails to provide a practical guide for newly qualified nurses who are attempting to navigate complex relational issues with nurses and other disciplines in healthcare teams. We next offer a re-framing of the concept of teamwork using a social capital framework that may offer useful insights about the norms and networks that influence your working relationship with others.

SOCIAL CAPITAL

Marx (1849) conceptualised the notion of *capital* as a value in terms of wealth, financial resources, assets or investments that were associated with the production and exchange of commodities and returns on monetary investments (Lin 1999). There is now a broader application of the term *capital* as a resource in human, cultural, educational, social, health and environmental areas (Cox 1995). All *capitals* are viewed as important resources contributing to the social, economic and cultural determinants of health (Wilkinson & Marmot 2003). There is an inter-relationship between *capitals*. For example, an individual's educational capital in the form of credentials/qualifications can lead to greater productivity or improved employability options. This means they can increase their economic capital as a measure of individual success (e.g. increased remuneration). As Portes (1998:6) explains, 'whereas economic capital is in people's bank accounts and human capital is inside their heads, social capital inheres in the structure of their relationships'.

Social capital is defined as the norms and networks that enable people to act collectively (Woolcock & Narayan 2000). Although various definitions of social capital exist, most coalesce around the idea that norms and networks play a part in achieving shared goals by fostering information dissemination, reducing opportunistic behaviour and fostering cohesive decision making (Nyhan Jones & Woolcock 2010, Ferlander 2007). Importantly, there is an assumption that teams with greater stocks of social capital are more likely to be productive and achieve better collective goals. Individuals collaborate to achieve team goals and outcomes that they could not achieve alone so, 'together everyone achieves more' (Murphy 2012:91). An individual's set of values and attributes shapes their engagement with others (e.g. expected norms of trustworthiness, cooperation, reciprocity) and is a vital ingredient in the development of social capital in groups and multidisciplinary teams.

Social capital dimensions

Given the importance of cohesive disciplinary and multidisciplinary healthcare teams, it would seem a natural extension to utilise social capital in team-building activities in healthcare workplaces. Social capital can be understood as the internal capacity for groups and teams to perform using networks and norms to cooperate by sharing resources (information, advice, favours) to solve problems (Ernstmann et al 2009, Ferlander 2007, Nyhan Jones & Woolcock 2010). As illustrated in Table 15.1, Grootaert and colleagues (2004:5) defined social capital into six dimensions for investigation, specifically:

1. Networks and groups

2. Norms of trust and solidarity

3. Collective action and cooperation

4. Information and communication

5. Social cohesion and inclusion

6. Empowerment.

TABLE 15.1
Operationalising social capital in multidisciplinary teams

Dimensions	Description	Social capital advantage in teams
1. Networks, Groups	• *Bonding* inward-looking ties to others 'like me'. • *Bridging* outward-looking ties with others with different social identity but comparable status. • *Linking* ties to others with dissimilar status, influence and resources.	• Teams with a range of members can access a wide range of useful resources. • Exchange of resources such as information, support, favours. • Valued norms include trustworthiness, reciprocity, cooperation, respect.
2. Trust Solidarity	• Trust (of family & familiar colleagues). • Generalised trust (of strangers, newcomers and organisations). • Willingness to help whoever needs it, not just friends. • Norms are expectations of behaviour	• Trust enhances cooperation. • Trust is the extent to which we can rely on others (familiar and strangers) to either assist us or (at least) do us no harm. • Communicate expectations.

Dimensions	Description	Social capital advantage in teams
3. Collective Action, Cooperation	• Whether and how effectively nurses work with others on common goals. • Cooperate with strangers to solve a problem or crisis.	• Cohesive multidisciplinary teams. • Reciprocity and cooperation between team members.
4. Information, Communication Exchange	• Influencing and leading to improve care. • Ways we receive and share research evidence, information and knowledge (considered to be resources) and for what outcomes.	• Communicate information and research knowledge within and across networks to improve care. Answer questions fully. • Consider who is excluded from information sources and the impact on their wellbeing and ability to provide safe and quality care.
5. Social Cohesion, Inclusion	• Be aware different ties and norms have the dual capacity to include or exclude individuals. • Inclusion promotes access to group resources such as support and information.	• Improved communication, resource exchange and cohesion. • Sanctions via exclusion will negatively impact wellbeing; ability to perform job; provision of quality healthcare services.
6. Empowerment	• Extent to which a nurse can influence processes directly affecting work–life and wellbeing and a preferred future.	• Personal efficacy, ability and capacity to make/influence decisions that can affect everyday activities and one's life. • Building resilience to cope in toxic teams.

Source: adapted from Ferlander 2007, Grootaert et al 2004, Hofmeyer 2012, Scott & Hofmeyer 2007.

Within each dimension, we can consider specific questions that allow us to understand the concept of social capital. For example, you may struggle to answer a question about how you could use social capital to access information from other nurses in the team. Conversely, if you were asked who you seek advice from in the team and why (e.g. their ties with you and their attributes), you would be able to reply.

We next review the six dimensions in greater detail to improve our understanding of social capital in multidisciplinary healthcare teams. The dimension of groups and networks examines the nature and extent of a nurse's participation in various networks and the diversity of resources exchanged to achieve common team goals. To understand forms of access and participation in different networks, it is important to identify the distinctions between *bonding, bridging and linking* (Gittell & Vidal 1998, Granovetter 1973, Nyhan Jones & Woolcock 2010) as illustrated in Table 15.2.

TABLE 15.2
Different forms of network ties: bonding, bridging and linking, strong and weak

Type	Network/Ties	Emphasis/ Awareness	Action
Bonding social capital	Refers to **strong interlocking horizontal ties** between close friends, family, work colleagues or groups 'like me' with similar status and social characteristics.	Places importance on identity and strategies for 'getting along'. Person's position in the networks influences their capacity to access resources to do their job.	**Strong** network **ties** can serve to replicate practice and preserve procedural status quo norms in teams. Implement strategies to mitigate exclusion of strangers, unpopular individuals or sanctioned due to violating group norms/expectations.
Bridging social capital	Refers to the strength of **weak horizontal ties** with close friends, family, work colleagues with different characteristics 'not like me'.	Places importance on open networks with expected norms to cooperate, collaborate, include and trust newcomers, accommodate difference and diversity. Reciprocity.	Recognise the value of **weaker ties** as vital to knowledge flow, diffusion and research uptake. Ties can provide strategies and opportunities for advancement in social and career relationships.
Linking social capital	Refers to **weaker vertical ties** that span power differences. Ties between people with different positions.	Places importance on connecting individuals to others in positions of power for 'getting ahead' and leveraging resources.	Mentor individuals (opinion leaders) with **weaker** cross-cutting network **ties** that operate on network/ team boundaries. Vital for diffusing new knowledge/evidence from other areas

Source: adapted from Hofmeyer 2012, Scott & Hofmeyer 2007.

Bonding networks refer to informal ties with others with similar social identity (age, occupation, education, income level, class, ethnicity) who can be called on for advice and assistance (Grootaert et al 2004, Nyhan Jones & Woolcock 2010). The nature of these ties can be nurturing and cooperative or serve to reinforce expected norms, loyalty and conformity between individuals (Portes 1998). The aim of the transactions in the network is to provide vital resources (information, job knowledge, advice, favours) so individuals can meet their job obligations. However, bonding network ties can also serve to exclude others outside the team from accessing vital resources. So it is critical to consider who is excluded or socially isolated in the team. Granovetter (1973) showed that a person's close colleagues and friends rarely knew more than they did, so strong bonding network ties (while possibly playing a greater role in emotional wellbeing) served to replicate practice and preserve the status quo. So we would be concerned if nurses only had bonding networks with nurses who were similar to themselves in profile and knowledge base. Typically such ties provide limited new information (Hofmeyer & Marck 2008).

Bridging networks refer to links with others with diverse and different experiences but similar in terms of status and power. The diversity of ties with other nurses is important to access different resources such as new clinical information. Linking networks refer to ties with others who are dissimilar in terms of their status and power so could be with leaders and wider links with external stakeholders. This is why successful teams feature a mix of bonding, bridging and linking networks, ethical norms and diverse resources. Questions also arise in this dimension about what characteristics are most valued by members in the networks. Trustworthiness, reciprocity, cooperation, honesty and respect dominate (Grootaert et al 2004, Nyhan Jones & Woolcock 2010).

The dimension of trust and solidarity is about the extent to which people feel they can rely on others to help them out or (at least) do them no harm (Grootaert et al 2004, Nyhan Jones & Woolcock 2010). Nurses need to feel confident that team members will be willing to help if needed and that individuals are competent. Some individuals limit trust to familiar colleagues who have proven to be trustworthy and competent. But in nursing teams with newcomers, trust needs to be extended to strangers, and newcomers in the first instance provide assurance that they can rely on others.

The dimension of collective action and cooperation is closely related to trust and solidarity. This dimension explores if and how individuals collaborate with others across the networks on collective team activities (Grootaert et al 2004). Collective action is a key component of resilient teams, but relies on adequate stocks of social capital in the team to be possible. Also of interest are the reasons why some nurses are more willing than others to work together, and if some nurses are more likely to exclude themselves or be excluded by the group. The social sanctions for violating the expected norms of participation and cooperation in the team can result in exclusion from the networks which can have dire consequences for an individual who may need support, favours or information from others. The importance of access to information cannot be underestimated for nurses in healthcare teams so the dimension of information and communication is critical. This dimension explores what information resources are available in the different networks, and the extent to which individuals can access information to do their job (Grootaert et al 2004, Nyhan Jones & Woolcock 2010). It is common practice to exchange information with colleagues. But if we have fragmented relationships with others, then we could be reluctant to ask questions to obtain information that might be crucial in planning and implementing safe care for patients.

The dimension of social cohesion and inclusion focuses on the tenacity of the ties between people and their two-fold capacity to include or exclude members of the group (Grootaert et al 2004, Nyhan Jones & Woolcock 2010). Inclusion promotes access to team identity, belongingness and resources. Recurring disagreements, divisions, everyday conflict and patterns of exclusion are often an indicator of low trust, serve to marginalise members of the team and limit access to needed resources. Murphy (2012:91) describes the notion of 'silent disengagement' first coined by Atul Gawande and expressed as 'that's not my problem'. A workplace with such disconnection is dangerous for multidisciplinary teams and patients. It is crucial to understand the impact of exclusion on individuals' wellbeing and work–life quality and to consider mechanisms by which conflict is managed (or not). The dimension of empowerment examines the application and outcome of social capital for individuals as a trans-formative process when they use their personal power to negotiate and influence decisions affecting their wellbeing, personal efficacy, sense of happiness and work-life (Grootaert et al 2004, Nyhan Jones & Woolcock 2010).

What we know

The concept of social capital is relevant to the formation and sustainability of effec-tive multidisciplinary healthcare teams because it provides a mutual way of talking about the expected norms of trust, cooperation, communication and knowledge exchange between newly qualified and more experienced professionals (Hofmeyer 2012, Hofmeyer & Marck 2008, Taylor 2012). The knowledge and resources to do our job are exchanged (or withheld) in the context of our networks (Hofmeyer & Scott 2007, Scott & Hofmeyer 2007). While the promise of inclusion and cooperation suggests 'value' in our social networks, it is important to be cognisant of resource-poor networks (lacking new information, support, favours) and the possibility of social isolation, exclusion and sanctioning (Portes 1998). A social capital framework offers a critical approach to examine use of power and exclusion in relationships and why some teams achieve collective goals better than other teams (Grootaert et al 2004, Hofmeyer 2012, Hofmeyer & Marck 2008, Sheingold et al 2012). Social capital accumulates where the process of working together is based on fairness and respect and professional practice (Cox 1995). Ethical principles are a component of a person's set of values and attributes, which is a vital ingredient in the development of social capital in multidisciplinary teams.

Social capital has intuitive appeal because it is based on the idea that social cohesion enhances wellbeing and 'relationships matter' (Field 2003:1). Moreover, Gopee (2002) claimed social capital can improve lifelong learning in the nursing workplace. Lifelong learning and professional development are associated with trust. Without trust, there is little social capital and organisational success. Kerfoot (1998) said that organisa-tional trust is the foundation upon which excellence and financial success can be built and depends on a trustworthy leader who is congruent, consistent, caring and competent. She said organisational effectiveness is dependent on human and social capital. Notably, Kerfoot (1998) linked social capital to economic advantage saying organisational trust among employees can increase reciprocity, optimise performance and improve healthcare. Our personal leadership and influencing style sets the scene in terms of norms—how we do things and engage with disciplinary and interdisci-plinary colleagues, patients and families. Different forms of leadership create different work environments and outcomes for nurses, the nursing workforce (Cummings et al 2010) and for patients (Wong & Cummings (2007) approaches to leadership; that is, building empathic, trusting, coaching and mentoring). Relational relationships with others to achieve common goals leads to lower staff turnover and higher job satisfac-tion; whereas pacesetting and commanding styles of leadership lead to staff burnout and turnover (Cummings et al 2010).

The leadership styles and practices of care unit managers can have a profound effect on the health of a team. When managers listen and respond to staff concerns, build strong, respectful relationships with staff and are interested in them as persons who bring expertise and knowledge to the workplace, nurse to nurse collaboration and teamwork is enhanced and patient outcomes are met (Cummings 2004, Cummings et al 2005).

It is timely to think critically about the enablers and barriers in work environments, levels of optimism and the resilience to deal effectively with change. This means having a willingness to foster positive relationships, collaborate and communicate across networks to enable the flow of new knowledge and take risks to implement new evidence in practice.

EDUCATION AND TRAINING FOR TEAMWORK

Of the scant teamwork studies in healthcare, most have investigated teamwork in the interdisciplinary context (Kalisch & Lee 2010, Kalisch et al 2007, Suter et al 2009). The ability to work effectively with professionals from other disciplines in interdisciplinary healthcare teams is one of the 21 competencies required for professional practice in the twenty-first century (O'Neill et al 1998). Collaborating with professionals in one's own discipline and in other disciplines was also strongly promoted in the landmark *Health21* Report (WHO 1999) that asserted:

> working alone with no regular exchanges of experience for mutual improvement can no longer be considered professionally satisfactory. Working in a team enables the professions to solve complex health problems that cannot be adequately dealt with by one profession alone.

However, the education and training of healthcare professionals has come under increasing scrutiny because it is deemed out of step with contemporary needs. Healthcare professionals are expected to work together in multidisciplinary teams, but are trained in separate disciplines (IOM 2003). The Institute of Medicine's (IOM) report, *To Err is Human*, states:

> most care delivered today is done by teams of people, yet training often remains focused on individual responsibilities, leaving practitioners inadequately prepared to enter complex settings ... the silos created through training and organisation of care impede safety improvements.
> (*Kohn et al 1999:146*)

In response, higher education institutions in Australia have sought to address the need for work-ready graduates by realigning academic education to build employability skills and competencies. Employability skills can be understood as: communication skills, effective interaction with colleagues and supervisors, conflict resolution and negotiation and creative problem solving, strategic thinking, team building and influencing skills (Abaidoo & Wachniak 2007, AQF 2011, Cumming 2010). Despite the significance of teamwork for quality and safety, there has been a limited increase in interprofessional curricula in baccalaureate programs to foster a disciplinary identity, teamwork training and employability skills to function in disciplinary and multidisciplinary teams (Hamman 2004, Neill et al 2012, Salas et al 2009, Suter et al 2009).

Respect for difference and disciplinary diversity is an essential team attribute. Different worldviews and values across disciplines can influence how individuals collaborate in the process of problem solving and making quality decisions about care. Strategies to facilitate effective teamwork include an open approach to critique by others and mentoring to develop professional and inter-professional identities. Standardised forms of communication can boost accurate knowledge exchange and common understandings between different disciplines to foster team building and effective team work (Vardaman et al 2012). Interventions to build resilient teams and skills using simulated learning approaches to improve staff engagement have also been examined (Kalisch et al 2007). Team-building activities have been shown to improve communication and clarity about different roles and increase cohesion and staff satisfaction (DiMeglio et al 2005). Hence there is a need to invest in team-building strategies in healthcare, addressing problems as they arise rather than letting them fester, raising different views and remaining on good terms with colleagues and leaders and mentoring nurses on problem-solving techniques and conflict resolution.

Reality of teamwork

The concept of teamwork is often presented in an erroneously Pollyanna way. It is promoted in an unrealistic and overly optimistic manner and assumed to be good in all contexts. We assert the reality of teamwork is somewhat different and often fraught with hierarchy, power and individual status interests that challenge meaningful negotiation. Similarly, Finn and colleagues (2010:1148) describe the 'evangelistic promotion of teamwork . . . the idea of teams is now widely accepted in our culture as something inherently positive'. A realistic way forward is to consider what values we bring to the team that shape our influencing and leading style and attributes such as personal resilience that are key to survival in dysfunctional healthcare teams.

BUILDING YOUR RESILIENCE TO THRIVE IN TEAMS

For some nurses, leaving a job or reducing team participation when the going gets tough in the team is an option for some but, for many, this is not a possibility. So what strategies can a nurse take to change and manage their work situation while building personal resilience and wellbeing to survive in workplaces marked by high workloads, conflict and fragmented relationships and dysfunctional team culture? There is a genuine need to develop mental toughness and physical stamina while maintaining a sense of purpose and meaning within a hectic and challenging pace of life. All of these elements contribute to building both personal and team resilience and cohesive teams. Trust relates to resilience because it fosters optimism and risk taking, which builds capacity within teams to respectfully solve problems and manage competing interests, dissent and diversity. Resilience is defined by Jackson et al (2007:3) as 'the ability of the individual to adjust to adversity, maintain equilibrium, retain some sense of control over their environment and continue to move on in a positive manner'. The concept of resilience and collegiality is about taking the lead to work respectfully and collaboratively across the generations. Find an ally and be an ally to others. Cummings (forthcoming) challenges us to view leadership as:

> being able to see the present for what it really is, see the future for what it could be, and then taking action to close the gap between today's reality and the preferred future of tomorrow.

Engaging others into seeing your vision of the future and to help build that future requires strong relationships and trust. Taking time out to recharge your spirit is crucial to foster positive emotions, happiness, work–life balance and resilience. This means actively pursuing a range of interests and connections with others who are caring and positive. Then we are more likely to be refreshed and able to contribute to a values-based innovative workplace culture and the pursuit of quality and excellence. Be mindful of your impact on others: a thoughtless word or careless response can have a devastating impact. The concept of emotional intelligence can increase resilience through its foundation of self-awareness and management of emotions at the time they are experienced (Goleman et al 2002). These foundational competencies allow individuals to then focus on others through a socio-political awareness of how decisions are made in the workplace and managing relationships with others in a way that supports trust, integrity and collective action to build a shared vision. Individual confidence and resilience supports team resilience.

Team building across generations

Understanding the generational and disciplinary diversity and differences that exist in healthcare workplaces is an important first step to fostering a climate of respect across generations and building effective teams. Leading those successful teams requires an understanding of how the motivational and value differences influence cooperation and teamwork with other disciplines. For example, GenXers born in the late 1960s and 1970s do not believe in 'paying their dues' in the workplace: they prioritise work–life balance to limit the work-creep into personal time, and are therefore reluctant to take on formal leadership roles. Gen Y, born between the early 1980s and early 2000s, change jobs regularly for new experiences, are technologically savvy and will not automatically respect age, authority or position (Benson & Brown 2011, Brunetto et al 2012, Scott-Young 2012). A social capital framework can guide an effective approach to inclusive team building and kindness across the generations. Bridging social capital networks can be fostered through active mentoring and coaching relationships and dialogue between all generations. The different generations of nurses can appreciate the diversity of knowledge, skills and perspectives of others, thus building norms of cooperation, tolerance, trust and inclusive cohesive teams. The key message is that all nurses can learn from each other and contribute to each other's transformation, wellbeing and lifelong learning, regardless of generational differences or hierarchy.

Resilient multidisciplinary teams

The characteristics of resilient teams mirror the dimensions of the concept of social capital. Bonding, bridging and linking networks and norms are foundational for cohesive teamwork, so we suggest the following actions could be adopted by managers and others to build social capital between team members:

1. Social capital networks and norms could provide a framework to begin dialogue about styles of leading and influencing, governance and social structures in organisations that will enhance teamwork between all generations of nurses, and be particularly inclusive of new graduate nurses.

2. Nurses working in multidisciplinary teams can foster bridging social capital and the exchange of new knowledge and information across the networks and teams through handovers and other informal teaching conversations underpinned by values.

3. Connected individuals can share new information to foster inclusive and effective multidisciplinary team relationships and networks for quality patient-centred care.

4. Building diverse networks and norms through team activities will strengthen teams and improve the flow of resources (advice, support, job knowledge). For example, graduate nurses may have strong bonding social capital networks with others like themselves, but have minimal bridging networks with more experienced nurses which would allow them to access different resources to improve their skills and ability to do their job.

5. Generations in the workplace. For example, managers could encourage Gen Y nurses to mentor others in areas such as technology and social media skills.

6. Managers can actively encourage and support nurses who are leading and influencing others in the multidisciplinary team to improve practice. They are typically caring, cooperative, well informed, articulate, approachable individuals who influence the uptake of research evidence into practice.

CONCLUSION

We conclude this chapter by asking you to take a moment to think about the characteristics of a person you admire, someone you would ask for advice, and feel confident they would answer fully. Consider that person's enduring set of values and beliefs that is visible in their interactions with others to build *social capital* in teams. Social capital can be understood as networks (bonding, bridging and linking) and norms of trust and cooperation that are visible in cohesive social relations, team spirit, belongingness and shared purpose (Hofmeyer 2003, Sheingold et al 2012). A social capital framework can explain how the quality of relationships between nurses can affect individual and multidisciplinary team outcomes. It is natural that we connect with some people more than others and forge lasting bonding ties because we may have shared significant experiences such as being first responders at a disaster or being relocated to another healthcare facility due to a hospital closure. This is why teams naturally comprise sub-groups of people who have bonding ties and affiliations. The critical issue is that these same individuals also have bridging social capital ties with newcomers and individuals from other sub-groups to access support, advice and favours. The concern arises when teams have a predominance of bonding social capital and callous disregard for the needs of others outside their network, such as in the earlier example of Unit B.

In the healthcare context, social capital is about the ability of different disciplines to develop genuine relationships with each other and work together to achieve desired outcomes. Nurses can lead the way by valuing individual diversity, cohesive relationships and teamwork that delivers better services for our communities. In the words of Westley and colleagues, 'in complex systems, relationships are key. Connections or relationships define how complex systems work; an organisation is its relationships not its flow chart' (2006:7). As coaching legend Vince Lombardi reminds us, 'individual commitment to a group effort—that is what makes a team work, a company work, a society work, a civilisation work' (Murphy 2012:91). This chapter calls for a re-valuing of relationships in multidisciplinary teamwork which is essential for integrated patient care. It highlights how to build your personal resilience and positive emotions to thrive in teams, which enhances your skills in leading and influencing throughout your career in nursing. Live as well as you can for yourself and others and be a nurse for the 21st century, promoting health for all those with whom you work and care for.

REFLECTIVE QUESTIONS

1. What values do you look for in other team members? What values do you bring to a team and where do you need to develop?

2. Where are the critical gaps in your personal and professional networks, and what actions could you take to build new links?

3. How do you feel when you are overloaded? What could you begin doing to build your resilience?

4. What are your core routines and habits that help you maintain a calm demeanour under pressure?

RECOMMENDED READINGS

Sheingold B, Hofmeyer A, Woolcock M 2012 Measuring the nursing work environment: can a social capital framework add value? World Medical and Health Policy 4(1):Article 3

Ferlander S 2007 The importance of different forms of social capital for health. Acta Sociologica 50(2):115–128

Cummings G G 2013 Your leadership style: how are you working to achieve a preferred future? Editorial, Journal of Clinical Nursing

REFERENCES

Australian Commission on Safety and Quality in Health Care (ACSQHC) 2011, September, National Safety and Quality Health Service Standards, ACSQHC, Sydney

Australian Nursing and Midwifery Council (ANMC) 2006 National competency standards for the registered nurse, 4th edn. Australian Nursing and Midwifery Council, Canberra. Online. Available: http://www.anmc.org.au/userfiles/file/competency_standards/Competency_standards_RN.pdf Accessed July 132012

Abaidoo S, Wachniak L 2007 Re-thinking graduate education: an imperative for a changing world. International Journal of Learning 14(5):205–214

Australian Qualifications Framework (AQF) 2011 Online. Available: http://www.aqf.edu.au/ Accessed 19 Feb 2012

Benson J, Brown M 2011 Generations at work: are there differences and do they matter? International Journal of Human Resource Management 22(9):1843–1865

Boyce R, Moran M, Nissen L, Chenery H, Brooks P 2009 Interprofessional education in health sciences. Medical Journal of Australia 190:433–436

Brunetto Y, Farr-Wharton R 2006 The importance of effective organisational relationships for nurses: a social capital perspective. International Journal of Human Resources Development and Management 6(2–4):232–247

Brunetto Y, Farr-Wharton R, Shacklock K 2012 Communication, training, well-being, and commitment across nurse generations. Nursing Outlook 60(1):7–15

Carter A J, West M A 1999 Sharing the burden: teamwork in the healthcare setting. In Firth-Cozens J, Payne R L (eds) Stress in Health Professionals. Wiley, Chichester, pp 191–201

Cox E 1995 A truly civil society. Australian Broadcasting Commission Annual Boyer Lectures ABC Books, Sydney, Australia

Cumming J 2010 Contextualised performance: reframing the skills debate in research education. Studies in Higher Education 35(4):405–419

Cummings G G 2004 Investing relational energy: the hallmark of resonant leadership. Canadian Journal of Nursing Leadership 17(4):76–87

Cummings G G (forthcoming) Your leadership style: how are you working to achieve a preferred future? Editorial, Journal of Clinical Nursing

Cummings G G, Hayduk L, Estabrooks C A 2005 Mitigating the impact of hospital restructuring on nurses: the responsibility of emotionally intelligent leadership. Nursing Research 54(1):2–12

Cummings G G, MacGregor T, Davey M et al 2010 Leadership styles and outcome patterns for the nursing workforce and work environments: a systematic review. International Journal of Nursing Studies 47(3):363–385

D'Amour D, Oandasan I 2004 IECPCP Framework: interdisciplinary education for collaborative, patient-centred practice. Research Report. Health Canada, Canada

DiMeglio K, Padula C, Piatek C et al 2005 Group cohesion and nurse satisfaction: examination of a team-building approach. Journal of Nursing Administration 35(3):110–120

Ernstmann N, Ommen O, Driller E et al 2009 Social capital and risk management in nursing. Journal of Nursing Care Quality 24(4):340–347

Ferlander S 2007 The importance of different forms of social capital for health. Acta Sociologica 50(2):115–128

Field J 2003 Social capital. Routledge, London and New York

Finn R, Learmonth M, Reedy P 2010 Some unintended effects of teamwork in healthcare. Social Science & Medicine 70(8):1148–1154

Gaboury I, Bujold M, Boon H, Moher D 2009 Interprofessional collaboration within Canadian integrative healthcare clinics. Social Science & Medicine 69:707–715

Gittell R, Vidal A 1998 Community organising: building social capital as a developmental strategy. Sage, Thousand Oaks, CA

Goleman D, Boyatzis R, McKee A 2002 The new leaders: transforming the art of leadership into the science of results. Little, Brown, London, England

Gopee N 2002 Human and social capital as facilitators of lifelong learning in nursing. Nurse Education Today 22(8):608–616

Granovetter M S 1973 The strength of weak ties. American Journal of Sociology 78(6):1360–1380

Grol R, Grimshaw J 2003 From best evidence to best practice: effective implementation of change in patients' care. The Lancet 362(9391):1225–1230

Grootaert C, Narayan D, Nyhan Jones V, Woolcock M 2004 Measuring social capital: an integrated questionnaire (SC-IQ).The International Bank for Reconstruction and Development/The World Bank, Washington DC

Hamman W R 2004 The complexity of team training: what we have learned from aviation and its applications to medicine. Quality Safety in Health Care 13(1): 172–179

Hofmeyer A, Marck P 2008 Building social capital in health care organizations: thinking ecologically for safer care. Nursing Outlook July/August 56:145–151.e2

Hofmeyer A 2012 Transition as a process for newly qualified nurses In: Fedoruk M, Hofmeyer A (eds) Becoming a nurse: making the transition from student to professional practice. Oxford University Press, South Melbourne, pp 35–50

Hofmeyer A, Scott C 2007 Final report: social capital in healthcare services. University of Alberta, Canada

Hofmeyer A 2003 Moral imperative to improve the quality of work-life for nurses: building inclusive social capital capacity. Contemporary Nurse 15(1–2):9–19

Institute of Medicine (IOM) 1990 Medicare: a strategy for quality assurance, volume I. National Academy Press, Washington, DC

Institute of Medicine (IOM) 2001 Crossing the quality chasm: a new health system for the 21st century. National Academy Press, Washington DC

Institute of Medicine (IOM) 2003 Health professions education: bridge to quality. Washington DC: National Academy Press

Jackson D, Firtko A, Edenborough M 2007 Personal resilience as a strategy for surviving and thriving in the face of workplace adversity: a literature review. Journal of Advanced Nursing 60(1):1–9

Kalisch B J, Curley M, Stefanov S 2007 An intervention to enhance nursing staff teamwork and engagement. The Journal of Nursing Administration 37(2):77–84

Kalisch B J, Lee K H 2010 The impact of teamwork on missed nursing care. Nursing Outlook 58(5):233–241

Kerfoot K 1998 Creating trust [On leadership]. Dermatology Nursing 10(1):59–60

Kohn L T, Corrigan J M, Donaldson M S (eds) 1999 To err is human: building a safer health system. National Academy Press, Washington, DC

Leonard M, Graham S, Bonacum 2004 Human factor: critical importance of effective teamwork and communication in providing safe care. Quality Safety in Health Care 13(1):85–90

Lin N 1999 Building a network theory of social capital. Connections 22(1):28–51

Marx K 1894 Capital: the process of capitalist production as a whole. International, New York

Murphy K K 2012 Together everyone achieves more. Journal of the South Dakota Medical Association 65(3):91

Neill D, Hammer J, Mims J 2012 Navigating the waters of interprofessional collaborative education. Journal of Nursing Education 51(5):291–293

Nyhan Jones V, Woolcock M 2010 Measuring the dimensions of social capital in developing countries. In: Tucker E, Viswanathan M, Walford G (eds) The handbook of measurement. Sage, Thousand Oaks, CA

O'Neill E H, The Pew Health Professions Commission 1998 Recreating health professional practice for the new century, 4th Report. Centre for the Health Professions, University of California, San Francisco CA

Portes A 1998 Social capital: its origins and applications in modern sociology. Annual Review of Sociology 24:1–24

Rafferty A M, Ball J, Aiken L H 2001 Are teamwork and professional autonomy compatible and do they result in improved hospital care? Quality and Safety in Health Care 10(2):ii32–37

Salas E, Almeida S, Salisbury M et al 2009 What are the critical success factors for team training in health care? The Joint Commission Journal on Quality and Patient Safety 35(8):398–405

Scott C, Hofmeyer A 2007 Networks and Social Capital: A Relational Approach to Primary Health Care Reform. Health Research Policy and Systems Available: www.health-policy-systems.com/

Scott-Young C 2012 What do you think of me? Move over, older workers, here comes Gen Y Cross Generational Management. UNISABusiness 2:22–23

Sheingold B, Hofmeyer A, Woolcock M 2012 Measuring the nursing work environment: can a social capital framework add value? World Medical and Health Policy 4(1):Article 3

Scott C, Hofmeyer A 2007 Networks and social capital: a relational approach to primary health care reform. Health Research Policy and Systems. Online. Available: http://www.health-policy-systems.com/

Sewell G 2005 Doing what comes naturally? Why we need a practical ethics of teamwork. International Journal of Human Resource Management 16(2):202–218

Suter E, Arndt J, Arthur N et al 2009 Role understanding and effective communication as core competencies for collaborative practice. Journal of Interprofessional Care 23(1):41–51

Taylor R 2012 Social capital and the nursing student experience. Nurse Education Today 32(3):250–254

Vardaman J M, Cornell P, Gonda M B et al 2012 Beyond communication: the role of standardised protocols in a changing healthcare environment. Health Care Management Review 37(1):88–97

Westley F, Zimmerman B, Quinn Patton M 2006 Getting to maybe: how the world is changed. Random House Canada, Toronto ON

Wilkinson R G, Marmot M 2003 Social determinants of health: the solid facts. World Health Organization, Copenhagen, Denmark

Wilson K A, Burke C S, Priest H A, Salas E 2005 Promoting health care safety through training high reliability teams. Quality and Safety in Health Care 14:303–309

Wong C, Cummings G G 2007 The relationship between nursing leadership and patient outcomes: a systematic review. Journal of Nursing Management 15: 508–521

Woolcock M, Narayan D 2000 Social capital: implications for development theory, research, and policy. World Bank Research Observer 15(2):225–250

World Health Organization (WHO) 1999 Health21: health for all policy framework WHO European region (European health for all series no. 6). WHO, Copenhagen

Xyrichis A, Ream E 2007 Teamwork: a concept analysis. Journal of Advanced Nursing 61(2):232–241

CHAPTER 16

Technology and professional empowerment in nursing

Alan Barnard

When you have read this chapter, you should be able to:

- explain the importance of technology for nursing practice and skills development
- describe characteristics associated with technology that are important for healthcare and clinical practice
- understand implications of technology for nursing care with specific reference to improving professional empowerment
- apply principles and values important for fostering excellence in nursing practice when associated with technology

KEY WORDS

Technology, empowerment, skill, person, nursing, technique, clinical, healthcare, caring, professional values, knowledge

NURSING AND TECHNOLOGY

This chapter considers the role and importance of technology for nursing practice, with specific reference to skill development and empowerment. Principles important to understanding technology are outlined and the implications of technology for nursing and healthcare are discussed, along with guiding principles and values important to appropriate integration of technology into clinical practice. It is argued that technology is important to our practice but is a phenomenon that must be understood adequately to address the many challenges it presents for current and future quality care.

Technology influences the practice of nursing both from the perspective of what we do and how we understand ourselves as practitioners. Nurses talk about technology, develop skills and knowledge to apply technology, interpret the health of our patients through application of technology, organise the workplace with the assistance of technology, praise the qualities of the latest advances and sometimes worry about loss of human contact and work in a changing workplace. Technology is used, for example, to deliver accurate treatment, to hold water, to cover patients and to observe the internal workings of the human body. Technology advancement is linked to shorter length of hospital stay, efficiency in care delivery, changing skills and knowledge, alteration to employment patterns, specialisation and standardisation of care (Locsin 2001, Rinard 1996, Sandelowski 2000). These outcomes of technological development combined with increasing legal liability and pressure on us to use increasing amounts of technology can often create a sense that nurses are embedded in healthcare practices that are focused on sameness, conformity, automation, safety, predictability and logical order.

Technology is significant to the history, contemporary practice and future of nursing. It has always been a part of nursing and in order to understand nursing as a discipline we need insight into the social, theoretical and practical implications that emerge as a result of our links with technology. Prior to the twentieth century, technical knowledge and skills developed by trial and error, and were passed down through generations via a practical and oral culture. Nurses relied on experience, intuition and faith. Technical skills included magical and aesthetic components that equated with moral and psychic life. Nursing practice relied less on scientific knowledge and explanation than on a personal and intuitive understanding developed and refined through practice (Barnard & Cushing 2001).

The rapid growth of scientific and technological knowledge in the twentieth century brought about enormous changes for nursing and healthcare, and technology has figured prominently as both a protagonist for development and an influential partner in our practice. Changes of significance have been our emerging role in the use of sophisticated technology to monitor patient progress, technological intervention through pharmaceutical administration and the use of technologies such as automated pumps and computers for recording and retrieval of information. Technology remains integral to healthcare and has significantly influenced our workplace, not only in terms of the artifacts (tools, machinery, automated equipment, etc.) and resources we use, but also how we do things, how we organise ourselves as nurses and what we value. In fact, 20 years ago Cooper (1993) warned that the process of technological change had advanced to such an extent that many areas of nursing practice had come to be defined by technology. For example, the haemodialysis machine is associated with renal nursing and the ventilator is associated with intensive care practice.

The warning has been confirmed further through, for example, the emergence of competency-based education and practice, which is linked directly to the safe integration and use of technology(ies). But regardless of whether the warning of Cooper is proving to be entirely accurate, it is acknowledged widely that nurses in all specialties are required to manipulate a significant amount of technology and accept increasingly complex roles and responsibilities associated with its ongoing importance in healthcare (Barnard & Locsin 2007, Daly et al 2009, Sandelowski 1997).

INTERPRETING TECHNOLOGY

The word technology (tech-nol-ogy) refers to the practical arts, specific implements and the knowledge and/or activity of a group (i.e. technologist). The phenomenon is subject to varied and sometimes inadequate explanation in nursing and is influenced by social status, culture, gender and politics (Barnard 2002, Pelletier 1989, Rinard 1996). First of all it is essential to recognise that technology is more than the sum of the things we use in healthcare. It has a characteristic that at one level includes the development of skills and knowledge but at another level is influential to perceived meaning and values (Feenberg 1999, Pacey 1999, Winner 2003).

One way to portray and interpret technology is as three concentric circles (see Fig. 16.1). Concentric circles highlight the characteristics that together emphasise a character-ological interpretation of the phenomenon. That is, the concentric circles try to show how each part of our practice can be interpreted in relation to the fundamental elements of technology. The interpretation is useful because it focuses our attention on not only the 'things we use in nursing' (located at the centre), but also their relations to other characteristics.

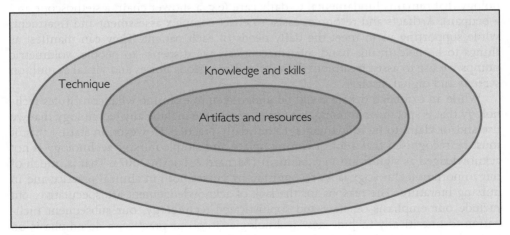

Technique

Knowledge and skills

Artifacts and resources

Figure 16.1
A character-ology of technology

Artifacts and resources

The smallest and central concentric circle depicted in Figure 16.1, artifacts and resources, is technology at its most obvious and refers to the integration, use and application of the 'things' of nursing. Rinard (1996) noted that in modern nursing there have been three key periods of change that have been significantly influenced by technology. The first period was 1950–65 and was characterised by new medical techniques and a significant introduction of pharmaceuticals to care. The second period was 1965–80 and was associated with greater use of sophisticated/automated technology and the emergence of new knowledge and specialisation. The third period was from 1980–90 and was associated with increasing technical control, streamlining and prediction of care as demonstrated by the emergence of automated pumps and monitoring equipment. A more recent fourth period, not identified by Rinard, could be explained as a period of rapid informational retrieval and computerised healthcare leading to rapid information gathering and care delivery at distance. There is a physical distancing such as the tendency for nurses to be located away from patients at the foot of the bed in surgical and ICU environments (Barnard & Sinclair 2006), or, for example, the distance that is created in tele-health environments.

We are required to include increasing amounts of technology in daily practice, and it is useful to clarify the various types of technology that are often found in our practice. We use simple, sophisticated, old, new, unique and commonplace technologies that continue to evolve in design and application. It can be observed that there are at least 12 different types of technologies that include clothes (e.g. shroud, pyjamas), utensils (e.g. bedpan, kidney dish), structures (e.g. hospital ward, isolation room), apparatus (e.g. Jordan frame, wheelchair, trolley), utilities (e.g. electricity, gas), tools (e.g. urinary catheter, syringe), resources (e.g. pharmaceuticals, sterile dressing), machines (e.g. intravenous infusion pump, ventilators), automata (e.g. computer, refrigerator), tools of doing (e.g. nurse's watch, stethoscope), objects of art or religion (e.g. nurse's uniform) and toys/games used for diversion (e.g. chessboard, dolls).

Although some machinery such as tools are new, increasingly accurate and powered by utilities such as electricity, it is worth noting that there is also a lot of simple technology that remains fundamental to daily care (e.g. a shower chair, a stethoscope and a bedpan). Artifacts and resources assist to enact complex assessment and treatment, while supporting us to meet the daily needs of each patient. They can manifest as things to be held in our hand, pharmaceuticals we dispense to people, volumetric pumps we use to assist treatment delivery and as various noises and visual stimuli on screens and digital displays.

While an extended debate could be undertaken to examine what constitutes technology that is specific to nursing, for our purposes we include any technology that we use and/or claim to be fundamental to our daily practice. However, in stating this, it must be recognised that a lot of commonplace and simple nursing technology is not acknowledged as significant (e.g. bedpan) (Barnard & Locsin 2007). That is, much of our important technology lacks recognition by nurses both in clinical practice and in nursing literature. The reasons for the lack of acknowledgement are speculative, but include our emphasis on new and sophisticated technology, our subsequent inclination to uncritically include new technologies into our practice, a de-emphasis on technology associated with the 'dirty work' of nurses, limited investigation into the historical development of nursing technologies and a lack of scholarship examining the phenomenon (Sandelowski 2000).

Knowledge and skills

The second or middle concentric circle in Figure 16.1 portrays technology as *knowledge and skills*. Artifacts and resources have associated professional meaning(s) that are in many ways determined by the knowledge and skills associated with their use (e.g. advanced technology of the ICU unit), their usefulness in terms of reliability and their functional design. Importantly, knowledge and skills contribute to the successful use of artifacts and resources, and are therefore as much technology as the objects themselves. Without required knowledge and skills for the use and application of technology, it has limited ability to meet the needs of nursing practice and care. For example, without the skills necessary to use a computer, it is not much more than plastic, metal and electricity, and will not assist daily practice. Without knowledge to interpret or efficiently fix a problem associated with technology (such as an alarm on an infusion pump) the technology is of little use and may well be a dangerous addition to patient care.

Nursing is a practical occupation and our knowledge is expressed most often through the way we perform our work. To this end, we focus often on what we do as practitioners and explain technology from perspectives that emphasise daily roles and responsibilities. For example, there has been debate concerning the increasing role of nurses in the use and maintenance of machinery and equipment. It has been argued that nurses have to fulfil the role of technician, and this is significantly distracting us from focusing on the experience of each patient (Boykin & Schoenhofer 2001).

Nurses rely on experience, continuing education, personal development and peer mentors to maintain and develop knowledge and skills that are associated with technology. Failure to establish and develop knowledge and skills is inadequate for practice and unhelpful to patient care, colleagues and the requirements of the healthcare sector. Knowledge takes many forms and relates to not only competencies related to nursing intervention, but also organisational policy, understanding scope of practice, interpreting quality and safety frameworks, and keeping up with changing evidence. These all form part of the development of technological competence, which is central to technology–nurse–patient relations and is vitally important for care.

The outcome of technological competence is not only the development of skills for technology use, but also our ability to know 'the other' (i.e. the person whom you nurse) as an individual. Thus when using technology in care we need to know and understand individual preferences, culture and beliefs. This significant part of caring is achieved as an outcome of purposefully seeking to know the person as an individual and through making appropriate use of technological data and resources for their benefit (Locsin 2001). This aspect of practice is an equally important component of technological competence. Patients trust that nurses will have the competence necessary to professionally use technology and demonstration of competence reduces anxiety and fear and increases the likelihood of successful care outcomes. Advances in organ transplantation, genetics, pharmaceuticals, microsurgery, virtual reality, e-health, telehealth and so on demand an equal ability on our part to update and adapt knowledge and maintain technological competence.

Knowledge and skills alter regularly, and thus an active interest in maintaining and advancing competence is a sign of a caring and responsible practitioner who is empowered to be accountable for the quality of their practice. Attitudes that reflect an offhand and neglectful interest in updating knowledge and skills are inadequate, and reflect a failure to value the importance of people for whom we care. It is a denial of the many possible contrary indicated outcomes that might arise from inadequate technology integration and is unprofessional.

Technology introduces options for care and can make clinical practice more efficient, quicker and more accurate. Skills alter as a result of technology, and this fact should encourage personal reflection on the nature, relevance and impact of change on individual and collective practice (Locsin 2001). For example, an automatic blood pressure monitor de-emphasises manual skills related to assessing a person's blood pressure, but demands new skills in terms of using the automated machine to obtain useful data. Many skills that were required previously for nursing are no longer necessary for contemporary practice and new skills emerge regularly to become part of daily care. For example, the practice many years ago of boiling urine in a test tube to analyse urine was replaced by the use of a coloured test strip, and the electronic blood pressure monitor often replaces the use of a hand-operated sphygmomanometer. We are engaged in an ongoing and regular process of deskilling and re-skilling in practice.

Thus the outcomes of technological change are associated with emerging technical complexity that must be integrated into the organisation of work. Technological sophistication is always about achieving greater efficiency and logical order, and relevant technological change should be associated with and judged against the achievement of better use of your time and resources and better patient care. For example, the intravenous infusion pump permits nurses to undertake 'other duties' while intravenous therapy is being delivered to their patient at a determined rate. However, the intravenous infusion pump de-emphasises skills associated with manually determining flow rate. An infusion pump is often a good thing for time saving and control in daily practice, but at a higher level we are reminded that an often unasked question in relation to technology and nursing is 'what skills need to be retained' and 'what skills can fall away' as a result of specific technological change(s).

These are important questions and are fundamentally necessary for current and future professional development. For example, although we have been proactive in acquiring new skills and knowledge for care, we are required sometimes to revisit older, less common ways of undertaking certain assessment(s) and treatment(s), especially in less resourced clinical areas.

But amidst all this change, some nurses interpret the process as a loss of caring and perceive human relationships as devalued or ignored. Rinard (1996) postulated that the evolution of technology and nursing is a story of de-skilling in which nurses have purposefully gendered nursing knowledge in line with vocational and societal expectations of what is (was) valued culturally as 'feminine', at the cost of serious analysis of skills.

De-skilling and re-skilling are issues worthy of analysis, but little has been undertaken within the profession. In fact, over the past 60 years nursing has seemingly been reluctant to critically analyse technological change within the contexts of skills alteration, societal trends and the changing nature of nursing work (Barnard 2002, Barnard & Cushing 2001, Fairman 1998, Rinard 1996, Sandelowski 1999b, 2000). Although new clinical activities have been added to the professional role of the nurse, these additions have been regarded often as secondary to a more generalised growth in the sophistication of nursing work.

Most technological development in nursing has arisen as a result of technology replacing older procedures with newer more efficient and reliable technology, and among this there are significant changes occurring to nursing labour. We do things more quickly, more efficiently, with more automation and at times with more accuracy, yet there is a clear disjunction between the social–scientific nature of nursing work, analysis of changing healthcare, theoretical interpretation of nursing and the realities of nursing work. The effects of technological change on the skill of each nurse have been analysed poorly, but at a practical level, changes are linked to increasing technical complexity, alteration to autonomy and a general sense of not ever having enough time to do everything.

Technique

The influence of technology on autonomy is most obviously illustrated in the third and most inclusive concentric circle in Figure 16.1, which highlights the concept of *technique*. The third circle extends our character-ology of technology to include the way systems, policy, politics, economics, ethics, organisational management and human behaviour are organised for the benefit of technology. The way nursing practice is organised for, as well as by, artifacts and resources is as much technology as the first and second levels of meaning. Technique is not a specific thing. Technique is a way of thinking, it is an attitude, it is a social and professional framework, that has an enormous influence upon each one of us.

Technique seeks to take naturally occurring phenomena such as reflective thinking, communication and human relationships and change them into organised and controlled phenomena. An example to illustrate technique might be the difference between a caring moment with a patient motivated by a nurse's compassion for another, versus the preplanned application of efficient communication strategies to construct a relationship based on predefined goals and outcomes. The latter has all the hallmarks of technique because there is emphasis, for example, on a 'one best way' to efficiently undertake the activity yet it can so often lack the humanness of personal commitment and connection. According to Lovekin (1991), technique is the consciousness that gives machines force, which sees everything else as machine-like or as needing to serve the machine-like, the ideal towards which technique strives.

Technique reduces the means of production, whether they be machines or us nurses, to that which is most technological (i.e. efficient and rational) in order to create a unified and predicable activity. Examples of technique in the management of healthcare services are economic rationalism, protocols, risk assessment, action planning, communication strategies, benchmarking, patient dependency models, systems theory, clinical pathways management and standardised care plans. A transformation is occurring in which many aspects of our practice that were once instinctive, reflexive, natural and particular to individuals and cultures are being transformed into rational method and instruction. In craft-based technology the worker is able to express themselves with a sense of creativity, pride in personal agency and autonomy in determining action and expression. In automated technology environments these values and experiences have a tendency to be replaced by a sense of dependency on predetermined actions, protocols and practice frameworks that permit partial exercise of personal ability and preference and knowledge that personal input can be replaced by another (Ferre 1995).

Technique is a complex phenomenon that is constituted by three subtle yet important characteristics. First, technique adheres to a *primacy of reason* to govern practice. It is a way of thinking, acting and living by which people attempt to control the internal, passionate and emotional world of everyday life via protocols, rules, evidence, frameworks and general observance to a logical order. Second, it requires a *desire for efficiency* in order to assist its goal and to justify its activity. The desire for efficiency is akin to the inventor or factory owner who seeks to streamline methods and actions in order to maximise outcomes. Efficiency seeks practical utility and a guaranteeing of results. There is a striving to reduce waste and the construction of systems that simplify and systematise previously uncontrolled or random activity. We nurses are free to engage in clinical practice, but this freedom is limited much like that of a clock. There is freedom for the hands to move around the clock face as long as nothing 'gets in the way'. The gears and springs move freely within the mechanism, yet there is a clear expectation that behaviour is determined and able to be repeated by each nurse.

It must be stressed that there is nothing wrong or dangerous per se with a desire for reasoned activity or efficiency. In fact, there is nothing new about rationality or efficiency as reasonable and worthwhile goals. They have both guided invention and activity throughout human history and, after all, who wants to be exposed to ineffective care?

However, the third characteristic of technique brings about new and different activity because it stresses primacy of efficiency in *every realm of human activity and thinking*. Technique has become so prevalent in society, organisations and nursing that people are increasingly incapable of thinking outside its boundaries in their search for meaning. A world has been created that has a tendency to override or minimise the importance of subjectivity and human experience. There is emphasis on control, efficiency, policy and order within a climate of litigation (Harvey 1997, Neuhaus et al 2002, Sinclair & Gardner 2001, Wagner 1992, 1994).

Technique reduces thinking and human-centred activities such as nursing to measurable and predictable outcomes. It has potential to change previously natural worlds of human experience to *other*. That is, technique brings about qualitative transformation(s) in care. Under these conditions nursing practice risks becoming a robotic-like activity that does not require its practitioners to be particularly caring, compassionate or necessarily understanding of the experiences of people (except if it is preplanned as an efficient activity). As a result of technique, a new struggle has emerged for nursing and we need to find ways to authentically respond to individual need(s), cultural difference(s) and personal choice.

TECHNOLOGY, NURSING AND PROFESSIONAL EMPOWERMENT

Empowerment can be measured at an individual, organisational and community level, and is associated with the ability to make independent decisions and maintain individual autonomy at a personal level (Masi et al 2003). It is characterised by a sense of control, goal attainment and competence. Professional empowerment is linked to ownership of knowledge, especially knowledge that is attributed to a specialist group or professional elite. It is obtained when each member of the professional group raises their status through autonomy, skill and competence, especially when related to the provision of care. This type of achievement reflects what Manojlovich (2007) refers to as the three available areas of empowerment for nursing, being: control over the content of our practice; the context(s) of practice; and competence.

Unfortunately, in nursing, power has arisen less often in association with ownership of knowledge and skills, because we have had difficulty confirming that which is specific to nursing, and nursing knowledge is associated with gendered skills of caring that are valued less by society and healthcare (Henderson 2003, Rinard 1996). Notwithstanding we continue to seek recognition as a discipline and seek to produce competent practitioners for clinical environments where technical performance is prized highly (Barnard & Locsin 2007).

In many clinical environments we have accepted new roles and responsibilities that have originated from the introduction of technology and the reassignment of duties from medicine (e.g. diagnostics and assessment). As a result, there is consistent reliance within healthcare sectors on our knowledge and skills, and this fact has been interpreted as a demonstration of our professional success (Almerud et al 2008, Sandelowski 2000). Nurses are often the only healthcare workers who possess necessary knowledge and skills required to operate particular machinery and tools in clinical environments. Technology cultivates for nurses enhanced respect, importance and uniqueness and, when it is used well, these qualities transfer to nursing as a profession (Fairman 1992, Sandelowski 1997).

However, it must be noted that despite the growth of knowledge and skills in nursing and the expansion of roles and responsibilities, the legal, clinical and political responsibility for technology continues to remain predominantly in the control of medicine. It is noted by Patel (2002) that even though physicians make up less than 10% of the workforce in the United States, they determine why, how, when and the frequency with which biomedical technologies will be used, not only in the diagnosis of patients, but also in their treatment. Nurses and other healthcare workers provide well-defined and restricted services that reflect a physician's orders or an agreed protocol. Doctors admit patients to hospital, order most diagnostic procedures and, by and large, have been the decision makers and gatekeepers who determine treatment(s) that patients will receive.

Future professional advancement must demand deeper insight into our relations with technology, and this growth will empower nurses because it will equip us to better engage in debate and decision making (Barnard & Sinclair 2006, Fairman 1998, Fairman & D'Antonio 1999). Expertise in clinical practice will be enhanced through our ability to: assess the suitability of technology for healthcare provision; advance person-focused care; sustain effective healthcare initiatives; and reinvigorate cultural, spiritual, moral and social values important to healthcare professions. Thus, it was encouraging to note that the United States Institute of Medicine in a 2001 report emphasised the need for patient-centred and performance-based care that is devised around healing relationships and the provision of healthcare founded on needs and values.

It is commonplace for nurses to interpret the overall effects of technology on nursing as either positive or negative (known commonly as the optimism versus pessimism debate) (Sandelowski 1997). Debates between nurses have been reliant upon whether, for example, technology is believed to have a determining feature which reduces menial work, increases comfort, emphasises a harmony between technology and caring and expands knowledge (optimism), or has a determining feature which undermines patient care, causes fragmentation of health services, fosters a lack of caring behaviour and deskills nurses (pessimism).

Either perspective (optimism or pessimism) is to some degree an expression of specialist and professional interests and value judgements concerning technological development. In reality, both perspectives contain elements of truth yet ultimately artifacts and resources are not in themselves inherently deterministic, but they do demand our attention. For example, problems related to enhancing a person-focused approach in high-technology areas reflect individual nursing experience(s), assumptions about the role of technology in clinical practice and the organisation of healthcare, rather than any essential or fundamental conflict between technology and nurses (McGrath 2008, Rudge 1999, Sandelowski 1999a). In a critical essay on the semiotics of the nursing–technology relationship, Sandelowski (1999a, 2000) highlighted the way(s) that language/depiction/sign within nursing has served to create a presumed problem between nurses and technology. It was argued that there is growing evidence that current representation of the relationship between nursing and technology does not support the development of practice informed by critical reflection, nor the development of strategies that best enable clinical decisions to be made about the appropriate use of technology.

The following principles express values that relate to a focused approach to thinking about technology and nursing. They are important for professional empowerment in practice, will equip you to engage in healthcare debate(s) and are suggested as important to reinvigorating social and public service.

Good healthcare matters because people matter

Healthcare and nursing practice must be guided fundamentally by principles that promote, establish and protect human dignity. Protection of dignity is central to all that nurses engage in, and is central to the utilisation and integration of technology in care. Each person and their family have intrinsic value. Their uniqueness and importance must be acknowledged in even the most sophisticated technological environments. Objectification and loss of human dignity have been linked with technology (Almerud et al 2008, Locsin 2001, Rinard 1996, Sandelowski 2000), yet so often an emphasis on the experience and uniqueness of the person is possible with foresight and courage. For example, Barnard and Sandelowski (2001) highlight that even during high-intervention experiences such as emergency resuscitation, clinical measures can be adopted in order to place human experience and dignity central to care. Good healthcare matters because people matter, and this moral value must be continually emphasised, especially within healthcare systems dominated increasingly by technique.

The right to quality care

Each person has a right to healthcare resources and quality nursing. Even though access to technology is sometimes restricted as a result of factors such as physical location and managed-care initiatives that place limitations on available resources (e.g. types of pharmaceuticals available in Australia and New Zealand), the dignity and worth of each life supports the view that we are responsible to effectively utilise and integrate appropriate technology.

Technology is political

The practice environment of a specialist unit, a community facility or a healthcare organisation will impact on the usefulness of technology. For example, a hospital unit that is designed poorly in terms of its layout or is resourced inappropriately is unsuitable to accommodate modern machinery and automata. Nurses can spend excess time and effort attending to technology and compensating for the inadequacies of poor resources. When resources do not foster adequately the use of technology, when they are defective or deficient and when support is not provided to foster skills and knowledge, the practice of nursing becomes difficult and stressful. Technology under these conditions becomes a burden to our practice. Funding, ward design, appropriate equipment and resources such as power and gas supply are crucial. When the practice environment is inadequate, the experience of integrating technology into care can be one of frustration, compromised health and safety for patients and staff, inadequate patient care and decreased efficiency and effectiveness (Lumley 1987, McConnell 1990, McGrath 2008).

Central to nursing practice is the need to create order in busy, demanding and complex clinical environments because practice alters regularly, policies and procedures are governed by external authorities and patients are very often acutely sick. Nurses can experience a lack of certainty in clinical practice (unpredictability, varying demands on time, numerous roles and responsibilities) due to the demands of busy and complex clinical practice environments, and we rely upon appropriate technology. In the following quotation a nurse explained her experience of technology and stated that:

> [T]echnology has so many advantages that if you are without it and you are busy, you do notice the difference. You tend to be more rushed and you don't have as much time to stop and chat … to your patients.
> (Barnard 1998:169)

When technology works effectively and is appropriately resourced in terms of its associated parts and repair, it provides substantial assistance to establishing safe and predictable patient care and can assist a nurse to coordinate various elements of clinical practice. Therefore, we need to be involved in determining the direction(s) of technological change and influencing decision making (Fairman 1996, Harding 1980, Hiraki 1992, McGrath 2008, Sandelowski 1997, 2000, Walters 1995). Decisions regarding access to particular technology, or the acquisition and use of machinery and equipment, are always political. Decisions related to technology will impact directly on the practice of each nurse, the organisation and the patients for whom we care. When new equipment arrives it has to be integrated not only in terms of its financial cost, but also in relation to skills and knowledge change. New technology means new skills to learn, new policy and another potential requirement to undergo further competency assessment. If new technology is essential, make sure everyone is doing everything they can to support its integration into your practice, through initiatives such as in-service and available expertise.

Technology reveals only part of each person's experience and condition
Sophisticated electronic and computerised technology emphasises a reliance on evidence that is made available for us as digital display, computer screens and printouts. Although technology offers real and worthwhile indicators as to the physical condition of a patient, an excessive reliance on technology can result in a tendency to accept quantitative evidence in preference to, and in spite of, the thoughts, experiences and feelings of the person. The following quotation from a nurse explains a typical scenario:

> [Y]ou've got this patient who is really grey, sinking in the bed, more and more you've got to be saying, what's happening? Is it just because of his oxygen saturation levels? Is there nothing else going wrong? Should I be checking other things? We've got to have faith in ourselves to go and check through and say, what is happening with this patient?
> (Barnard 1998:189)

It is unprofessional to replace patient assessment skills with a singular reliance on information from machinery and equipment. Excessive focus on information from technology without adequate consideration of a patient's total physical and emotional condition can result in treatment and intervention that is inappropriate and insensitive.

Technology is not a neutral object and nurses are not its master

Technology assists to achieve care outcomes that are complex and significant. However, technology is not neutral to care and sometimes overrides consideration of cultural, spiritual, emotional, physical and psychological needs as it strives to bring about efficient outcomes (Almerud et al 2008, Barnard 1997, McGrath 2008, Sandelowski 2000). That is, technology always has a seen and unseen impact upon our activity, goals and outcomes. It does not lead always to treatment outcomes acceptable for patients, but it is not a demonic force leading always to uncaring nurses in inhospitable wards. Technology will assist you to reach care outcomes across a range of possibilities from positive to negative, and therefore expertise in practice needs to be based upon a holistic framework that informs awareness and planning. Holism emphasises the centrality of the person and by extension the values, choices and individual lives that come into our care and management. The increasing emphasis within healthcare upon, for example, standardisation, protocols and integrated systems to manage healthcare delivery, whilst often extremely beneficial, have to be balanced against a willingness to advocate for the values and expectations of the person for whom we profess to care.

Technology to a greater or lesser extent alters our capacity to determine and accomplish individual goals, professional approaches to care and principles of nursing practice. It influences what Walters (1994) described as the ability of each nurse to *focus* his or her energies on the person and their ability to *balance* technology with the qualities of caring. Technology can positively and negatively influence a nurse's available time to establish a nurse–patient relationship and be involved in personal care. For example, technology in a clinical environment that malfunctions often will not save time nor release a nurse to concentrate on practice principles that place the person at the point of primary concern. These conditions will not necessarily deliver the treatment your patient wants, can cause distress and uncertainty and will restrict the daily delivery of care. Poorly integrated technology will make the daily practice of nursing more demanding, time consuming and distracted. In addition, when clinical practice is dominated by excessive policies, protocols and limited resources, as well as constant demands to check equipment, administer drugs and respond excessively to inappropriate alarms, technology becomes a compelling and sometimes annoying influence upon a nurse's time, physical commitment and intellectual attention.

The demands of technology will sometimes intervene independent of strategies used to ensure the smooth operation of a clinical area. Choice of technology affects people's lives and requires users to formulate different ways to do things. It is not surprising that when problems arise from technology it can affect available time to, for example, care for a person's body (e.g. mouth care, hygiene, bathing). We are required to manage the effective integration of technology sometimes at the cost of other roles and responsibilities. The demands of telephones, buzzers and equipment checking can draw us away from the other things we need to do. In the following quote from a nurse, the experience is explained:

> All those alarms and monitors, they're geared to catch your attention aren't they? I mean, that's why they have alarms. So the first thing you do when you have alarms is go to it. It's like telephones at home. The first thing that you do when the telephone rings, it doesn't matter how busy you are, you drop everything to go and answer

the phone, instead of saying, it's just a phone, leave it ring. I mean you put telephone answering machines on telephones these days, because the phone has to be answered doesn't it? We're geared these days to attend to noises and equipment before we attend to people.
(*Barnard 1998:193*)

You cannot use technology without also, to some extent, being influenced by its use. Our ability to display many of the caring behaviours associated commonly with nursing (i.e. a focus on personal experience, empathy, compassion) can be challenged, not often by a lack of compassion, empathy or desire to be involved more with people, but by the influence of technology on roles and responsibility. It is extremely important to recognise that the amount of technology in nursing practice does not alter our ability to feel compassion for the experience of others. It is simply not true to claim that the majority of nurses do not desire to engage in patient-focused practice founded on compassion and concern. It is true, however, to claim that sometimes technology and the way(s) we use it gets in the way of our ability to express the desire.

CONCLUSION

When technology is used appropriately in clinical practice it improves the effectiveness and efficiency of nursing, empowers carers and establishes predictable measures, assessment and behaviour. It assists greatly in our ability to understand the physical condition of the patient, and saves time by making patient assessment increasingly accurate and potentially reliable. These advantages are extended further when we properly integrate technology into personalised care and our practice is one of expertise and competence. Importantly, technology–nurse relations are more than just being able to manage equipment. Nursing practice continues to change in association with technology. Changes influence the practice of nursing from the perspective of what we do, how we think and how we understand ourselves as practitioners. There is nothing minor or insignificant about technology as it will continue to have a major role in changing healthcare (Barger-Lux & Heaney 1986, Barnard 2002, DeVries & Barroso 2000, Sandelowski 2000).

Nurses are increasingly responsible for technology and we work within administrative and bureaucratic structures that influence our roles, responsibility and frameworks that assist us to know the scope of our practice. Knowledge and skills associated with nursing practice have altered over time, the ends to which we find ourselves working have changed and clinical practice continues to broaden despite a lack of understanding and explanation about ongoing changes to arise from technology. Gordon (2006) highlighted that emerging literature and practice demonstrates a clear and apparent disjunction between the technical aspects of care and the embodied experience of people. Nursing discourse increasingly highlights an emphasis on mechanistic and reductionist explanations that focus on technical aspects of care without an equal emphasis on the experience and personal nature of the healthcare experience for each patient (person). Gordon describes the situation as a new Cartesianism: a new dualism in which the technical is separated from the embodied and experiencing person.

More scholarship and research is needed that addresses technology and nursing from perspectives that examine how we use artifacts and resources in practice, the relationship of clinical practice to theoretical models of nursing and caring, competency development and a range of philosophical and sociological issues associated with power, gender, human experience and discipline development. Finally, the question remains, what do we do about technique in our clinical practice in order that we might begin to empower ourselves and the people for whom we care? The answer to the question lies probably in political action, individual activism and advocacy, planning care based on each person's needs and being willing to create a certain detachment from the imperatives that technique engenders. We should not underestimate the challenge that is before us.

Technique is integrated within the socio-cultural context of society and nursing, and person-focused practice(s) is a freedom to be won. Our duty is to occupy ourselves with the dangers, errors, advantages, difficulties and temptations of technology for the benefit of people. In undertaking this duty, we empower ourselves as significant contributors to healthcare.

REFLECTIVE QUESTIONS

1. What does this chapter tell us about the relations between nursing, technology and professional empowerment?

2. What important issues and values need to be understood in order to appropriately integrate technology in clinical practice?

3. Reflect on your clinical experience noting how often and under what circumstances the values outlined in this chapter are achieved.

4. What future research and development could be initiated in clinical practice to better achieve the professional principles and values expressed in this chapter?

RECOMMENDED READINGS

Barnard A, Sandelowski M 2001 Technology and humane nursing care: (ir)reconcilable or invented difference? Journal of Advanced Nursing 34:367–375

Nelson S, Gordon S (eds) 2006 The complexities of care: nursing reconsidered. Cornell University Press, London

Sandelowski M 2000 Devices and desires: gender, technology and American nursing. University of North Carolina, Chapel Hill

REFERENCES

Almerud S, Alapack R, Fridlund B, Ekebergh M 2008 Caught in an artificial split: a phenomenological study of being a caregiver in the technologically intense environment. Intensive and Critical Care Nursing 24(12):130–136

Barger-Lux M J H, Heaney R P 1986 For better or worse: the technological imperative in health care. Social Science Medicine 22(12):1313–1320

Barnard A 1997 A critical review of the belief that technology is a neutral object and nurses are its master. Journal of Advanced Nursing 26:126–131

Barnard A 1998 Understanding technology in contemporary surgical nursing: a phenomenographic examination. Unpublished PhD thesis, University of New England, Armidale

Barnard A 2002 Philosophy of technology and nursing. Nursing Philosophy 3:15–26

Barnard A, Cushing A 2001 Technology and historical inquiry in nursing. In: Locsin R (ed) Advancing technology, caring and nursing. Auburn House, Westport, pp 12–21

Barnard A, Locsin R (eds) 2007 Technology and nursing practice. Palgrave-Macmillan, London

Barnard A, Sandelowski M 2001 Technology and humane nursing care: (ir)reconcilable or invented difference? Journal of Advanced Nursing 34:367–375

Barnard A, Sinclair M 2006 Spectators and spectacles: nurses, midwives and visuality. Journal of Advanced Nursing 55(5):578–586

Boykin A, Schoenhofer S O 2001 Nursing as caring: a model for transforming practice. National League for Nursing, Massachusetts

Cooper M C 1993 The intersection of technology and care in the ICU. Advances in Nursing Science 15(3):23–32

Daly J, Speedy S, Jackson D 2009 Contexts of nursing: an introduction, 3rd edn. MacLennan & Petty, Sydney

DeVries R, Barroso R 2000 Midwives among the machines: recreating midwifery in the late 20th century. Online. Available: www.stolaf.edu/people/devries/docs/midwifery.html

Fairman J 1992 Watchful vigilance: nursing care, technology, and the development of intensive care units. Nursing Research 41:56–60

Fairman J 1996 Response to tools of the trade: analysing technology as object in nursing. Scholarly Inquiry for Nursing Practice: An International Journal 10:17–21

Fairman J 1998 The nurse–technology relationship in the context of the history of technology. Nursing History Review 6:129–146

Fairman J, D'Antonio P 1999 Virtual power: gendering the nurse–technology relationship. Nursing Inquiry 6:178–186

Feenberg A 1999 Questioning technology. Routledge, New York

Ferre F 1995 Philosophy of technology. University of Georgia Press, London

Gordon S 2006 The new cartesianism. In: Nelson S, Gordon S (eds) The complexities of care: nursing reconsidered. Cornell University Press, London, pp 104–121

Harding S 1980 Value laden technologies and the politics of nursing. In Spicker S F, Gadow S (eds) Nursing: images and ideals, New York, Springer, pp 49–75

Harvey J 1997 The technological regulation of death: with reference to the technological regulation of birth. Sociology 31(4):719–736

Henderson S 2003 Power imbalance between nurses and patients: a potential inhibitor of partnership in care. Journal of Clinical Nursing 12:501–508

Hiraki A 1992 Tradition, rationality, and power in introductory nursing textbooks: a critical hermeneutics study. Advanced Nursing Science 14(3):1–12

Locsin R (ed) 2001 Advancing technology, nursing and caring. Auburn House, Westport

Lovekin D 1991 Technique, discourse and consciousness: an introduction to the philosophy of Jacques Ellul. Associated University Press, New Jersey

Lumley J 1987 Assessing technology in a teaching hospital: three case studies. Paper presented at the 'Technologies in health care: policies and politics conference', Canberra

Manojlovich M 2007 Power and empowerment in nursing: looking backward to inform the future. The Online Journal of Issues in Nursing 12(1):Manuscript 1

McConnell E A 1990 The impact of machines on the work of critical care nurses. Critical Care Nursing Quarterly 12(4):45–52

McGrath M 2008 The challenges of caring in a technological environment: critical care nurses' experiences. Journal of Clinical Nursing 17(8):1096–1104

Masi C, Suarez-Balcazar Y, Cassey M et al 2003 Internet access and empowerment. Journal of General Internal Medicine 18:525–530

Neuhaus W, Piroth C, Kiencke P et al 2002 A psychosocial analysis of women planning birth outside hospital. Journal of Obstetrics and Gynaecology 22(2):143–149

Pacey A 1999 Meaning in technology. MIT Press, Cambridge

Patel K R M 2002 Health care policy in an age of new technologies. M E Sharpe, New York

Pelletier D 1989 Health care technology: sharpening the definition and establishing aspects of the social context. Australian Health Review 12(3):56–64

Rinard R 1996 Technology, deskilling, and nurses: the impact of the technologically changing environment. Advances in Nursing Science 18(4):60–70

Rudge T 1999 Situating wound management: technoscience, dressings and 'other' skins. Nursing Inquiry 6:167–177

Sandelowski M 1997 (Ir)reconcilable differences? The debate concerning nursing and technology. Image: Journal of Nursing Scholarship 29:169–174

Sandelowski M 1999a Culture, conceptive technology, and nursing. International Journal of Nursing Studies 36:13–20

Sandelowski M 1999b Venous envy: the post-World War II debate over IV nursing. Advances in Nursing Science 22(1):52–62

Sandelowski M 2000 Devices and desires: gender, technology and American nursing. University of North Carolina, Chapel Hill

Sinclair M, Gardner J 2001 Midwives' perceptions of the use of technology in assisting childbirth in Northern Ireland. Journal of Advanced Nursing 36(2):229–236

Wagner M 1992 Appropriate birth care in industrialised countries. Paper presented at the 'Future birth conference', Sydney

Wagner M 1994 Pursuing the birth machine. Ace Graphics, Sydney

Walters A J 1994 An interpretative study of the clinical practice of critical care nurses. Contemporary Nurse 3:21–25

Walters A J 1995 Technology and the lifeworld of critical care nursing. Journal of Advanced Nursing 22:338–346

Winner L 2003 Social constructivism: opening the black box and finding it is empty. In: Scharff R C, Dusek V (eds) Philosophy of technology: the technological condition. Blackwell, Oxford, pp 233–244

CHAPTER 17

Nursing and informatics: a transformational synergy

Jen Bichel-Findlay and Cathy Doran

LEARNING OBJECTIVES

At the completion of this chapter, the reader should be able to:

- define nursing informatics
- identify the skills required for nurses to be competent in informatics
- outline the benefits of informatics for nurses
- differentiate between data, information, knowledge and wisdom
- describe the challenges of achieving an information-literate nursing workforce
- outline the benefits of an electronic health record
- describe the articulation of nurses with the PCEHR.

KEY WORDS

Nursing informatics, health informatics, medical informatics, knowledge worker, information literacy, electronic health record

INTRODUCTION

Despite being an information-intensive discipline, the healthcare system is prone to tremendous inefficiencies because of inadequate communication infrastructure and practices. While information technology is advancing in other sectors of most industrialised countries, healthcare systems operate in an information environment that is inefficient, fragmented, often inaccessible, devoid of technical standards and ease of interoperability and interfacing, 'mired in a morass of paper records and bills, fax transmittals and unreturned telephone messages', and endangers the lives and health of its constituents (Goldsmith et al 2003:45). Rifkin (2001) asks health professionals to consider the modern-day irony of emergency clinicians having an easier time accessing a patient's bank account (using their automatic teller machine card) than they would finding critical medical history, as information about medical conditions, electrocardiograms, response to previous treatment, current drug therapy and identified drug allergies are typically stored on paper and often inaccessible in emergencies.

It cannot be disputed that healthcare has lagged behind in the adoption of information technology. There has been a sudden explosion of health information technology (HIT) adoption in the last decade, due to worldwide health reform, the ageing population, the increase in chronic illnesses, the need for patient-centric care and the need to improve healthcare quality and safety. This has led to a call for a more coordinated approach to patient care and the need to share information between care providers using electronic health records and patient-controlled health records. The current Australian healthcare workforce is hoping that the not-too-distant future will bring them access to lifelong computerised patient records. These records would be created by linking multiple encounters, be easily and quickly accessed from remote locations and offer decision support in all aspects of healthcare delivery. Clinicians wanting access to patient information will no longer be limited by environment (ward, unit, department) or time (after hours, weekends) boundaries, as the record will always be available.

The current health service environment expects clinicians to use technology to integrate more and more information from more and more diverse sources, and convey this information to more and more people (Westby & Atencio 2002). Information technology is also expected to play a significant role in developing more informed and less passive healthcare consumers, triggering a shift in the roles of patient and clinician, of which the impact has yet to be fully established. A transformation in information technology is currently taking place in healthcare systems worldwide, and the resulting communication paradigm shift associated with this transformation will change how clinicians use clinical information to treat their patients.

Whilst increasing the level of control over various functions and fortifying the quality of care delivered to patients, it is anticipated that these systems will transfer clinicians to a virtual surreal world of healthcare perfection by preventing medical errors at the point and time of care, improving efficiency and reducing healthcare costs (Blumenthal & Glaser 2007, Fett 2000). This technology has the potential to enhance nursing practice and add to the development of nursing science in this coming information processing era (Sewell & Thede 2013). Informatics itself will not only create new roles for nurses, but will also enable nurses who are experiencing substantial pressure from their already high workloads to access a range of relevant information in an expedient manner. Nurses will need to be more discriminate users of information in the future, and identify and develop new ways of using technology to support the practice of nursing. The discipline of nursing must acknowledge the interactive and synergistic effect that exists between nursing informatics and nursing practice if it is to play a central role in supporting strategic goals of healthcare in the future.

ORIGINS OF NURSING INFORMATICS

The delivery of healthcare is information-intensive, and this considerable amount of information management of healthcare data is an indispensable aspect of contemporary healthcare organisational infrastructure. In order to deliver quality healthcare to consumers, clinicians need to acquire, evaluate, interpret and generate relevant information from the data they have gathered, recorded and communicated. It has become increasingly difficult for health professionals in all facets of clinical practice and healthcare management to deliver their services without employing existing information technologies, and this challenge will only continue as consumers expect and demand increasing quality of healthcare services. Informatics is the scientific discipline that employs information technology to deal with the capture, storage, retrieval, communication and optimal use of data, information and knowledge (Sewell & Thede 2013). More simply, it is 'the science and art of turning data into information' (Hebda & Czar 2013:6).

This discipline of health informatics is over half a century old, having evolved from medical informatics, however it has only secured a prominent position in healthcare since the 1980s. The term *informatics* is thought to have derived from the Russian term *informatika*, which is an adaptation of the French word *informatique*, originally signifying a combination of computer and information science (Ball et al 2000, Hebda & Czar 2013, Sackett & Erdley 2002). Current definitions, however, encompass a broader scope of responsibility. Health informatics is the science and practice around information in health that leads to informed and assisted healthcare, where 'informed' means the right information about the consumer, patient or population together with relevant health knowledge available at the right time in a useable form, and 'assisted' means the activities of the clinician are made safer and easier and the health consumer is supported in their decisions and actions (Health Informatics Society of Australia 2012).

While the first medical informatics conference (Medinfo) was held in Stockholm in 1974, the term 'nursing informatics' was not used until the 1980 Medinfo conference in Tokyo. Nearly a decade later, Graves and Corcoran (1989) published the seminal definition of nursing informatics that combined three sciences (computer, information and nursing) to support the management and processing of nursing data, information and knowledge to sustain the practice of nursing and the delivery of nursing care. Managing information pertaining to nursing is the focus of nursing informatics, allowing the identification of relationships between interventions and outcomes, the reduction of documentation duplication and the availability of data to researchers to expand evidence-based nursing knowledge.

Nursing informatics essentially dates back to Florence Nightingale, who realised not only the importance of data and its relationship to patient outcomes and quality nursing care, but also how data could promote innovation in health service delivery (McBride 2006). It can also be argued that nursing data has not always been valued, given that nursing documentation was not initially incorporated into the patient record but was placed in a separate repository. The advent of the nursing process in the 1970s provided nursing with a framework to document interventions and activity, and this improved the type of information recorded about the patient. Despite these improvements, however, nursing information recorded in a paper-based patient chart in reality tended to disappear following discharge of a patient. This significantly impacts on nursing knowledge, as information not easily accessed cannot be learned from, and therefore wisdom cannot be expanded (Sewell & Thede 2013).

It is important to understand the relationship between data, information, knowledge and wisdom. Data is the collection of numbers, characters or facts (generally numeric or alphabetic code) that are gathered according to some perceived need for analysis and possibly action at a later point in time, such as vital signs, length of stay, and so on (Hebda & Czar 2013). The focus of data is naming, collecting and organising (Saba & McCormick 2011). Information is the collection of data that has been interpreted, such as temperature readings plotted and compared with normal values, or data that has been examined for patterns and structure (Hebda & Czar 2013). The focus of information is organising and interpreting (Saba & McCormick 2011). Knowledge is the synthesis of information derived from a number of sources to produce a single concept or idea, and is based on logical processes of analysis, providing order to thoughts and ideas – validation of the information provides knowledge that can be used again (Hebda & Czar 2013). The focus of knowledge is interpreting, integrating and understanding (Saba & McCormick 2011). Wisdom arises when knowledge is used appropriately to manage and solve problems, and results from cumulative experiences, learning skills and ways of thinking (Hebda & Czar 2013). The focus of wisdom is understanding, applying and applying with compassion (Saba & McCormick 2011).

Since the 1990s various professional nursing organisations in the United States (US) have urged nursing faculties to master and teach informatics skills and knowledge to undergraduate nurses who will work in a healthcare system reliant on information technology. The American Nurses Association recognised nursing informatics as a subspecialty of nursing in 1992, and currently all nursing education programs in the US incorporate nursing informatics as a core competency (Sewell & Thede 2013). The International Council of Nurses also recognises the importance of informatics, with its fact sheet stating that nursing informatics is a critical component of healthcare, effective decision making and high-quality nursing practice (International Council of Nurses 2005). It can also ensure nursing's visibility in local, national and international healthcare data sets, thereby empowering nurses with information to influence policy and promote nursing research (International Council of Nurses 2005). The National League for Nursing in the US asserts that universities should be building informatics capacity in undergraduate nurses so they can practise evidence-based care in an information-rich environment (National League for Nursing 2008, Skiba & Thompson 2007). Visionary leadership will ensure that tomorrow's nurses possess the skills to use information technology and the expectation of its availability (Simpson 2008). In fact, Saba and McCormick (2011) highlight that in some US hospitals, there are nurses currently being employed who have never charted on paper.

Undergraduate nursing informatics programs will not assist the existing nursing population. Nurses currently working in health services will need support and training to become competent in basic computer skills and information literacy, ensuring that they can work effectively in an electronic healthcare environment (Hart 2008). 'Professional bedside nurses must attain and maintain a level of informatics competency that can serve as the bedrock to their practice, strengthening their clinical decision making, enhancing the patient experience, and helping to improve health outcomes' (Schleyer et al 2011:173).

All Australian higher education institutions offering nursing include education for students on computer use and health and nursing informatics, largely due to a 1997 government report on health information management and telemedicine that proposed all Australian universities take a leading role by integrating information and communication technologies into nursing curricula (Smedley 2005). By 2002, the National Review of Nursing Education recommended online education and the use of information and communication technologies as essential for sustainable education practices and the functioning of nurses in the workplace, and most nursing laboratories now provide the same computer equipment that is currently available in hospital environments (Smedley 2005). New Zealand undergraduate nursing programs share a similar approach as Australia. In particular, the University of Auckland embeds health informatics into every subject in the entire undergraduate nursing degree providing graduate nurses with the informatics skills required to support clinical practice (Honey 2006).

The Australian national competency standards for registered nurses also highlights the significance of information, in relation to using best available evidence and demonstrating analytical skills in accessing and evaluating health information and research evidence (Australian Nursing and Midwifery Council 2006). The Nursing Council New Zealand identifies that nurses require information management and communication competencies but does not go as far as to indicate that these skills are related to either health informatics or computer technology (Honey & Westbrooke 2012).

A study undertaken in 2005 in Australia indicated that undergraduate nurses were offered basic computer training, however information literacy and management was not included in coursework (Smedley 2005). Another study conducted in 2007 in Australia found that nurses were generally poorly prepared to engage with information technology in their practice, and that very few nurses had any formal information technology training (Australian Nursing Federation 2008). According to Foster and Bryce (2009), Australia is lagging behind in the development of competencies for undergraduate nurses and all practising nurses, with validated informatics competencies currently not existing.

A national project to develop, validate and publish informatics competency standards for the nursing profession in Australia has commenced, funded by the Australian Department of Health and Ageing and managed by the Australian Nursing Federation (Foster & Bryce 2009). This project will 'ensure the continued development of a skilled, capable and informed nursing workforce, able to use the tools that technology provides for the delivery of safer and better integrated patient care' (Australian Nursing Federation 2008). The informatics competency standards will 'provide a basis for the provision of appropriate contemporary curricula for informatics education and continuing education that is appropriate for the workplace' (Australian Nursing Federation 2008). The Australian Nursing Federation (2008) stress that not only is it essential to build workforce capacity in health informatics that will support and advance healthcare initiatives for the benefit of all Australians, it is also vital that a national approach to the development of competencies in informatics for nurses and integration of these into nursing curricula is a priority.

Other countries are more advanced in the development of nursing informatics competencies to ensure that nurses can practise in an HIT environment. Europe has established certification programs that define the skills and competencies necessary to be a proficient user of a computer and common computer applications—European Computer Driving Licence (ECDL) and the International Computer Driving Licence (ICDL). The ECDL is known as ICDL outside of Europe, and both programs have specialist modules for health informatics systems users. Finland, Norway and Italy have adopted the ECDL for all nurses, and Great Britain makes available the ICDL for all nurses to ensure basic computer skills (Gugerty & Sensmeier 2010).

Informatics will become even more critical in the current reformed health service environment within Australia, with the Council of Australian Governments supporting the National Health Reform Agreement in August 2011. Whilst providing for the most sustainable funding arrangements for Australia's health system and attempting to improve health outcomes for all Australians, this agreement supports a data-driven health service environment through the establishment of the National Health Performance Authority (improve accountability and performance reporting) and the Independent Hospital Pricing Authority (improve transparency and efficiency of services) (Australian Government Department of Health and Ageing 2012b). The progressive introduction of activity-based funding commenced in 2012 aims to capture consistent and detailed information on hospital sector activity and accurately measure the costs of delivery, as well as providing incentives for hospitals to treat more patients more efficiently and in the most appropriate setting. Capturing consistent and detailed information will only be achieved with informatics tools as part of an information infrastructure.

INFORMATICS SKILLS FOR NURSES

Staggers and Thompson (2002:260) proposed that 'the goal of nursing informatics is to improve the health of populations, communities, families, and individuals by optimizing information management and communication'. Ten years later, this statement is even more salient, as informatics is the enabler that supports nursing care, with the nurse as the primary interface between information technology and the patient, and often between the patient and the healthcare system. In this crucial position, nurses need to be more discriminating users of information, and extend their scope beyond gathering data and using information, to using and building knowledge (McGonigle & Mastrian 2012).

Nursing staffs' attitudes towards technology, particularly computers, has been studied extensively for a variety of reasons. First, collecting and processing most patient data has historically been the responsibility of nursing and, even today, they rely primarily on labour-intensive methods to record, retrieve and manipulate information (Patel & Currie 2005). Secondly, nurses contact nearly every other healthcare provider, and their attitudes and perceptions significantly influence the perception of these other providers (McLane 2005). Lastly, nurses are quite often the resource other clinicians approach or access when they have questions about the use of computerised systems (McLane 2005).

The need for nurses to increase their knowledge of computers was recognised as early as 1988 by the National League for Nursing in the US, who suggested that practising nurses ought to have four informatics competencies—documenting nursing practice, accessing information, using the data and information from a computer system and coordinating information flow (Liu et al 2000). All nurses were expected to reach informed user level, most professional nurses should reach proficient user level and those nurses with advanced training ought to become developers of systems (Grobe, cited in Liu et al 2000). Training programs for nurses were developed, and included a range of topics such as computer hardware, software, vocabulary, applications relevant to nursing, word processing skills, system security and limitations of computers (Liu et al 2000, Saranto & Leino-Kilpi 1997).

In 2002 the American Nurses Association developed recommendations for the computer and information literacy skills of novice and experienced nurses (Hobbs 2002). Novice nurses should use computer technology to accomplish tasks, and have skills in the use of a word processor, database and spreadsheet, in using applications to give/document patient care or communicate via email (Hobbs 2002). Experienced nurses should have the knowledge, attitude and skills to support their major area of practice, and see relationships among data elements and make judgements based upon data trends and patterns (Hobbs 2002).

In 2005, nursing leaders in the US established a vision for the future of nursing that bridged the quality chasm with information technology, and the Technology Informatics Guiding Educational Reform (TIGER) initiative was established (DuLong & Ball 2010). TIGER aimed to facilitate more engagement of practising nurses and nursing students in the evolving digital era of healthcare, ensuring all nurses were educated in using informatics and were empowered to deliver safer patient care (DuLong & Ball 2010, Skiba et al 2010). This group determined that using informatics was a core competency for all clinicians, and that unfortunately many nurses lacked information technology skills (McGonigle & Mastrian 2012). The model identifies three competency areas—basic computer skills, information literacy and information management (Saba & McCormick 2011). This reform initiative moved into a second phase in 2007, where nine key collaboratives were established to engage the nursing community more deeply into the realm of informatics (Saba & McCormick 2011). Currently, TIGER III is creating a champions group as well as a virtual learning environment, specifically addressing four of the nine phase II key collaboratives—competencies, staff development, education and usability (Saba & McCormick 2011). TIGER initiatives are being established in other countries, and this will augment the integration of informatics into daily nursing activities.

Another major initiative also occurred in 2005, with the Health Information and Management Systems Society (HIMSS) developing the Impact of Health Information Technology (I-HIT) Scale to measure the impact of HIT on the nursing role and on interdisciplinary communication occurring in hospitals in the United States (Dykes et al 2010). The scale addresses the general advantages of HIT, the workflow implications of HIT, the information tools to support communication tasks and the information tools to support information tasks (Dykes et al 2010). In 2007, six additional countries were added to the survey—Australia, New Zealand, England, Scotland, Ireland and Finland—under the auspices of the International Medical Informatics Association—Nursing Informatics (IMIA-NI) Special Interest Group (Dykes et al 2010). This study provided valuable insight into the uptake of HIT and the impact HIT has on nurses across the globe.

Australian respondents revealed that nurses recognise the importance of HIT and have access to HIT tools, such as patient administration systems and results reporting, but they do not have the tools that would assist with communication and care coordination such as clinical documentation and care planning (Dykes et al 2010). This affected their overall satisfaction with HIT across the survey. In response to the question of how satisfied are you with the HIT applications/tools currently available in your hospital, Australia, England, Ireland and Scotland were more dissatisfied than satisfied, and the US, Finland and New Zealand were more satisfied than dissatisfied. Finland was extremely satisfied (over 80%) and England was the least satisfied (approximately 30%) (Dykes et al 2010).

In response to the statement that HIT allows for patient/family participation in care, Australia recorded the strongest level of disagreement (over 70%). Australia recorded the least agreement with the statement that HIT facilitates my efficiency in practice (65%), and only 40% of Australian respondents supported the statement that HIT decreased the time they needed for end of shift handover (Dykes et al 2010). Australia recorded the least levels of agreement with the statements that HIT applications available at my facility helps me access information necessary for safe patient care (78%) and I know how to access the applications available in the electronic medical record system (under 70%) (Dykes et al 2010). The survey also found that HIT changed the nurse's role in multidisciplinary communication as more information was available via HIT (Dykes et al 2010). On the positive side, over 75% of Australian respondents considered that they had information tools to support communication tasks including patient tracking, and nearly 70% had access to applications that supported both patient care and administrative processes (Dykes et al 2010). The authors, however, were concerned that more than 75% of Australian respondents had not participated in implementing HIT at their facility, believing this to impact on perceptions as well as utilisation of HIT (Dykes et al 2010). The Australian component of this study showed that HIT has the potential to assist nurses with the information that is needed to improve patient care.

The study in Ireland and Scotland was not as successful as Australia, due to poor adoption rates of HIT within hospitals (Dykes et al 2010). The New Zealand study was problematic and difficult to validate as there was a poor response rate, however it did identify that the HIT currently available was 'not nursing-focused and nurses use the system for accessing laboratory and radiology results' (Dykes et al 2010). Overall, the international study provided a baseline for future measurement on how HIT impacts nursing practice, as well as highlighting the lack of HIT systems that can currently support nursing care and the capacity for nurses to fully adopt HIT. Marin & Lorenzi (2010:50) claim that 'nurses, more than other health professionals, must blend this new technology into their care processes'. Nurses need to be competent in HIT in order to blend technology into nursing practice.

Regardless of what setting a nurse is providing care in, and at what level the nurse is engaging with patients, it should be acknowledged that two roles essentially exist in informatics for nurses—a clinician who is an informatics specialist and, more commonly, a healthcare provider who must use information technology in their delivery of care. Nursing informatics specialists are generally expert clinical nurses who have informatics qualifications and exceptional communication skills, who represent the nursing stakeholders in decisions that have an impact on clinical systems in the practice setting (HIMSS Nursing Informatics Awareness Task Force 2007). These nurses take on many roles including project management, business analysis, trainers, business case developers, requirements gatherers and managers of health information systems (HIMSS Informatics Awareness Task Force 2007). It is the nurse informatics specialists that ensure that the clinical nurses' requirements and workflows are included in the development of clinical systems. On the other hand, nurses caring for individual patients need to be able to access evidence-based information and patient data at the point of care to inform their patient encounters. In turn, patient data that nurses enter during the process of documenting their patient encounters needs to be entered in a way that can lead to aggregation of data to inform future patient encounters (McGonigle & Mastrian 2012).

Sewell & Thede (2013) identify four levels of informatics competencies for nurses— the beginning nurse who possesses basic information management and computer skills (accesses data and uses a computer, basic desktop software and decision support systems); the experienced nurse who is highly skilled in using information management and technology to support major areas of practice such as making judgements on trends and patterns and suggesting improvements in nursing systems; the informatics nurse specialist who integrates and applies information, computer and nursing sciences; and the informatics innovator who conducts informatics research and generates informatics theory. HealthWorkforce Australia (2012) is currently investigating the health informatics workforce in order to identify the issues and pressures faced by this group in the current healthcare environment, as well as examining and quantifying the current and future demand and supply. The project will also assess the extent of any gaps, and inform education and training strategies (HealthWorkforce Australia 2012). A skilled informatics workforce will certainly be needed in Australia in the next decade, given the substantial state and federal government investment in electronic health information systems.

The ability to use computers has generally been referred to as 'computer literacy', however current authors prefer the term 'computer fluency'. Literacy is seen as a temporary state, whereas fluency is able to increase one's ability to effectively use a computer when needed (Sewell & Thede 2013). Information literacy refers to the ability to recognise pertinent information for retrieval and discovery of knowledge (Sewell & Thede 2013). Nurses are currently expected to be information-literate professionals who possess clinical judgement based on scientific evidence and technological development (Skiba 2005). They are now viewed as knowledge workers, who are immersed in knowledge dissemination, acquisition, generation and processing (McGonigle & Mastrian 2012).

INFORMATICS BENEFITS TO NURSES

More than a decade ago, Ball et al (2000) claimed that technology development occurs in three stages—substitution, where technology is substituted to automate or perform functions without a change in the nature of the data processing; innovation, where technology is combined with existing functions that facilitate a generation of new functions or tasks; and transformation, where technology is used to transform the nature of work (such as radiology practices). At that time, the authors (Ball et al 2000) highlighted that nurses had been in the substitution stage of information technology acceptance for over three decades, as the profession was only using part of the technology's capability. Elfrink (1996) was also perplexed at why nurses were willing to learn about other technologies such as complex life-saving machines and complicated life-sustaining procedures, yet the mastery of information technology had been considered a low priority, resulting in nursing practice remaining entrenched in inefficient and dated approaches to communication. Despite technology offering nursing greater scope for managing information and developing knowledge to support current and future practice, it could be argued that nurses in many countries, including Australia, have still not formulated a culture that encourages acceptance and use of information technologies as fundamental tools for information management and exchange.

Informatics, particularly electronic health records, has the potential to influence many activities in healthcare delivery—reduce medical errors and duplication of tests, improve communication and access to current and comprehensive patient information, expand the quality of data collections to support decision making, provide transparency around increasing costs, strengthen patient record security and assist healthcare workers in coping with a reduced workforce and increasing demand (Australian Health Informatics Education Council 2011). A major advantage of using technology is that data are entered once, but can be retrieved and used many times, and automation techniques facilitate the sharing of these data and information for quality measurement, quality improvement, regulatory compliance, research and education (Hebda & Czar 2013, McGonigle & Mastrian 2012, Sewell & Thede 2013). This will also increase the time devoted to patient care and create a lifelong clinical record, often referred to as a 'womb to tomb' approach to health history.

From a clinical nursing perspective, informatics has the potential to augment practice and add to the development of nursing science in a number of ways. A major benefit of technology for nurses is to improve documentation and reduce the time devoted to documentation. This is significant given that studies estimate 15–25% of nursing time is spent documenting patient care (Gugerty et al 2007). It is hoped that duplication will be substantially reduced, given that nurses currently enter data on an observation or flow sheet and repeat this entry in the patient record or nursing notes, or enter patient allergies on a plethora of forms. Having to enter the same data twice or more wastes time and also increases the potential for error through inaccurate transcribing. Utilising electronic systems to capture information about the patient also ensures consistency and completeness in entry, as well as requiring data and information to be structured. Automation facilitates efficiency in activities such as medication administration, decision support system alerts, worklist reminders and prompts, discharge instructions, nursing care plans and clinical pathways and medication information (Hebda & Czar 2013, Sewell & Thede 2013). The time saved can be directed towards other activities such as planning, patient and carer/family education, risk assessments and so on.

Informatics applications can also assist the clinical nurse with professional networking, allowing them to communicate with colleagues worldwide and to remain aware of best practice methods (Sewell & Thede 2013). The vast array of online communication tools includes interactive networking such as Web 2.0 and 3.0; instant messaging, chat and Twitter; voice over the internet protocol (VOIP); teleconferencing via the internet—web conferencing, webcast, webinar; collective intelligence tools; wikis; cloud computing; folksonomies and tagging; blogs; RSS feeds; mashup; group discussion forums; grass roots media; podcasts and vodcasts; and email (Sewell & Thede 2013). As previously indicated, nurses are knowledge workers, and therefore are lifelong learners. It is estimated that knowledge workers devote at least 50% of their time searching for and evaluating information (McCormick 2009). Increased access to real-time data and information at the point of care will improve currency and comprehensiveness of knowledge that can be readily applied to patient care.

Informatics applications can assist the nurse manager to automate staffing rosters, track shift vacancies and subsequent filling by overtime, casual or agency staff; review and examine nursing practice activities in relation to standards and competencies;

assist in the dissemination of information about clinical guidelines and standardised care activities; address quality improvement and outcomes analysis; undertake cost and trend analysis for budgetary purposes; develop business cases for unit improvements based on current and comprehensive data and information; participate in action research activities to patient care issues; and devise new models of nursing care delivery (Hebda & Czar 2013).

Nurse educators can use technology to deliver and support web-based, distance and online education; provide remote access to library and internet resources; facilitate online course registration and scheduling; assist in the preparation of and access to education session slides and handouts; administer online examinations, streamline the recording of compliance with mandatory education requirements; track information about students' classroom and clinical performance, particularly comparing individuals with group norms; and communicate with students about course objectives, recommended readings, assessment activity and so on (Hebda & Czar 2013). As previously discussed, educators must also prepare nursing students to handle data and assess and retrieve information (Hebda & Czar 2013).

There is an obvious association between informatics and nursing research, and informatics can play a large part in expanding the scientific base of the profession. Technology can significantly streamline literature searching; enhance the collection of data related to clinical interventions; locate trends in aggregate data from small- to large-scale data sets; perform statistical analysis; facilitate the application of nurmetrics; allow for research in real-time; and facilitate research collaboratives with nurses in multiple geographic locations (Hebda & Czar 2013, Sewell & Thede 2013). Technology will also ensure a shift in knowledge acquisition for nurses from historical avenues such as tradition, authority, borrowed theory, trial and error, personal experience, role modelling, reasoning and research to an approach based on data analysis and best practice evidence supported by research (Hebda & Czar 2013).

ELECTRONIC HEALTH RECORD

Early informatics applications were designed to overcome four problems that still exist in the current healthcare arena—lack of care coordination, reliance on memory, lack of recorded logic of delivered care and lack of an effective feedback loop (Sewell & Thede 2013). The informatics application that most countries are currently trying to deploy nationally into their healthcare environment, with varying degrees of success, is an electronic health record or EHR. An EHR is a longitudinal electronic record that captures episodic patient-focused summary information from multiple clinical systems that traverse general practitioner, community, hospital (emergency inpatient and outpatient) and specialist patient care. Governments are committed to EHRs in an attempt to address the rising cost of healthcare, the ageing population, increased health disorder chronicity amongst the population and to meet consumer expectations. Transforming a health service from using a paper-based clinical record to a fully electronic system does not happen overnight, and nurses are required to use both systems concurrently using a hybrid medical record. Nurses are expected to know intuitively which system holds the latest and most up-to-date information for their patients.

Every year, on average, Australians visit a general practitioner four times, obtain 12 prescriptions, and visit a medical specialist three times (Australian Government Department of Health and Ageing 2012a). Often the care provided is disjointed, due to the lack of communication between care providers, and results in duplication of services. Authors of a recent major study addressing Australian healthcare encounters also reveal that appropriate care is only provided to 57% of patients and, for some common conditions, only 32% of patients receive the recommended care (Runciman et al 2012). These authors highlight the need for national agreement on clinical standards and improved structuring of health records to encourage the delivery of more appropriate care (Runciman et al 2012).

The EHR journey in Australia started in 1999 when the commonwealth and state governments formed a taskforce to develop an electronic health record for Australia (Cook & Foster 2010). The taskforce recommended a health information network for Australia and was subsequently endorsed in 2000 by the state and commonwealth health ministers (Cook & Foster 2010). Australia's EHR was created under a health policy act known as HealthConnect (Commonwealth of Australia, cited in Cook & Foster 2010). Even though several of the HealthConnect pilot projects were successful, the EHR did not proceed beyond the state pilot projects (Cook & Foster 2010). The National E-Health Transition Authority (NeHTA) was established in 2005 to 'focus on e-health informatics standards and integrating infrastructure' (Cook & Forster 2010:536). Since that time, NeHTA has developed the building blocks for a national EHR, including standards such as health identifiers, event summaries and privacy, consent and access control policies (Cook & Foster 2010).

In 2009, the National Health and Hospitals Reform Commission (NHHRC) made recommendations for e-health, which has catapulted the development of a 'Personally Controlled Electronic Health Record' (PCEHR) under the legislative framework of the Personally Controlled Electronic Health Records Bill 2011 (Commonwealth of Australia 2009). NeHTA is the governing body for overseeing the rollout of the PCEHR, including the development of design specifications. The PCEHR rollout is restricted to three wave I sites and nine wave informatics sites. From July 2012, all Australians have been able to choose to register for an electronic health record, and the consumer controls what information will be held on the PCEHR and who can access the information from the PCEHR (NeHTA 2012).

The PCEHR will deliver a secure, electronic record of a patient's medical history that will be stored and shared in a network of connected systems. Information such as discharge summaries, event summaries from emergency departments, pathology reports, shared health summaries, and so on will be readily available to health professionals/organisations that the consumer determines should have access to their information (NeHTA 2012). From NeHTA's perspective, providing access to a PCEHR results in treatment being faster (less time searching for past treatment information), safer (more information readily available such as allergies, vaccinations and past treatment) and easier (less reliance on memory regarding medication history and ordered tests) (NeHTA 2012).

From a nursing perspective, the PCEHR has the potential to assist care in emergency departments. Patients registered with the PCEHR will have their health history available for registered organisations providing that the patient gives consent. In the case of a life-threatening illness or injury, clinical staff will also be able to access the patient's health history. It will also improve communication and access to shared clinical information between hospital and primary healthcare providers, public and private healthcare providers, different state and territory healthcare providers and organisations and different healthcare professionals delivering care to the same patient. A patient's record could also be flagged to monitor potential risks, facilitating early intervention. Access to this array of information will benefit emergency nurses greatly, as critical healthcare information does not generally follow the patient when they move between geographic locations, local health districts and healthcare providers.

With the exception of the Eastern Sydney Connect Wave 2 pilot, where nurse-initiated discharge summaries are sent to the PCEHR (McDonald 2012), the role that nurses play as communicator, coordinator, educator and facilitator of patient-centric care will not be visible in the PCEHR. Nurse leaders and informatics specialists need to ensure that nursing information captured electronically is considered as a vital component of the PCEHR.

CONCLUSION

While the issues of quality of care, access to care, cost of services and allocation of limited resources have been evident in healthcare for some time, new and complex challenges are confronted in the implementation, utilisation, evaluation and development of new technologies in an antiquated and imperfect healthcare delivery system. A major reengineering of the healthcare delivery system will be needed if major progress is to be made, which will necessitate changes in technical, sociological, cultural, educative, financial and other important factors (Ortiz et al 2001). In order to deliver quality healthcare to consumers in this information processing era, clinicians need to acquire, evaluate, interpret and generate relevant information from the data that they have gathered, recorded and communicated. It has become increasingly difficult for health professionals in all facets of clinical practice and healthcare management to deliver their services without employing existing information technologies, and this challenge will only continue as consumers expect and demand increasing quality of healthcare services. The delivery of healthcare is information-intensive, and this considerable amount of information has to be handled by clinicians who are experiencing substantial pressure from their already high workloads. Information management of healthcare data is an indispensable aspect of contemporary healthcare organisational infrastructure, and information technology must play a major part if significant improvements in quality are to be realised.

Nurse informatics specialists understand the progression from data to information to knowledge, and finally to wisdom, as well as the use of computers and programs to process data and information. They can help restructure the healthcare delivery system through their ability to collect, aggregate, organise and re-present information in a useful way. Nurses need to become innovators of technology rather than adopters of technology, as informatics is no longer an option for nurses and other clinicians, but rather a requirement (Skiba et al 2010). Nursing graduates need to be technologically competent and information literate, and optimise the value of their intellectual capital by shifting their focus from critical thinking to critical synthesis (Haase-Herrick & Herin 2007, Simpson 2007). While information technology is not a panacea, it is an integral component to transforming the delivery of healthcare from a task-based to a knowledge-based discipline (Haase-Herrick & Herin 2007). The healthcare environment is information and knowledge intensive, and nurses are the largest group of knowledge workers in the system. Nurses who understand the current and evolving technology and can identify the beneficial potential that technology has in relation to managing and processing nursing information will assist the nursing profession as a whole to assume a leadership position in health reform. Table or surface computing, which will eliminate the need for a mouse or keyboard, is not far from being deployed, and this technology application will provide nurses with even more scope to improve and streamline patient care. Nurses who are aware of the potential of informatics can actively participate in delivering efficient, transparent and safe care to patients in an environment where data, information and knowledge are successfully managed to guarantee that wisdom directs all nursing activities.

REFLECTIVE QUESTIONS

Choose one or more of the following areas of healthcare and then answer the seven questions that follow:

Clinical

Management

Education

Research

1. What are the major issues that could be enhanced by the deployment of informatics solutions?

2. What are the benefits (to the patient and to the nursing staff) associated with the use of these informatics solutions?

3. What are the risks/problems associated with the use of these informatics solutions?

4. What are the likely challenges in accepting the deployment of these informatics solutions?

5. How would you evaluate whether the informatics solutions were successful (for the patient and for the nursing staff)?

6. What strategies are needed to facilitate the uptake of nursing informatics solutions in these four areas?

7. What is needed to encourage nurses in these areas to be actively involved in the development of informatics solutions?

REFERENCES

Australian Government Department of Health and Ageing 2012a eHealth: Healthcare professionals – FAQs. Online. Available: http://www.ehealth.gov.au/internet/ehealth/publishing.nsf/Content/faqs-hcp/$FILE/HCP-FAQs.pdf

Australian Government Department of Health and Ageing 2012b National Health Reform: activity based funding and the Independent Hospital Pricing Authority. Online. Available: http://www.yourhealth.gov.au/internet/yourhealth/publishing.nsf/content/nhra-brief-qa-abf#5

Australian Health Informatics Education Council (AHIEC) 2011 Health informatics: scope, careers and competencies Version 1.9. AHIEC, Sydney

Australian Nursing and Midwifery Council (ANMC) 2006 National competency standards for the registered nurse. ANMC, Canberra

Australian Nursing Federation (ANF) 2008 Green light for national IT competencies project. Professional News July 2008. ANF, Canberra

Ball M J, Hannah K J, Douglas J V 2000 Nursing and informatics. In: Ball M J, Hannah K J, Newbold S K, Douglas J V (eds) Nursing informatics: where caring and technology meet, 3rd ed. Springer-Verlag, New York City, NY, pp 6–14

Blumenthal D, Glaser J P 2007 Information technology comes to medicine. New England Journal of Medicine 356(24):2527–2534

Commonwealth of Australia 2009 Australian Government Department of Health and Ageing National Health Reform: a healthier future for all Australians final report. Commonwealth of Australia, Canberra

Cook R, Foster J 2010 Case Study 19D Australia: Developing the electronic health record, a continuing nursing challenge. In: Weaver C A, Delaney C W, Weber P, Carr R L (eds) Nursing informatics for the 21st century: an international look at practice, education and EHR trends, 2nd ed. Health Information and Management Systems Society (HIMSS), Chicago, IL, pp 535–540

DuLong D B, Ball M J 2010 TIGER: Technology Informatics Guiding Educational Reform – a nursing imperative. In: Weaver C A, Delaney C W, Weber P, Carr R L (eds) Nursing informatics for the 21st century: an international look at practice, education and EHR trends, 2nd ed. Health Information and Management Systems Society (HIMSS), Chicago, IL, pp 17–24

Dykes P C, Brown S, Collins R W et al 2010 The impact of health information technology (I-HIT) survey: results from an international research collaborative. In: Weaver C A, Delaney C W, Weber P, Carr R L (eds) Nursing informatics for the 21st century: an international look at practice, education and EHR trends, 2nd ed. Health Information and Management Systems Society (HIMSS), Chicago, IL, pp 69–88

Elfrink V 1996 The information technology frontier: a call for pioneers. Computers in Nursing 14(2):82–83

Fett M 2000 Technology, health and health care. Occasional Papers: Health Financing Series, Volume 3. Commonwealth Department of Health and Aged Care, Canberra

Foster J, Bryce J 2009 Australian nursing informatics competency project. In: Saranto K, Brennan P, Park H-A et al (eds) Proceedings of the 10th International Congress on Nursing Informatics: connecting health and humans. IOS Press BV, Helsinki, pp 556–560

Goldsmith J, Blumenthal D, Rishel W 2003 Federal health information policy: a case of arrested development. Health Affairs 22(4):44–55

Graves J R, Corcoran S 1989 The study of nursing informatics. Journal of Nursing Scholarship 21(4):227–231

Gugerty B, Sensmeier J 2010 Informatics competencies for nurses across roles and international boundaries. In: Weaver C A, Delaney C W, Weber P, Carr R L (eds) Nursing informatics for the 21st century: an international look at practice, education and EHR trends, 2nd ed. Health Information and Management Systems Society (HIMSS), Chicago, IL, pp 129–143

Gugerty B, Maranda M J, Beachley M et al 2007 Challenges and opportunities in documentation of the nursing care of patients: a report of the Maryland Nursing Workforce Commission, Documentation Work Group. Maryland Nursing Workforce Commission, Baltimore, MD

Haase-Herrick K S, Herrin D M 2007 The American Organization of Nurse Executives' guiding principles and American Association of Colleges of Nursing's clinical nurse leader: a lesson in synergy. Journal of Nursing Administration 37(2):55–60

Hart M D 2008 Informatics competency as development within the US nursing population workforce: a systematic literature review. CIN: Computers, Informatics, Nursing 26(6):320–329

Health Informatics Society of Australia (HISA) 2012 About HISA. Online. Available: http://www.hisa.org.au/?about

Health Information and Management Systems Society (HIMSS) Nursing Informatics Awareness Task Force 2007 Informatics Nursing Management, March. Online. Available: www.nursingmanagement.com

HealthWorkforce Australia 2012 Speciality workforce studies. Online. Available: http://www.hwa.gov.au/work-programs/information-analysis-and-planning/specialist-workforce-studies

Hebda T, Czar P 2013 Handbook of informatics for nurses and healthcare professionals, 5th ed. Pearson, Boston, MA

Hobbs S D 2002 Measuring nurses' computer competency: an analysis of published instruments. CIN: Computers, Informatics, Nursing 20(2):63–73

Honey M 2006 Case Study 17B Bringing technology into the classroom. In: Weaver C A, Delaney C W, Weber P, Carr R L (eds) Nursing informatics for the 21st century: an international look at practice, education and EHR trends. Healthcare Information and Management Systems Society (HIMSS), Chicago, IL, pp 202–203

Honey M L L, Westbrooke L A 2012 Nursing Informatics in New Zealand: from history to strategy. In: Proceedings of the 11th International Congress on Nursing Informatics, AMIA. Online. Available: http://proceedings.amia.org/29tjqn/29tjqn/1 p 173

International Council of Nurses 2005 Nursing matters: what is nursing informatics? International Council of Nurses, Geneva

Liu J, Pothiban L, Lu Z, Khamphonsiri T 2000 Computer knowledge, attitudes, and skills of nurses in People's Hospital of Beijing Medical University. Computers in Nursing 18(4):197–206

Marin H D F, Lorenzi N M 2010 International initiatives in nursing informatics. In: Weaver C A, Delaney C W, Weber P, Carr R L (eds). Nursing and informatics for the 21st century: an international look at practice, trends, and the future, 2nd ed. Healthcare Information and Management Systems Society (HIMSS), Chicago, IL, pp 45–51

McBride A B 2006 Informatics and the future of nursing practice. In: Weaver C A, Delaney C W, Weber P, Carr R L (eds). Nursing and informatics for the 21st century: an international look at practice, trends, and the future, 2nd ed. Healthcare Information and Management Systems Society (HIMSS), Chicago, IL, pp 5–12

McCormick J 2009 Prepare for the future of knowledge work. Information Management. Online: Available: http://www.informationmanagement.com/infodirect/2009_121/knowledge_worker_information_management_ecm_content_management-10015405-1.html?zkPrintable=true

McDonald K 2012 Sydney connects with shared health record. Pulse IT (26) February:58–60

McGonigle D, Mastrian K G 2012 Nursing informatics and the foundation of knowledge, 2nd ed. Jones & Bartlett Learning, Burlington, MA

McLane S 2005 Designing and EMR planning process based on staff attitudes towards and opinions about computers in healthcare. CIN: Computers, Informatics, Nursing 23(2):85–92

National League for Nursing 2008 Position statement: preparing the next generation of nurses to practice in a technology-rich environment: an Informatics agenda. National League for Nursing, New York City, NY

National E-Health Transition Authority (NeHTA) 2012 PCEHR Lead sites. Online. Available: http://www.nehta.gov.au/ehealth-implementation/pcehr-lead-sites

Ortiz E, Meyer G, Burstin H 2001 The role of clinical informatics in the Agency for Healthcare Research and Quality's efforts to improve patient safety. Proceedings – AMIA Annual Symposium 508–512

Patel V L, Currie L M 2005 Clinical cognition and biomedical informatics: issues of patient safety. International Journal of Medical Informatics 74(11–12): 869–885

Rifkin D E 2001 Electronic medical records: saving trees, saving lives. Journal of the American Medical Association 285(13):1764

Runciman W B, Hunt T D, Hannaford N A et al 2012 CareTrack: assessing the appropriateness of health care delivery in Australia. Medical Journal of Australia 197(2):100–105

Saba V K, McCormick K A 2011 Essentials of nursing informatics, 5th ed. McGraw-Hill, New York City, NY

Sackett K M, Erdley W S 2002 The history of health care informatics. In: Englebardt S, Nelson R (eds). Healthcare informatics from an interdisciplinary approach. Mosby, St Louis, MO, pp 453–477

Saranto K, Leino-Kilpi H 1997 Computer literacy in nursing: developing the information technology syllabus in nursing education. Journal of Advanced Nursing 25(2):377–385

Schleyer R H, Burch C L, Schoessler M T 2011 Defining and integrating informatics competencies into a hospital nursing department. CIN: Computers, Informatics, Nursing 29(3):167–173

Sewell J, Thede L 2013 Informatics and nursing: opportunities and challenges, 4th ed. Wolters Kluwer Health, Philadelphia, PA

Simpson R 2007 Information technology: building nursing intellectual capital for the information age. Nursing Administration Quarterly 31(1):84–88

Simpson R 2008 Chief nurse executives: creating nursing's future with IT. Nursing Administration Quarterly 32(3):253–256

Skiba D J 2005 Preparing for evidence-based practice: revisiting information literacy. Nursing Education Perspectives 26(5):310–311

Skiba D, Thompson B 2007 Report of the NLN survey on informatics competencies in the curriculum. A paper presented at Evolution or Revolution: Recreating Nursing Education. The National League for Nursing's Annual Education Summit. Sep, Phoenix, AZ

Skiba D J, DuLong D, Newbold S K 2010 TIGER collaborative and diffusion. In: Ball M J, Douglas J V, Walker P H et al (eds) Nursing informatics: where technology and caring meet, 4th ed. Springer-Verlag, New York City, NY, pp 35–50

Smedley A 2005 The importance of informatics competencies in nursing: an Australian perspective. CIN: Computers, Informatics, Nursing 23(2):106–110

Staggers N, Thompson C 2002 The evolution of definitions for nursing informatics: a critical analysis and revised definition. Journal of the American Medical Informatics Association 9(3):255–261

Westby C, Atencio D J 2002 Computers, culture, and learning. Topics in Language Disorders 22(4):70–87

CHAPTER 18

Healthy communities: the evolving roles of nursing

Anne McMurray

LEARNING OBJECTIVES

When you have completed this chapter, you will be able to:

- explain the conceptual foundations of community health
- discuss the importance of primary healthcare to maintaining health in a community
- develop a working knowledge of community assessment
- be prepared to undertake public health surveillance for a range of issues compromising the health of people living in the community
- identify risks and opportunities in promoting the health of a community
- explore a range of contexts and roles for community nurses
- establish a set of realistic goals for maintaining the health of a given community.

KEY WORDS

Community health, public health, community nursing, primary healthcare, social determinants of health, health promotion

INTRODUCTION

As others have argued in this text, nursing is a contextualised activity. What nurses do, how they think about what they do, the research evidence that informs what they do and the responses of those they care for are all dependent on the context or situation. The community is one of the most interesting contexts of nursing practice; one that requires comprehensive and sophisticated assessment skills as a basis for planning interventions for various population groups and the community itself. In the community nurses require self-confidence, an attitude of inquiry, adaptability to different situations and the leadership skills to develop processes and programs. These characteristics are invaluable to community nurses as their role involves anticipating needs beyond the immediate health issue and setting. In many cases they are also the only health professional on site, which may be a person's home, workplace, school or recreational facility, day care centre or clinic. Community nursing is therefore multidimensional. The caring role is distinctive in being carefully and systematically tailored to the needs of each different community and the diversity of its people.

Caring for a community may involve joining advocacy movements to promote such things as healthy environments, services, accessible food and safe water, conducting research studies to identify risks and opportunities to shape people's access to health and health services, or helping community residents access the knowledge and skills to change or sustain the community themselves. Caring for the citizens of a community can involve home visiting, monitoring the health of population groups, such as farmers or inner city dwellers, or providing services for various groups across the age continuum from children to older persons. Each type of community nursing provides inordinate rewards, particularly when the outcomes to health and wellbeing are recognisable as having resulted from nursing work. This chapter explores the various community contexts within which nurses foster personal health and wellbeing, and community health and vibrancy.

CONCEPTUALISING COMMUNITY

Most people consider their community in terms of geography. We all live somewhere, even those whose lives are transient, including the homeless. A geographical community can be defined by a city, town or rural area, the region, country or continent. These geographies shape people's lives in sometimes predictable ways, and often determine the extent to which they have access to health services, adequate resources for living and care when it is needed. But closer examination of any particular geographical context reveals numerous variations. Planning care for residents of any community must accommodate the different needs and resources of men and women, young and older persons, people who are healthy, ill or living with a disability and those whose lives are affected by education, employment, financial resources, family and cultural factors and access to neighbourhood supports (CSDH 2008). These constitute the social determinants of health (SDH), and they are crucial to conceptualising 'community'. Although each person has individual biological and psychological characteristics, we are all social beings, and our social interactions occur in the communities that define our lives. If a given community is unable to provide jobs, education or culturally appropriate care and support, the challenges inherent in living healthy lives or providing care for community residents are much greater than when these factors are accommodated. The social determinants (listed in Box 18.1) are therefore central to

Box 18.1

The social determinants of community health

- Personal factors: biology, gender, genetics, health and developmental status, coping skills, health practices, health literacy
- Family factors: culture, social status, financial resources, generational changes
- Social networks: social supports, neighbourhood assets, social changes
- Employment opportunities, working conditions
- Educational opportunities and supports
- Physical resources, climate, geographical features, developments and hazards.

the context of community health, as they are the key to building community capacity for health and wellbeing (CSDH 2008).

Another construct related to the social determinants of community health is the social ecology of community health. Healthy communities are the product of interactions between people and their environments, a synthesis of actions and interactions in the spaces people inhabit and the resources they use (McMurray & Clendon 2011). Baisch (2009:2467) describes this as evolutionary: 'a dynamic and evolving process' that creates community health. The ecological perspective also means that relationships between people and their environments are reciprocal. The interactions and exchanges that occur in any given community therefore benefit both the residents and the community itself. The dynamic nature of community health is essential to community vitality. In the community context, people are better able to achieve positive health outcomes when their health is understood as part of the overall ecology of their lives; when they live, work, play, study, worship or shop with a sense of belonging, in a safe, supportive and sustainable place. The ecological perspective demonstrates the close relationship between health and place. Health is created and maintained in places with relatively high assets for capacity building and relatively low community risks to health (McMurray & Clendon 2011).

As outlined above, communities can be conceptualised as geographical entities, a set of influential social determinants of health, the ecological relationships that arise from interactions between health and place and a set of assets or risks to capacity building. In addition, communities are influenced by change. Changing circumstances can create threats and/or opportunities for people whose lives are affected by such physical characteristics as global warming, natural disasters, fires or extreme weather events. Cultural changes also affect families, and therefore their communities (McMurray & Clendon 2011). For example, certain expectations or group norms can change over time, so that the current generation may behave in ways that differ from their forebears. These changes are evident in contemporary society in relation to such things as the acceptance of out-of-home care for young children and non-traditional roles for women. Other changes may arise from government policy decisions to develop or withdraw certain essential services people need to live healthy lives, or to create redevelopments or industries that either promote or inhibit living opportunities or employment. Most of these policy changes have a profound effect on family life. For example, providing a baby bonus or other subsidy scheme for child support can encourage some people to increase the size of their family. Changing the age at which older people are eligible to receive a government pension influences the workplace by encouraging some people to retire at a certain age (McMurray & Clendon 2011). Providing disability insurance coverage to all families may have an effect on the workforce by freeing up home carers to return to paid work.

Most changes occur because of the interaction between a number of factors; for example economic factors, natural events such as climate change and policy responses to these changes (McMurray & Clendon 2011). One example of this type of change is evident in rural communities, where many farming families have found their livelihood threatened by the changing fortunes of producing certain agricultural products. Some have diversified their farms to produce goods that attract government subsidies determined by trade agreements with other governments, while others have simply downsized their properties and their productivity (McMurray & Clendon 2011). Many rural families have experienced dramatic health issues related to their changing fortunes, which have been exacerbated by the reduction of health and other services in rural areas. Another community change that has had a major impact on family life is the new wave of Fly-in-Fly-Out (FIFO) workers. The FIFO workforce has arisen from the resources boom in many Australian communities, which has seen many workers (mostly fathers) FIFO to mining sites, in some cases contributing to an erosion of family social life. Fathers spend inordinate time in isolation from services and social supports and the spouse or partner left behind (typically mothers) has had to adjust to living a large proportion of their lives as single parents, with little hands-on support for child rearing. These changing community conditions require people to adapt, to find supports outside the family and to become resilient in ways they may not have anticipated in previous stages of their relationships (McMurray & Clendon 2011).

Global changes such as the Global Financial Crisis and other economic problems have also changed urban communities. With the increasing trend towards inner city living in many capital cities, a large number of older city dwellers have found their lives disrupted by redevelopments that have left them unable to remain in their previously safe, predictable, affordable neighbourhoods. With the resultant need to relocate, many have had to access healthcare and other services that may not be quite as appropriate to their needs as they had experienced in the past. Since the information revolution and the rapid escalation of communications technologies, younger people tend to access health information from the internet and social media. However, the new technologies are often difficult for older people, who may have relied on health professionals for health information throughout their lives. In contemporary society there is a need for everyone to become health literate to make sound health decisions in everyday life (McMurray & Clendon 2011). A health literate community is one 'where people are not only aware of the things that keep them healthy, but they feel confident and comfortable making choices that influence their health, and they are comfortable working with health professionals to improve their health and the health of their community' (McMurray & Clendon 2011:16). The implications for nurses and other caregivers are important, as it is more time consuming to provide guidance and health education where people have little understanding of their condition, and there may be a need for repeated home visits and referrals to ensure that they receive adequate and appropriate care. A further factor that affects the pervasiveness of health literacy in a community is the extent to which communities promote an ethos of participation. When community members are encouraged to participate in assessing their needs and planning strategies to address these needs there is a greater likelihood of successful outcomes. Without input from community residents, there is always the risk that service planning and therefore effectiveness of care may not achieve its intentions. This issue is important for all care providers and a critical element of primary healthcare.

PRIMARY HEALTHCARE

Primary healthcare (PHC) is a pathway to achieving health for all people. The principles of PHC revolve around social justice and the shared expectations of health professionals and the public (De Vos et al 2009). Clearly, this is an inclusive approach, where all members of the population are considered equal in terms of their right to health. In all contexts of care, but particularly in the community, nurses use a PHC philosophy to guide their work by recognising people's right to equitable social circumstances, equal access to healthcare, self-determination and participation in all aspects of life (McMurray & Clendon 2011, World Health Organization (WHO) 2008). Because of this focus on inclusiveness there is an expectation that community members, rather than health professionals, have control over the decisions about priorities and resources that affect their health. In this respect, a PHC approach is empowering for the community (McMurray & Clendon 2011). What PHC means for nurses is that their role is to act as a resource for community decision making, encouraging health literacy among the population, and providing direction for people to achieve their self-defined goals. In many cases, the role translates into coordinating care. However, in other situations, the focus may be on health education targeted to a specific health problem such as care during a chronic illness; or a family's need for guidance in preventing illness such as immunising a child or preventing falls in older persons. Even while providing education, there remains a focus on self-determination.

New Zealand was one of the first countries in the world to formalise a national commitment to PHC through government policy (Ministry of Health New Zealand [MOHNZ] 2001). Nurses and midwives throughout New Zealand have readily adopted the principles and practices of PHC to demonstrate their professional commitment to better health through PHC. The objective of nursing within a PHC framework is to accommodate people's preferences and choices while ensuring that they have sufficient and appropriate information to make informed choices and the resources to support these choices (McMurray & Clendon 2011). Assessing their health, their information needs and the type of assistance they require can help foster self-determination when it is undertaken collaboratively, from a position of partnership. Partnerships between different sectors also lead to better planning. For example, when health, education and transportation personnel are all involved in planning services there is a greater likelihood that the right people will use the right services for the right reasons with the right outcomes. Partnerships between health and other professionals and those who need their services will help develop realistic solutions that not only are accessible and appropriate in the local community, but also suit the timing, conditions, social and cultural expectations of the individual or family requiring assistance (McMurray & Clendon 2011). From a healthcare system perspective, tailoring solutions to family and community conditions enhances efficiency and effectiveness, including use of appropriate, locally available technologies. These factors underline the importance

309

of context in community care. Within a PHC framework, plans are developed for the longer term, beginning with a focus on preventing illness or injury in the community, restoring people to good health once they have become ill, disabled or injured and arranging the structural conditions in their homes and communities to support their return to normal living. This comprehensive approach embodies health promotion, wherein the goal is to promote the structures, supports and decisions for good health (McMurray & Clendon 2011).

PUBLIC HEALTH IN THE COMMUNITY

Like PHC, the public health approach is also aimed at preventing disease and promoting the health of a given population. Public health initiatives are typically based on population-level data such as the rates and distribution of disease in a given population. An important public health focus is therefore on measuring and analysing certain diseases or conditions that may place a population at risk of illness or injury. The information is then used to plan interventions that will either treat the disease or condition, or prevent it from spreading further. This is an epidemiological approach: studying the risks of various diseases; accessing surveillance information on apparent or imminent epidemics; and identifying signs of vulnerability in a population. The object of public health interventions is to ensure the highest level of health for the greatest number of the population (McMurray & Clendon 2011). Like PHC the overarching goal is to work with communities to achieve equitable, accessible care that promotes health through culturally and socially appropriate community participation. Both PHC and Public Health are therefore aimed at encouraging people to become healthy, maintain health and wellbeing and control their health destinies.

ASSESSING THE COMMUNITY

There are numerous models, tools and guidelines for assessing community capabilities and existing levels of community health, some of which are compared in Table 1. One approach is to follow carefully prescribed rules for analysing assessments as a basis for planning care and promoting health. For example, the Epidemiological Model is based on a Web of Causation, whereby assessment includes defining the Agent (an infectious

Table 18.1
Community Assessment

Model	Categories of Assessment
Web of Causation	Agent, Host, Environment
Health Belief Model	Individual Perceptions, Modifying Factors, Likelihood of Action
Health Promotion Model	Cognitive-Perceptual Factors, Modifying Factors, Participation in Health Promoting Behaviours
Lewin Model	Unfreezing, Change, Refreezing
PRECEDE-PROCEED	Predisposing, Reinforcing, Enabling Factors
Big Picture Planning	People, Place, Health Patterns, Gatekeepers

organism, for example); the Host (individual or group health status or behaviours such as the rate of immunisation); and the Environment, which includes the interactions between the agent and host (Valanis 1988). Another model is the Health Belief Model, which guides identification of a person's perceptions about their susceptibility to disease or the seriousness or severity of a disease, modifying factors such as age, social class, knowledge or prior contact with the disease and the likelihood of action—their perceptions of benefits or barriers to taking steps to prevent disease or maintain health (Becker 1974). The model has been adapted for nursing in Pender's Health Promotion Model, which further explained individual perceptions as cognitive perceptual factors. Cognitive perceptual factors include the definition, importance of and control over health (rather than a focus on disease) and acknowledgement of situational and interpersonal influences on whether or not people modify their health behaviours (Pender & Pender 1987). Both Becker and Pender models guide identification of lifestyle factors and behaviours that may either be positive in triggering preventative actions, or have a negative effect in that they increase the risk of ill health or injury.

Another model for assessment that can be used to guide community change is Lewin's (1951) three-step Unfreezing, Changing (Moving) and Refreezing model. Lewin developed the model on the assumption that we all live in a life space composed of experiences that are valued as positive, negative or neutral. Assessing and weighing up the driving and restraining forces that influence either complacency or a willingness to change and communicating goals and expectations clearly can help 'unfreeze' habits, and help people move their position to create sustainable change.

Green and Kreuter (1991) developed the PRECEDE-PROCEED model. This model begins with gathering diagnostic information: first, a social diagnosis, including such issues as education, community crime, population density, unemployment and other variables similar to the SDH. This phase is followed by an epidemiological diagnosis, intended to reveal rates of morbidity, mortality, disability and fertility. Next, a behavioural and environmental diagnosis is undertaken. Included are indicators such as dietary patterns, preventative actions such as safe sexual behaviours, self-care indicators and coping skills. The environmental diagnosis includes economic and geographic indicators of community health and services. Analysis of these factors is complemented by an educational and organisational diagnosis to reveal Predisposing, Reinforcing and Enabling factors that could lead to behavioural and environmental change. Predisposing factors include knowledge, attitudes, values and perceptions that may hinder or facilitate motivation for change. Reinforcing factors include the attitudes and behaviours of others. Enabling factors are those skills, resources or barriers that could help or hinder the desired changes. Following this phase, an administrative and policy diagnosis is conducted to examine the community's capabilities and resources to respond to needs. With this level of assessment, implementation of changes can begin, based on careful evaluation of each of the previous aspects of the model (Green & Kreuter 1991).

The most effective assessments are those that consider the multidimensional and dynamic nature of community life as well as individual and family strengths and constraints. Accurate assessments should therefore include the known SDH in the population and be aimed at tailoring interventions to the community's specific needs. The SDH may be embedded in the Health Belief and Health Promotion Models as Modifying Factors, and in the PRECEDE-PROCEED Model as part of the various stages of diagnosing community problems. In many cases, community nurses are guided by their knowledge and familiarity with the community employing them to identify health issues and develop strategic plans for health promotion and intervention.

Some nurses like to adhere to the type of guidelines for assessment mentioned in the previous paragraphs. However, a slightly less structured approach such as the 'Big Picture Assessment' can also reveal information that may not correspond to the strict categories identified in the traditional models. This model is particularly useful when the focus is on visible indicators of community life and information on people-place relationships as well as health issues provided by community residents.

The 'Big Picture' assessment or 'Lay of the Land' approach often begins with the nurse conducting a 'windscreen survey', driving around the community to gain the 'lay of the land'—a big picture of life in that context. Such a survey can yield information about spaces for recreation, transportation and access, child care services, the location of schools, clinics, hospitals and other health services, places of employment, the state of available housing such as whether there are affordable homes or whether certain sections of the community seem to be in decline. This type of information can also be confirmed by speaking to various community groups or by analysing records of community activities such as immunisation rates, public health indicators and data from other policy documents that indicate activities of the local council or other authorities (fitness programs, elder day care facilities). Community assets, strengths and risks can also be identified by being attentive to people's visible health behaviours such as observing people out walking, older persons engaging in T'ai chi and/or parent get-togethers.

In addition to the 'big picture', talking to people often yields a wide range of information that shows the demographic 'mix' in the community—how many people in which population groups may require certain specific services (e.g. older persons, young children); the mix of cultures in the community; what people think about their lives; opinions about environmental strengths that may support healthy lifestyles or barriers to health. Once this information is gleaned, step two involves mapping resources—trying to understand the capacity for supporting health, the assets and support systems that may be mobilised for certain interventions. Phase three is aimed at identifying the key players who may help in establishing and supporting resources for health, while phase four involves identifying people and place relationships. In the final phase, assessment can take the form of a SWOT analysis to identify strengths, weaknesses, opportunities and threats to community health. A systematic approach to this type of assessment is outlined in Box 18.2 on the next page.

COMMUNITY NURSING ROLES
Home visiting
As mentioned above, there is a wide range of nursing roles in the community context. Perhaps the most well known of these is home visiting, which distinguishes nursing in the community from most hospital-based roles (St John et al 2007). Home visits are integral to 'domiciliary nursing', where a nurse may be employed by a government health department or private agency to provide care in either a person's home or a group residence, such as aged care facility. The objective of this type of nursing is to maintain continuity of care for those who have been discharged from hospital following illness or injury, or to prevent hospitalisation or re-hospitalisation for those at risk of exacerbation of illness. In many cases continuity of care relies on caring for the caregivers, whose burden is often substantial, particularly where a family member is

Box 18.2

An example of big picture assessment

PEOPLE

- demographic and psychosocial characteristics
- family caregivers
- communication networks
- professional and volunteer support systems
- community leaders
- community cultures, ethnic mix
- people–place relationships, connections

PLACE

- community geography (urban, rural, regional, remote)
- natural resources, access to land, water, food
- unique structural features
- community development capacity, formal and informal supports
- access to welfare, housing, home ownership, transportation, schools

HEALTH PATTERNS

- local burden of disease and disability
- social determinants of health
- access, availability, affordability of health and disability services
- local patterns of service utilisation

GATEKEEPERS

- intersectoral coalitions vs barriers to collaboration
- local, state, national health policies and priorities
- distribution of health professionals
- global factors (social, economic, developmental)

in the latter stages of life (Ward-Griffin et al 2012). Home visits are therefore focused on identifying and addressing the needs of all family members. Because of the need for family-centred care it is important for the home visiting nurse to understand health across the lifespan. In-depth understanding of developmental needs at each stage of life will help ensure appropriate assessments to assist people across all age groups, including new parents, their infants and/or other children, adolescents, adults and older persons (Mitchell & Ellis 2011, O'Connor & Alde 2011).

The home visiting nurse role is also a feature of some general practice (GP) clinics where nurses are employed by either the practice or a specialist surgeon to assist them with pre-surgical or post-treatment assessments and follow-up. These roles do not have specific designations, instead they tend to be negotiated by the nurse and the employing medical practitioner or surgeon. For example, a cardiac surgeon may employ a part-time nurse to conduct a pre-operative home visit to prepare the client for surgery, assess their home environment to ensure adequate support for them on returning home post-operatively and provide any health education and guidance required by the client and family. Similarly, some general practitioners employ nurses to conduct home assessments and specific health teaching for chronic conditions such as diabetes, cardiac conditions or any other issue that may require ongoing monitoring, as outlined under practice nursing (below).

Historically, home visiting has been mainly concerned with assessments and minor treatments under medical instructions for such things as maternal and child care, child development concerns, chronic conditions such as wounds, diabetic or cardiac indicators or activities of daily living (Mitchell & Ellis 2011, O'Connor & Alde 2011). The home visit has always focused on holistic assessments, encompassing identification of physical, psychological, social and environmental needs and resources. However, in the contemporary healthcare context, the role of home visiting nurses has been extended to include a greater emphasis on the diagnostic role and provision of acute care in the home. Many home visiting agencies provide programs such as Hospital in the Home (HITH), and offer a range of services from diagnostic tests to treatments that can include intravenous injections, pump infusions and a range of complex treatments (Duke & Street 2003). The breadth and protracted nature of these programs have shifted the focus from a public health orientation of surveillance and monitoring in the home to treatment and extended PHC planning which, in turn, requires advanced practice skills as well as technological skills, including expertise in information technologies.

Community nurses providing advanced care typically find this level of practice rewarding, particularly with the level of autonomy that comes with being a sole practitioner responsible for rapid and critical decision making. However, being a sole practitioner can also be daunting, and requires ongoing skill and knowledge development to inform clinical decision making and appropriate guidance for members of the community. In the home visiting context there are also unique concerns about nurse-client relationships. In the first instance, entering a person's home or residential domain of any kind is a privilege rather than a right, and must be carefully planned. Balancing client needs with the demands of the organisation is another consideration. Home visiting nurses typically have a daily caseload based on the mix of clients assigned to their care. Employers usually set a standard for time management of visits to ensure they are able to cover the type and number of client needs and allow sufficient time for the nurse to travel between visits and establish or maintain the nurse–client relationships. Time management techniques include maintaining adequate planning knowledge of the issues to be encountered in the home, with careful documentation of the goals of the visit and any preliminary plans for care (St John et al 2007).

Home visiting requires sensitivity to a multitude of circumstances. The invitation to enter a home needs to be respected, and often there are situations that have to be accommodated before assessments or treatments can begin. Sometimes the visit involves innocuous but important relationship negotiations such as sharing a cup of tea or sitting with a person until they are ready to disclose health issues. In other cases there may be a threat to the nurse's safety. In the latter case the nurse must be aware of the need to follow all agency safety guidelines (St John et al 2007). These typically include learning to 'read' the home situation for any threats to personal safety, wearing visible agency identification but refraining from wearing any jewellery or items that may attract unwanted attention, ensuring the vehicle and mobile phone are maintained and that there are no barriers to leaving the home quickly if any threat arises. The latter situation involves staying in communication with the agency, and maintaining mobile phone access, especially to emergency numbers, at all times.

Once the visit has been completed, accurate documentation is essential. Documentation is usually completed using the agency proforma to identify the individual(s) assessed and/or treated, and the outcomes, extent and effectiveness of the intervention. Also documented are comments about client satisfaction with care or requests for changes, any diagnostic information including health status, new needs and/or services including those from other care providers, identification of resources and referrals and plans for continuing care. In addition to these formal categories of information, home visiting nurses often mention any preferences or features of the home or situation that may help the next nurse in conducting subsequent home visits.

Community child health nursing

Although there are some differences in titles across states (child health, maternal child health, child and family health), the role of the child health nurse in the community is relatively similar throughout Australia. In New Zealand child health nurses practise as 'Tamariki Ora' nurses or, for those employed by the New Zealand Plunket Society, 'Plunket' nurses (McMurray & Clendon 2011). In both countries, child health nurses are specialists who provide holistic care to children and their families in either clinics or home visits. Some child health nurses provide a range of services in primary schools, especially where there is no designated school nurse, including student screening, health education for teachers and parents and community engagement activities. Another type of specialised child health practice involves acting as the expert resource person in special schools for children with disabilities (McMurray & Clendon 2011).

In the clinics, child health nurses conduct developmental assessments on infants and children, but their practice also encompasses considerable health promotion activities. The role includes assessing and responding to individual needs, case management, home assessments, early identification and primary intervention of clients with psychosocial and mental health issues, group facilitation and multidisciplinary team functions to support parenting (Borrow et al 2011). Some nurses work in outreach programs that are aimed at developing parenting capacity, while others are attached to early learning centres. Most also conduct parenting groups, acting as family advocates and promoting family networks to share common issues and knowledge of local resources (Munns et al 2004). Throughout all of these activities the child health nurse maintains a focus on the community to promote community development and capacity building in partnership with parents and other members of the community (Borrow et al 2011). In the context of these activities a major goal is health literacy, enabling parents to develop the knowledge and skills they need to nurture their children through the developmental continuum and to maintain current and practical knowledge of supportive processes and structures in the community (McMurray & Clendon 2011). This embodies the advocacy role enacted by most community nurses.

School health nursing

School nursing is a multidimensional role combining child health, mental health, case manager, occupational health and team coordinator (Brooks et al 2007, Smith & Firmin 2009). School nurses (SN) in both Australia and New Zealand assess students' developmental needs, promote their health and wellbeing and intervene when they have health problems, all while advocating for a healthy environment in the school community that will also support school staff members. SNs' roles are slightly different for primary and secondary school. In Australian primary schools the role is focused on ensuring students are safe, healthy and ready to learn, and this includes developmental screening for conditions affecting learning, such as vision and hearing (McMurray & Clendon 2011). They also respond to children's needs for support in relation to diet, behaviours at school, issues related to the home environment and coping with stress. Like child health nurses, SNs working in schools where young people have disabilities often act as the mediator between the health and education systems. This aspect of the role includes liaising with teachers, parents, peers and others affected by the child's journey along the health and development continuum (McMurray & Clendon 2011). An important aspect of the SN role is screening and surveillance for infectious diseases and developmental problems, which can also include administering immunisations. Careful documentation is a large part of this type of surveillance and monitoring, and is essential to organising referrals to specialist services when necessary and maintaining clear and sensitive communication between parents, other health professionals and education staff (Wallis & Smith 2008).

High school nurses tend to deal with student needs that revolve around adolescent psychosocial issues such as problems with parental relationships and other issues that affect students' mental health. These can include issues related to sexuality, risky behaviours or other areas where peer pressure causes conflict between the young person's struggle for identity formation and family or group norms (McMurray & Clendon 2011). Included is the need to help students deal with bullying, stress-related illnesses, obesity and prevention of chronic conditions. Nurses are also called on to work collaboratively with staff for vulnerable students, some of whom may have social issues such as family crises, immigration or refugee-related problems, poverty and violence or substance abuse, family relationship challenges or major personal issues such as pregnancy and/or sexually transmitted infections or a risk of suicide (Barnes et al 2004, Brooks et al 2007).

Some SNs also teach health education classes, either alone or in partnership with the relevant school staff member. Most SNs gain enormous satisfaction from the role, a substantial part of which is based on a trusting, socially inclusive relationship with students. Relationship building is seen as the key to supporting young people, being there at the right time to help them make positive choices when they are confronted with social issues (McMurray & Clendon 2011). A cornerstone to building this type of relationship is the need to maintain current knowledge of adolescent behaviours, and sensitivity to the changing nature of their social world, whether this lies inside or outside the school; for example, in the context of their social media interactions (McMurray & Clendon 2011). SN practice is therefore philosophically aligned with primary healthcare. It requires a balance between close engagement with particular students and promoting health and capacity development in the entire school community, which can be achieved by maintaining extensive networks with a wide range of personnel, family members and community resources (Smith & Firmin 2009, Wainwright et al 2000).

Occupational health nursing

Occupational health nursing carries the primary healthcare philosophy into the workplace, focusing on education, health promotion, clinical services, case management and other industry-specific innovations to keep the workplace and its workers safe and healthy (Guzik et al 2009, Marinescu 2007). Occupational health nurses (OHNs) practise in partnership with workers and their employers to maintain healthy and safe working practices and a healthy and safe environment. The role requires diplomacy, especially in situations where the nurse participates with others in lobbying for safe working conditions, which may be costly to the employer. OHNs therefore need high-level communication skills, in-depth understanding of interpersonal and industrial relations and familiarity with professional and government standards and legislation. Other factors influencing OHN practice include knowledge of environmental issues, the context and expectations of the employing organisation, in-depth understanding of employer and union philosophy and policies, budgetary restraints and familiarity with the boundaries of OHN practice (McMurray & Clendon 2011).

In some cases, OHNs are responsible for safety in the workplace, while in others there may be safety specialists to provide first aid and develop injury surveillance and prevention programs. Irrespective of the extent of the safety team, nurses need to have sufficient environmental knowledge and assessment skills to conduct surveillance and monitoring of workplace hazards (McMurray & Clendon 2011). Ergonomic assess-ments are also important to understand the fit between the worker and their interface with the work environment. Ergonomic risks can include boredom, glare, repetitive motion, poor workstation–worker fit, lifting heavy loads or tasks that require the worker to assume an abnormal position. Physical hazards can include such things as extremes of temperature, noise, radiation or poor lighting. Biological hazards include exposures to chemical or various biological agents. Psychosocial hazards are those that produce inordinate stress, such as shiftwork, or negative interpersonal relationships on the job, such as bullying and incivility. Other employee assessments can include pre-employment health examination and updates during periodic health assessments. As with other nursing roles mentioned previously, careful documentation is a pivotal part of the OHN role, particularly when disputes arise over differences in expectations by employers and employees (McMurray & Clendon 2011).

Like school nursing, a large part of the role is in dealing with stress. OHNs can help monitor worker stress, providing education, counselling, worksite stress reduction programs or referrals to specialist services (Wallace 2009). Another workplace issue revolves around disaster planning, which requires close collaboration with emer-gency services, other health professionals and workplace health and safety personnel (Lobaton Cabrera & Beaton 2009). The OHN also needs to maintain current and high-level skills in first-aid procedures, crisis intervention and trauma management, including threats from workplace violence. For employees with chronic conditions or disabilities, the OHN provides liaison between the employee, their GP, PN, specialists, social worker, physiotherapist or other health professional, particularly as workers recover from injury or illness (Aziz 2009). Some OHNs maintain a range of health intervention programs to engage workers while they are recovering from an illness episode or injury. These include employee assistance for those with substance abuse problems, corporate smoking cessation, and workplace health and fitness programs. In many cases, successful implementation of rehabilitation or health promotion programs also relies on having an extensive referral network, which brings in the necessity to maintain intersectoral collaboration, a feature of PHC.

Practice nursing

Practice nurses (PN) are those employed by a general practice, but also includes New Zealand nurses attached to Primary Health Organisations. As mentioned above some PNs are employed specifically to conduct home visits, but most work collaboratively alongside the GP in the practice. Some undertake practice management roles and quality improvements as well as clinical roles (Walker 2010). Because general practice is mainly concerned with providing primary care rather than primary healthcare (which has a broader focus on health promotion) many PN roles revolve around such primary care activities as chronic illness management (Halcomb & Hickman 2010). In Australia assessment, health promotion and monitoring of those with chronic conditions has evolved as an important part of PN practice, particularly since 2010, when Commonwealth policies began to fund PN activities through Medicare and Practice Incentive Payments (PIP). As a result, GPs now receive remuneration for practice nurses to undertake immunisations, provide wound care, cervical screening, assessments of older persons and management of conditions such as asthma, diabetes and mental health through the Chronic Disease Management Initiative (Halcomb et al 2005, Keleher et al 2007, Porritt 2007). Historically, the PN role was up to the employing general practitioner, but in response to government subsidisation of GP practices and a growing awareness of the knowledge and skills of PNs approximately 60% of general practices now employ a PN (Australian General Practice Network 2010). The scope of their practice varies according to the nurse's expertise and experience, practice arrangements, the GP's understanding of the role and the needs of the local population (Halcomb et al 2005, Keleher et al 2007). In rural areas, where there are acute shortages of GPs, the number of PNs is expanding and this is expected to demonstrate improvements to the health of the rural population. As PNs become more prevalent, one would expect greater clarity of their role for clients, GPs and other health professionals. Together with specialisation and accredited systems of education, this could help promote greater interdisciplinary collaboration and ultimately better access to quality healthcare for a broader segment of the population (Walker 2010).

Nurse practitioners

Nurse practitioners (NP) have been practising in Australia and New Zealand only since 2001, but this role is gaining legitimacy, as more NPs complete advanced education and clinical specialisation (Duffield et al 2009). In New Zealand some NPs work within the PHOs, while others are attached to agencies that require specialist services such as child health, family planning, sexual health or wound care. The focus of the NP role is on health promotion, education and extended practice, including limited prescribing, initiation and interpretation of diagnostics, referral to medical specialists and, in some states, admitting and discharging patients as well as approving absence from work certificates (Lee & Fitzgerald 2008). A growing number of NPs specialise in emergency nursing to help alleviate the pressure on emergency departments, and they have been found to improve efficiencies and quality of care in that setting (Searle 2007). Others work as gerontological NPs in residential or community settings, meeting the needs of underserved older persons (Caffrey 2005), and some NPs work in general practice settings. NPs are invaluable in rural areas, sometimes being the only health professional for vast distances.

Rural and remote area nursing

In Australia rural nurses are usually employed by state health departments or specific agencies, such as occurs in remote Indigenous areas, where the employer may be Aboriginal Medical Services (AMS). New Zealand rural nurses have developed special rural nurse services for Māori such as 'By Māori for Māori' as well as a number of nurse-led clinics that serve rural populations (McMurray & Clendon 2011). The nurses in these New Zealand clinics are called 'iwi providers', and their services to vulnerable people in the rural settings are an integral part of New Zealand's initiatives within the national PHC strategy. In all countries remote area nursing is challenging, particularly in terms of the isolation, which means the nurse, like others in the community, must deal with being at a great distance from friends, services and resources. Although there are financial incentives to practise in remote areas, this type of nursing requires broad knowledge of healthcare, including emergency care, as well as in-depth understanding of people, their physical, cultural and psychosocial needs and their strong connection to community (the people–place relationship) (McMurray & Clendon 2011). Remote area nursing typically means being the sole practitioner and treating a wide range of conditions from critical injuries to chronic conditions and the disabilities of ageing. Because remote areas often have limited choices for healthcare and restricted access to goods, services and opportunities for social interaction, the nurse is often placed in a multidimensional role as emergency nurse, mental health counsellor and community development manager (Allan et al 2007, Greenhill et al 2009, Wong & Regan 2009). These roles require advanced clinical skills, comprehensive knowledge of family and people–place relationships and a level of familiarity with cultures that will enable the nurse to act as a 'culture broker' or intermediary between people who hold various cultural beliefs about health and health care. Home visiting is usually an integral part of the role. In many cases, remote area and rural nurses also need technological skills for communication, particularly if they are expected to use telehealth systems (McMurray & Clendon 2011).

In both remote and rural nursing, working closely with the community where a nurse is on call 24 hours a day can be stressful, given that in small communities there is little separation between a person's personal and professional life. Where there may be more than one health professional, maintaining relationships with colleagues outside of work can have an effect on the work dynamic as well as social relationships (Mills et al 2010). Some nurses relish this close engagement with community members and the opportunity to practise in a primary healthcare context, but the added responsibilities of managing a health clinic and supervising health workers who often leave after short periods of time can also be tiring (Hegney et al 1999). For this reason most employers make sure that nurses from other geographic areas who work 'out bush' have periods of respite to get back to their friends and families at least once a year.

CONCLUSION

In planning for the health of any community and its population there are a number of goals common to each of the roles outlined above. These goals are aimed at any activities that can create and maintain high levels of population health as well as fostering an 'enabling community', guided by the principles of PHC. They include the following:

- Encouraging empowerment of the population by adopting an inclusive, partnership approach to planning, ensuring authentic communication that will help people make their views, goals, preferences and priorities understood.

- Adopting a culturally safe and appropriate approach to planning, which requires knowledge of your own and others' cultural preferences, norms and conventions.

- Basing plans on comprehensive assessments as a basis for promoting equity of access to healthcare and to community capacity building.

- Being mindful of health promotion principles: assisting people to become health literate while helping them rearrange the structures, supports and policy decisions for good health.

- Using appropriate technologies so that interventions are affordable, achievable and fit for the population.

- Including other sectors such as education, transportation and environmental plans in planning for community health.

- Acting as an advocate for the community in all nursing activities.

In addition to these common goals, effectiveness in community health nursing requires political advocacy; knowledge of the government and non-government structures that will help people achieve and maintain health. To help a community through such a multilayered, multidimensional role exemplifies the notion that high-quality, safe care for communities and the people who live there can only be achieved when the context of care is carefully considered in conjunction with the specific health issue being addressed. This geographic, cultural and socially embedded nature of community nursing makes it one of the most rewarding and inspiring roles in nursing.

REFLECTIVE QUESTIONS

1. Describe the role of nurses in establishing and sustaining healthy communities.
2. What are the key aspects of a community assessment?
3. What strategies would you use to promote a healthy community?
4. How would you use primary healthcare principles to guide community assessment?
5. How are community health nurses able to achieve public health goals?

RECOMMENDED READINGS

Baisch M 2009 Community health: an evolutionary concept analysis. Journal of Advanced Nursing 65(11):2464–2476

Barnes M, Rowe J 2008 Child, youth and family health. Churchill Livingstone, Sydney

McMurray A, Clendon J 2011 Community health and wellness: primary health care in practice, 4th edn. Elsevier, Sydney

Talbot L, Verrinder G 2005 Promoting health: the primary health care approach, 4th edn. Elsevier, Sydney

Walker L, Patterson E, Wong W, Young D 2010 General practice nursing. McGraw Hill, Sydney

REFERENCES

Allan J, Ball P, Alston M 2007 Developing sustainable models of rural health care: a community development approach. Rural and Remote Health 4(7):1–13

Australian General Practice Network 2010 National practice nurse workforce survey report 2009. AGPN, Canberra

Aziz B 2009 Making more of nurses. Occupational Health 61(5):22–23

Baisch M 2009 Community health: an evolutionary concept analysis. Journal of Advanced Nursing 65(11):2464–2476

Barnes M, Courtney M, Pratt J, Walsh A 2004 School-based youth health nurses: Roles, responsibilities, challenges, and rewards. Public Health Nursing 21(4): 316–322

Becker M 1974 The health belief model and personal health behaviour. Charles B. Slack, New Jersey

Borrow S, Munns A, Henderson S 2011 Community-based child health nurses: an exploration of current practice. Contemporary Nurse 40(1):71–86

Brooks F, Kendall S, Bunn F et al 2007 The school nurse as navigator of the school health journey: developing the theory and evidence for policy. Primary Health Care Research & Development 8:226–234

Caffrey R 2005 The rural community care gerontologic nurse entrepreneur: role development strategies. Journal of Gerontological Nursing 31(10):11–16

Commission on the Social Determinants of Health (CSDH) 2008 Closing the gap in a generation. Health equity through action on the social determinants of health, Final report of the Commission on the Social Determinants of Health, WHO, Geneva

De Vos P, Malaise G, De Ceukelaire W et al 2009 Participation and empowerment in primary health care: from Alma Ata to the era of globalization. Social Medicine 4(2):121–127

Duffield C, Gardner G, Chang A, Catling-Paull C 2009 Advanced nursing practice: a global perspective. Collegian 16:55–62

Duke M, Street A 2003 Hospital in the home: constructions of the nursing role – a literature review. Journal of Clinical Nursing 12:852–859

Green L, Kreuter M 1991 Health promotion planning: an educational and environmental approach. Mayfield Publishing Company, Mountain View

Green L, Kreuter M 2005 Health promotion planning: an educational and ecological approach. McGraw-Hill, New York

Greenhill J, Mildenhall D, Rosenthal D 2009 Ten ideas for building a strong Australian rural health system. Rural and Remote Health 9(1206):1–7

Guzik A, Nivison Menzel N, Fitzpatrick J, McNulty R 2009 Patient satisfaction with nurse practitioner and physician services in the occupational health setting. American Association of Occupational Health Nurses Journal 57(5):191–197

Halcomb E, Davidson P, Daly J et al 2005 Nursing in Australian general practice: directions and perspectives. Australian Health Review 29(2):156–166

Halcomb E, Hickman L 2010 Development of a clinician-led research agenda for general practice nurses. Australian Journal of Advanced Nursing 27(3):4–11

Hegney D, McCarthy A, Pearson A 1999. Effects of size of health service on scope of rural nursing practice. Collegian 6:21–42

Keleher H, Joyce C, Parker R, Piterman L 2007 Practice nurses in Australia: current issues and future directions. Medical Journal of Australia 187(2):108–166

Lee G, Fitzgerald L 2008 A clinical internship model for the nurse practitioner programme. Nurse Education in Practice 8:397–404

Lewin K 1951 Field theory in social science. Harper & Row, New York

Lobaton Cabrera S, Beaton R 2009 The role of occupational health nurses in terrorist attacks employing radiological dispersal devices. American Association of Occupational Health Nurses Journal 57(3):112–119

McMurray A, Clendon J 2011 Community health and wellness 4e: Primary health care in practice. Elsevier, Sydney

Marinescu L 2007 Integrated approach for managing health risks at work – the role of occupational health nurses. American Association of Occupational Health Nurses 55(2):75–87

Mills J, Birks M, Hegney D 2010 The status of rural nursing in Australia: 12 years on. Collegian 17:30–37

Ministry of Health New Zealand [MOHNZ] Primary health care. 2001. MOHNZ, Wellington

Mitchell C, Ellis I 2011 Promoting family and child health, In: Kralik D, van Loon A (eds) Community nursing in Australia, 2nd edn. John Wiley & Sons, Milton, Qld, pp 314–351

Munns A, Downie J, Wynaden D, Hubble J 2004 Changing focus of practice for community health nurses: advancing the practice role. Contemporary Nurse 16(3):208–213

O'Connor M, Alde P 2011 Older persons' health and end-of-life care. In: Kralik D, van Loon A (eds) Community nursing in Australia, 2nd edn. John Wiley & Sons, Milton, Qld, pp 354–386

Porritt J 2007 Policy development to support nurses in general practice: an overview. Contemporary Nurse 26(1):56–64

St John W, Fraser K, Bennett E 2007 Home visiting. In: St John W, Keleher H (eds) Community nursing practice: theory, skills and issues. Allen & Unwin, Crows Nest NSW, pp 230–248

Searle J 2007 Nurse practitioner candidates: shifting professional boundaries. Australasian Emergency Nursing Journal 11:20–27

Smith S, Firmin M 2009 School nurse perspectives of challenges and how they perceive success in their professional nursing roles. Journal of School Nursing 25(2):152–162

Valanis B 1988 The epidemiological model in community health nursing. In: Stanhope M, Lancaster J (eds) Community health nursing: process and practice for promoting health, 2nd edn. Mosby, St Louis

Wainwright P, Thomas J, Jones M 2000 Health promotion and the role of the school nurse: a systematic review. Journal of Advanced Nursing 32(5):1083–1091

Walker L 2010 Practice nursing. In: Walker L, Patterson E, Wong S, Young D 2010 General Practice Nursing. McGraw Hill, Sydney pp 2–23

Wallis K, Smith S 2008 Developmental screening in pediatric primary care: the role of nurses. Journal for Specialists in Pediatric Nursing 13(2):130–134

Wallace M 2009 Occupational health nurses – the solution to absence management? American Association of Occupational Health Nurses Journal 57(3):122–127

Ward-Griffin C, McWilliam C, Oudshoorn A 2012 Relational experiences of family caregivers providing home-based end-of-life care. Journal of Family Nursing 18(4):491–516

Wong S, Regan S 2009 Patient perspectives on primary health care in rural communities: effects of geography on access, continuity and efficiency. Rural and Remote Health 9(1142):1–12

World Health Organization (WHO) 2008 World Health Report 2008 Primary health care, now more than ever. WHO, Geneva

Young J, Eley D, Fahey P et al 2010 A nurse-led model of chronic disease management in Australian general practice: health-related quality of life outcomes. Australian Practice Nurses Association, Golden Opportunities, Gold Coast, Qld Australia, 6–8 May

CHAPTER 19

The challenges of rural and remote nursing

Marie Hutchinson and Leah East

LEARNING OBJECTIVES

In this chapter we introduce the nature of rural and remote nursing. When you complete this chapter you should be able to:

- identify the nature of rural communities and the major factors that influence their health status
- outline some of the challenges of providing healthcare in rural and remote locations
- describe the characteristics of rural and remote nursing and the challenges and rewards of the role
- identify the continuing challenge for nursing in addressing the health needs of rural and remote communities.

KEY WORDS

Nursing, rural and remote, communities, Indigenous, health, healthcare

RURAL NURSING

The health of rural and remote communities and the challenges of providing healthcare in locations that are often long distances from major urban centres has gained much Government attention in recent decades (Australian Government Department of Health and Ageing 2008, Commonwealth of Australia 2012). Though rural and remote healthcare has increasingly become the focus of policy makers and governments, with attention often upon recruiting and retaining General Practitioners (GPs) (Commonwealth of Australia 2012), nurses have a long tradition of providing care in rural and remote locations. Nurses and midwives represent by far the largest group of health professionals in the rural workforce (Wakerman et al 2007). In many rural and remote communities nurses are recognised as the backbone of healthcare and are 'expert generalists' who provide for the breadth of healthcare needs of their community ranging from health promotion, school health nursing, occupational health and safety, midwifery, chronic and aged care to emergency and crisis intervention (Mahnken 2001). Meeting the healthcare needs of rural and remote communities remains a continuing challenge for the nursing workforce.

Distance from urban centres and population sparsity are frequently used to define the concept of rurality. These are useful concepts to initially understand what it means to be residing in a remote region; however, there are various degrees of rurality and remoteness, and these types of geographic interpretations fail to fully capture the meaning of living in a rural community and the cultural and social nuances of rural life. The concept of rurality is not one dimensional; instead, location, history, culture, economic policy, place and identity feature strongly in any attempt to know what it means to be rural or live in a rural location. For nurses working and living in rural or remote locations, the nature of their practice is strongly influenced by all of these factors, making rural nursing one of the more challenging and rewarding fields of nursing practice.

INTRODUCING RURAL AND REMOTE POPULATIONS

Approximately one-third of Australians live outside of major urban settings and, of these, 12% reside in outer regional and remote locations. Likewise, close to 14% of New Zealanders live in locations classified as remote (Australian Institute of Health and Welfare [AIHW] 2012b, Ministry of Health 2012). Within Australia and New Zealand, rural and remote places are determined primarily by geographic location, urban influences and reliance on employment within city and urban centres (Commonwealth of Australia 2012, Statistics New Zealand 2007). Reflecting their distance from urban centres, Australian settings are described as either being Inner or Outer regional, Remote or Very Remote areas (Commonwealth of Australia 2012). Similarly, in New Zealand settings are classified into rural areas of either high, moderate or low urban influences and reliance, or highly rural/remote areas that have relative independence for employment from urban centres (Statistics New Zealand 2007).

Understanding what it means to live in rural and remote regions can be challenging, particularly when we consider the multifaceted dimensions used to define these communities and the ambiguity of these terms. Despite the distance from urban centres or locations, communities and people classified as rural or remote are not a homogeneous group (AIHW 2012b). They are diverse in population and form a vital part of society. Nonetheless, traditionally rural and remote communities have been portrayed through stereotypical images of living in the sticks and farming the land, with the perceptions of the rural population including being backward or conservative (Liu et al 2001). In stark contrast to these assumptions, country people do not necessarily live on a farm and they are not inevitably rustic or conservative; instead they live in many different places and are characterised by great diversity and innovation. Rural and remote communities can include farming, coastal and rainforest regions, communal living and tourist islands or mining towns that are characterised by their unique cultural and philosophical beliefs (AIHW 2012a, Baldwin & Bentley 2012).

People living outside of urban settings often have strong cultural, spiritual or generational ties that can exist to the land, traditions and the people. These ties shape their sense of personal and community identity. For many rural people, ties to country are strong; for example Indigenous peoples' identity is inextricably linked to community, person, land, spirituality and place, creating complex relational bonds and reciprocal obligations (AIHW 2012a). Exploring young people's narratives of rural and urban differences, Holt (2010) reported how rural young people experienced their rurality as a relational understanding of place and of identity.

As nurses, when we attempt to understand what it means to live in or come from the country we must move beyond defining rural and urban in simple geographic, consumerist or material terms. Instead, it is important to give attention to understanding the subjective, deep-rooted and shared social understanding of association and identification that shape rural character and culture (Lenthall et al 2011). Understanding the health of rural and remote people requires that we consider the relationship between people, place and identity. In rural identity, the sense of connection to place is so strong that for many, being removed or relocated away from their place of country can cause considerable distress (Bernoth et al 2012).

REFLECTION

Think of a rural or remote location that is familiar to you—describe the characteristics of the people living in this community. What has shaped your impression?

The tyranny of distance and population sparsity

In rural and remote contexts, distance creates particular challenges. The cost of delivering services to rural and remote areas is higher per capita when compared with that of the city (Wakerman et al 2007). As a result, resources are often spread sparsely across large areas. On average, rural and remote people are disadvantaged in their access to goods and services, and in some areas may also experience issues in access to basic necessities, such as clean water and fresh food (AIHW 2008). For these communities, the tyranny of distance is also compounded by the tyranny of population numbers. In many instances the population of these communities may be too small to generate sufficient demand to sustain viable services (Humphreys et al 2008) and decline in population can set in place a cycle of decay. Shrinking populations lead to a fall in demand, which in turn leads to decreased employment and a continued drain on the population as people leave the community, particularly younger adults who may leave in search of work (Commonwealth of Australia 2012).

Recent decades have seen significant demographic and economic change in rural and remote communities, with many in decline while others have experienced growth (Australian Bureau of Statistics 2012). The impact of population decline in rural communities has been more marked as a result of economic and resource-driven models of service provision and urban-centric approaches to education, transport and health policy (Liu et al 2001). These approaches tend towards cost effectiveness and the centralisation of services. In rural communities, this has seen the redesign or loss of healthcare facilities, schools and other essential services such as banks; this change is said to have exacerbated economic decline and population drift (Grzybowski et al 2011, Liu et al 2001). As a consequence of population decline and economic and social policy that favours urban populations, the nature of resources and services provided to rural and remote communities has evolved to be less than that offered to their city counterparts (Townsend 2008).

Many rural communities have experienced the simultaneous redesign or withdrawal of services, population decline, growing unemployment and a deterioration in their living conditions (Commonwealth of Australia 2012). This change has had a profound effect on the social circumstances of people living in these communities. In contrast to this picture of decline, some rural and remote communities have experienced economic and population growth. The movement of retirees to regional and rural coastal towns has been a driver of change in coastal fringes and the migration of younger families has occurred in some larger rural centres (Commonwealth of Australia 2012). These shifts in population mean that, in some communities, the distinction between rural and urban identity is no longer as clear cut as it may have been in the past, with once rural country towns becoming large regional centres.

THE HEALTH OF RURAL AND REMOTE COMMUNITIES

People living in rural and remote communities face many challenges; in the main they experience more health disadvantage, are less healthy and experience greater illness and mortality than their city counterparts (AIHW 2012b). The deeply embedded economic and social disparity experienced in rural and remote communities equates to lower incomes and fewer healthcare and educational opportunities (Bureau of Infrastructure 2008). These disparities are compounded by limited access to services and, as a result, contribute to the higher rates of illness and mortality among people who reside in these communities (AIHW 2008). Refer to Box 19.1 for a summary of current information related to the state of health in rural and remote populations.

The limited access to healthcare services can be exacerbated by differing attitudes to health and illness between people in rural and remote regions and those in the city. Elliot-Schmidt and Strong (2008) suggest that rural people are more likely to delay seeking healthcare and are more concerned as to how illness or disability affects their productivity. In a study of 467 rural residents, the study findings suggested that stoic attitudes together with high levels of self-efficacy may act as a barrier, particularly for men, in health-seeking behaviour and mask problems when they do present for healthcare (Judd et al 2006). Furthermore, rural people may face issues in disclosing their health concerns to professionals who live in their community, or alternatively when seeking care from distant services are concerned their cultural or behavioural differences may result in them being misunderstood (Mills et al 2007).

Throughout Australia and New Zealand, rural and remote communities are often recognised to be Indigenous communities (inclusive of Aboriginal, Torres Strait

---

Box 19.1

The state of health in rural and remote populations

- Compared with populations in major cities in Australia, the people in regional areas have a life expectancy 1–2 years lower, and in remote areas this gap increases to 7 years (AIHW 2008).

- Residents of highly remote areas of New Zealand have fewer educational qualifications than the national average (Statistics New Zealand 2007).

- In Australia over 60% of Indigenous peoples live in rural and remote areas, and on the whole their life expectancy is about 17 years lower compared with that of other Australians (AIHW 2008).

- Māori-Indigenous New Zealanders residing in rural areas have a lower life expectancy of approximately 9.5 years compared with their non-Indigenous counterparts (Ministry of Health 2012).

- Rates of death by injury and suicide are higher in rural and remote areas, particularly among men (AIHW 2010).

- The overall rates of people living with disabilities are on average about 20–30% higher in rural and remote communities (AIHW 2008).

- Rural and remote communities are less connected to the digital age and have suboptimal infrastructure to support, for example connection to the internet (Statistics New Zealand 2007).

Islanders and Māori individuals) with their health being an important part of the fabric of rural life. However, this group has continued to have poorer health status compared with that of urban dwellers, which contributes to the higher rates of morbidity and mortality in rural and remote communities (AIHW 2008, Ministry of Health 2012). Indigenous people residing in rural areas have a lower life expectancy, an increased rate of low birth weight and infant mortality, higher interpersonal violence and an increased risk of suicide (AIHW 2012a, Ministry of Health 2012, O'Brien & Jackson 2007).

Ageing is another factor that is affecting rural and remote communities, with projections that by mid-century the shortfall in residential aged care places will be most noticeable in non-urban areas (Liu et al 2001). Little is known about how growing older may be different in urban and rural areas. For many older people in rural and remote locations, needing help at home may mean relocating away from family and friends either temporarily or permanently. Given the strong association with community and sense of place in rural people, moving away to supportive accommodation is particularly problematic. Anderson (2012) notes that in some communities the elderly may be relocated to residential aged care facilities up to 12 hours' distance from their rural home community. Such a situation places considerable burden on families and carers who must travel to provide support and care. Drawing attention to this dislocation, Anderson conducted interviews with the family of rural elderly relocated for residential care; the resulting social dislocation from friends, relatives and rural communities was described as being 'in exile' (Anderson 2012).

THE CHALLENGE OF PROVIDING HEALTH SERVICES IN RURAL AND REMOTE LOCATIONS

When regional, rural and remote locations are compared with urban centres they often have lower levels of access to health services and the profile of the health workforce varies significantly (Health Workforce Australia 2011). In general, there is a misdistribution of the health workforce between urban centres and rural and remote communities (Australian Government Department of Health and Ageing 2008) and attracting experienced healthcare professionals to these locations is a constant challenge (Commonwealth of Australia 2012). Both Australia and New Zealand have relied extensively on overseas trained healthcare professionals to fill this void (Commonwealth of Australia 2012, Health Workforce New Zealand 2011). In light of this reliance, government initiatives, including financial schemes and training programs, are continually being developed to attract healthcare professionals, including nurses, to staff regional and remote healthcare positions (Health Workforce New Zealand 2011).

In the face of increasing difficulty in recruiting and retaining a health workforce, sustaining hospitals, residential aged care and other health services remains a challenge in many rural and remote communities that impacts on the delivery of healthcare. A number of specific models of health service have been developed to meet this challenge—these include: Indigenous health services which are often community-controlled organisations; multi-purpose services that provide integrated services such as aged care, medical or community services; the Royal Flying Doctor Service which provides emergency and primary care outreach services, outreach medical and allied health services, and on-call primary care services staffed by GPs and nurses (Australian Government Department of Health and Ageing 2008, Birks et al 2010).

The presence of a hospital is an important factor in influencing the adequacy of health services in rural or urban communities and it is an important factor in the decision for a health professional to live and work in a community (Australian Bureau of Statistics 2012). In Australia, New Zealand and internationally, recent decades have seen the downgrading and closure of many rural hospitals and an increase towards care and services provided in the home (Barnett & Barnett 2003, Liu et al 2001). In 2007, approximately 130 rural maternity services had been closed in Australia (Dietsch et al 2008). These healthcare reforms provide particular challenges for the equitable provision of services to people living in rural and remote locations (Mahnken 2001).

The closure of hospitals or the downgrading of services has exacerbated the need for people living outside major urban centres to travel large distances or temporarily relocate to regional or city areas for treatment not available in their community. The need to travel considerable distance for healthcare means that vulnerable people, often from the most socioeconomically disadvantaged areas of the country, have to find the financial and support resources to cope with this dislocation. The extent of the inequity experienced by rural and remote communities in accessing hospital and other health services has been described as one of the principal human rights issues for people living in rural and remote areas (The Human Rights Commission 2000).

The challenge of providing health services in rural and remote communities not only shapes the services available, it has a major impact on the practice of health professionals. Imagine a serious accident over 500 km from a major health facility and 150 km to the closest town with a small hospital, and we begin to understand the challenge of providing healthcare in rural and remote contexts. In many settings, nurses will be required to respond to such an accident and, in the more isolated locations, may have little immediate support or back-up.

REFLECTION

Identify a rural town and conduct an internet search to identify health services available to residents.

Do you think the service is equitable to residents in a major urban city?

Imagine you are a nurse in this community. Where might you work and what other services would be available to support you in your role?

THE NATURE OF RURAL AND REMOTE NURSING

Rural and remote nursing is dynamic in nature and offers immense opportunity for professional and personal development. Nurses working in these locations describe their work as more diverse than their urban counterparts do, and the varied nature of this work provides opportunities and challenges unique from other nursing experiences (Yates et al 2012). In these settings, nurses are broad generalists who may or may not hold specialisations and often deal with a wide range of issues that require advanced practice knowledge and skills (Howie 2008).

Rural and remote nurses are often somewhat embedded within the community in which they work. They establish strong relationships with community members and are frequently perceived as being a part of the community to whom they provide care (Kulig et al 2008) and for whom they care for throughout the lifespan (Yates et al 2012). The experience of nursing in a rural or remote context is often characterised by the development of deep and effective relationships in the communities nurses serve (Mills et al 2010b), with a sense of connection to the place and the people which engenders a rich understanding of holistic care (O'Brien & Jackson 2007).

In their dual role of nurse and community member, rural and remote nurses will often personally know or have knowledge about most people in their community (Kulig et al 2008). Relationships and communication networks in small communities also mean that little that occurs is not known by others (Mills et al 2007). This lack of anonymity, entwinement of personal and private lives and the high level of visibility create particular challenges for nursing practice. When a nurse in an urban hospital provides care, few but the immediate family of the patient know the details of the care provided. In contrast, the actions of rural nurses are more visible and known to the community (Kulig et al 2008). This high level of visibility can be a difficult work life challenge for nurses who take up employment in rural and remote communities (Place et al 2012). Maintaining privacy and confidentiality in this context require that nurses establish clear boundaries between their private and work life and strategies to ensure patient confidentiality (Kenny & Allenby 2012).

Scope of practice

When compared with nursing in urban settings, rural and remote nursing is characterised by a high degree of responsibility and autonomy, considerable flexibility and a requirement for extended or advanced skills (Baldwin & Bentley 2012). In more geographically isolated areas nurses are likely to be the principal clinician on site, working at a distance from the multidisciplinary team (Lenthall et al 2011). By necessity, rural and remote nursing practice is generalist in nature, meaning that nurses address the health needs of their entire community (Francis & Mills 2011).

As broad generalists, rural and remote nurses practise across the lifespan and their work includes prevention, primary care, rehabilitation and acute interventions. The scope of practice of rural and remote nurses has often been described as extended, advanced and expanded (Cant et al 2011, Mills et al 2010a). While the scope of practice of nurses working in these settings varies according to the needs of the population and the range of other services available, it includes comprehensive assessment, diagnosis and case management, interventions such as suturing, plastering, prescribing and/ or supplying medication, as well as involvement in health education and screening, public health initiatives and health promotion (Cant et al 2011, Mills et al 2010a).

In outer regional and remote locations additional multidisciplinary services are provided by outreach services and various forms of telecommunication support consultation. This means that nurses in these settings must establish and maintain effective working relationships with other team members who are often at a considerable distance (Mills et al 2010b). Furthermore, nurses and Indigenous health workers areas are often the mainstay of health services in remote areas, with the most common interprofessional relationship being between the two (Kulig et al 2008). This working relationship provides the 'cultural mentorship' that nurses require working in such a demanding environment, and helps ensure the care they provide is culturally appropriate (Mills et al 2010b).

Extended, advanced and solo nursing roles

As remoteness increases, there are a decreasing number of healthcare professionals available within communities and the scope of practice of nurses becomes more extended or advanced. For many nurses in outer regional and remote locations their practice extends across the scope of registered nurse practice to include the full spectrum of care, from the provision of primary healthcare at one end to frontline emergency care at the other (Kulig et al 2008). Working as a nurse in remote locations requires not only experience, but also extensive knowledge, specialised skills and the ability to adapt to changing health scenarios (Baldwin & Bentley 2012, Kulig et al 2008, Mills et al 2010a). For example, imagine providing diabetic education in the morning and by the afternoon you are providing frontline critical care to a patient who has been involved in a motor vehicle accident.

Although small numbers of doctors live in Indigenous and remote communities, the majority are based in towns or regional centres which are attached to hospitals and/or outreach emergency services (AIHW 2008). Providing on-call services is a feature of outer regional and remote locations and nurses work in partnership with doctors or, in instances where there is no doctor available, nurses are the mainstay of healthcare and on-call coverage for the local community. In New Zealand, one small study in the Opotiki district revealed that on-call nurses with GP back-up provided a sustainable service to a community with high levels of socioeconomic deprivation and a high proportion of Māori who were more likely to require out of hours service, which was primarily provided by nurses (Scott-Jones et al 2008).

While the majority of nurses working in regional communities work within small multidisciplinary teams, nurses working in very remote areas often do so on their own. A 2011 study has indicated that of 301 very remote settings in Australia, 59 of these sites were primary healthcare clinics with a nurse being the sole provider of care (Lenthall et al 2011). In a number of remote Indigenous communities, fly-in mine sites or small isolated towns, solo nurse clinics operate to provide the only form of onsite healthcare. These nurses live and work in physically difficult circumstances, are required to undertake high levels of on-call work, have heavy workload demands and report a high level of safety risk and personal violence (Hegney et al 2002). Nurses working in these settings are often unable to take leave and are on 24-hour call for long periods of time (Yates et al 2012). Remote area nurses report that, even when the on-call roster is shared with other team members, they may often be called instead as they are seen as the community resource (Birks et al 2010, Scott-Jones et al 2008). High staff turnover resulting from these pressures increases the workload for remaining nurses. These issues have been of long-standing concern to remote area nurses, with a growing consensus that solo nurse services should be abandoned in favour of teams of nurses with suitable qualifications and experience to undertake this role (Haines & Critchley 2009).

Even though university courses and government initiatives have been introduced to support the rural nursing workforce, and some nurses working in remote communities have expanded their knowledge and undertaken postgraduate qualifications, the literature suggests that many are still ill-equipped and poorly prepared for the demands of extended and advanced practice roles (Coyle et al 2010, Lenthall et al 2011, Mills et al 2010a). Literature also suggests that there is a decline in rural and remote nurses undertaking specialised skills such as those associated with women and child healthcare (Lenthall et al 2011), which is an essential component of primary healthcare in rural communities. The consequences of lack of training, skills and support among rural and remote nurses can not only result in increased stress but also has the potential for adverse health outcomes for communities as a result of nurses providing care outside their scope of practice (Mills et al 2010a).

To meet the demands of unserviced healthcare needs in the community, remote nurses fulfil advanced practice roles far wider than that of the Nurse Practitioner, often with minimal formal preparation for the role and outside of the legislated boundaries of registered nurse practice (Mills et al 2010a). A continued criticism of Australian rural health policy has been an almost exclusive policy focus on medical workforce supply issues (Harvey 2011, Pearson 2008, Wakerman et al 2007). While it is important to acknowledge the importance of doctors, any solution to the critical problems faced by rural and remote communities must also address nursing workforce issues.

REFLECTION

What do you think the differences would be in working in a remote community such as Broken Hill in Australia or the Gisborne region of New Zealand as either a registered nurse or an undergraduate nurse compared with working in a large metropolitan referral hospital in a capital city?

Have you or would you consider undertaking a clinical placement in a remote community? Why or why not?

The challenge of sustaining the rural and remote workforce

Remote area nurses are reported to suffer particularly high levels of occupational stress. The demands of working in rural and remote settings is said to be compounded by inadequate staffing, poor management, staffing issues, workload and work responsibilities, and limited professional development and support (Opie et al 2010). In the face of these challenges, rural and remote area nurses can experience considerable role stress (Yates et al 2012). Furthermore, workplace violence and concerns for personal safety are reported to be correlated with psychological distress and emotional exhaustion among remote area nurses (Opie et al 2010).

In one study examining work stress among 349 nurses working in remote areas, findings indicated this group reported higher than average levels of psychological distress and emotional exhaustion when compared with other samples of nurses, human service workers and Australian Police Officers (Opie et al 2010). Although rural and remote nursing is characterised by many challenges that increase the likelihood of experiencing psychological distress, these frustrations are in the most part related to management and system issues rather than the communities or individuals (O'Brien & Jackson 2007, Opie et al 2010).

Recruiting and retaining a health workforce is a significant issue across Australia and New Zealand. As a strategy to provide a rural healthcare workforce and services in rural and remote regions, educational providers have developed a range of undergraduate clinical placement initiatives to expose students to practice in rural and remote settings (Health Workforce Australia 2011). These programs are based on the premise that rural placement programs and a rural background can provide opportunities associated with graduate employment choices in rural or remote settings (Playford et al 2006). Undergraduate rural clinical placement provides for unique clinical experiences and influences more positive views about future work in such areas (Webster et al 2010). However, for students, living and studying in rural communities can create particular challenges. Pront et al (2012) report that preceptors may struggle to make themselves available to students due to work demands and the small number of staff available at any one time, while students in this study reported that learning in an environment characterised by more community engagement was an enriching aspect of their placement.

New graduates in rural areas have the added challenge of transitioning to work roles that demand a wide knowledge base and a broader range of generalist skills. Ostini and Bonner (2012) report on findings from a study of new graduates in a large regional facility. The study demonstrated that, with adequate support, graduates can successfully transition to practise in a regional acute care facility. Positive aspects of the program were reported to include the slower pace and increased opportunities for learning, as well as supportive colleagues and ongoing employment opportunities (Ostini & Bonner 2012). A number of initiatives are also in place to attract graduates to rural areas. However, these are largely, but not exclusively, targeted towards medical graduates. These initiatives include salary incentives to work in areas of greatest need, bonded scholarships and a range of non-financial incentives for graduates (Health Workforce Australia 2011).

CONCLUSION

Nursing has a long-established tradition of providing healthcare in rural and remote locations, often in the face of great adversity. The determinants of health for people living in rural and remote locations are poorer than their urban counterparts. This disadvantage arises from a complex interplay of geographic, economic, social and policy factors. This disadvantage impacts not only on the people living in these communities and seeking healthcare, but also on the healthcare workers who support these communities. In recognising these challenges, educational programs and government support and incentives are continually being implemented to foster growth, safety and improved working conditions among rural and remote nurses and to facilitate optimal care for people residing in rural and remote communities. Despite these challenges, rural and remote nursing is a highly rewarding career that offers unique and rich experiences that can be both professionally and personally fulfilling.

REFLECTIVE QUESTIONS

1. Consider the health status of rural and remote Australia or New Zealand. What are the major health issues? Identify strategies to improve this situation. How might nurses implement or incorporate these strategies in their practice?

2. Working in a rural setting means nurses often work autonomously with few immediate supports. What type of supports could be introduced to assist rural and remote nurses and reduce burnout?

3. Reflecting back on your undergraduate preparation, what additional skills would you need to work in a rural and remote location? What type of education do you think would prepare you for the role of a beginning rural or remote area nurse?

RECOMMENDED READINGS

Australian Institute of Health and Welfare (AIHW) 2012 Australia's health: the thirteenth biennial health report of the Australian Institute of Health and Welfare. Canberra. Online. Available: http://www.aihw.gov.au/publication-detail/?id=10737422172

Cramer J 2005 Sounding the alarm: remote area nurses and Aboriginals at risk. University of Western Australia Press, Perth

Health Workforce New Zealand 2011 Health Workforce New Zealand: retention initiatives. Wellington

Lenthall S, Wakerman J, Opie T, et al 2011 Nursing workforce in very remote Australia, characteristics and key issues. The Australian Journal of Rural Health 19:32–37

Ministry of Health 2012 Mātātuhi Tuawhenua: health of Rural Māori 2012. Wellington. Online. Available: http://www.health.govt.nz/publication/matatuhi-tuawhenua-health-rural-maori-2012

REFERENCES

Anderson K 2012 Working rural and remote: rewards and challenges. Australian Nursing Journal 19(7):22–25

Australian Bureau of Statistics 2012. 3218.0 – Regional Population Growth, Australia, 2009–10. Online. Available: http://www.abs.gov.au/ausstats/abs@.nsf/Products/3218.0~2009-10~Main+Features~Main+Features?OpenDocument

Australian Government Department of Health and Ageing 2008 Report on the audit of health workforce in rural and regional Australia. Commonwealth of Australia, Canberra, Australia

Australian Institute of Health and Welfare (AIHW) 2008 Rural, regional and remote health: indicators of health system performance, Rural Health Series, Number 10. Australian Institute of Health and Welfare. Online. Available: http://www.aihw. gov.au/publication-detail/?id=6442468150

Australian Institute of Health and Welfare (AIHW) 2010 A snapshot of men's health in regional and remote Australia, Rural health series no. 11. Australian Institute of Health and Welfare, Canberra, Australia

Australian Institute of Health and Welfare (AIHW) 2012a Australia's health: the thirteenth biennial health report of the Australian Institute of Health and Welfare, Canberra, Australia. Online. Available: http://www.aihw.gov.au/publication-detail/?id=10737422172&tab=3

Australian Institute of Health and Welfare (AIHW) 2012b Rural health demography. Online. Available: http://www.aihw.gov.au/rural-health-demography/

Baldwin A, Bentley K 2012 Rural and remote nursing. In: Berman A, Snyder S J, Levett-Jones T, Dwyer T, Hales M, Harvey N, Luxford Y, Moxham L, Park T, Parker B, Reid-Searl K, Stanley D (eds) Kozier and Erb's Fundamentals of nursing, 2nd edn. Pearson, Frenchs Forest, pp 157–171

Barnett R, Barnett P 2003 'If you want to sit on your butts you'll get nothing!' Community activism in response to threats of rural hospital closure in southern New Zealand. Health & Place 9(2):59–71

Bernoth M A, Dietsch E, Davies C 2012 Forced into exile: the traumatising impact of rural aged care service inaccessibility. Rural and Remote Health 12(1):1924. Online. Available: http://www.rrh.org.au

Birks M, Mills J, Francis K et al 2010 Models of health service delivery in remote or isolated areas of Queensland: a multiple case study. Australian Journal of Advanced Nursing 28(1):25–34

Bureau of Infrastructure, Transport and Regional Economics (BITRE) 2008 About Australia's regions. Department of Infrastructure, Transport, Regional Development and Local Government, Canberra, Australia. Online. Available: http://www.google.com.au/#sclient=psyab&hl=en&tbo=d&q=About+australia+regions&oq=About+australia+regions&gs_

Commonwealth of Australia 2012 National strategic framework for rural and remote health. Canberra, Australia

Cant R, Birks M, Porter J et al 2011 Developing advanced rural nursing practice: a whole new scope of responsibility. Collegian 18(4):171–182

Coyle M, Al-Motlaq M A, Mills J et al 2010 An integrative review of the role of registered nurses in remote and isolated practice. Australian Health Review 34(2):239–245

Dietsch E, Davies C, Shackleton C et al 2008 'Luckily we had a torch': contemporary birthing experiences of women living in rural and remote NSW. Charles Sturt University. Online. Available: http://bahsl.com.au/old/pdf/birthing-in-rural-remote-NSW.pdf

Elliot-Schmidt R, Strong J 2008 The concept of well-being in a rural setting: understanding health and illness. Australian Journal of Rural Health 5(2):59–63

Francis K L, Mills J E 2011 Sustaining and growing the rural nursing and midwifery workforce: understanding the issues and isolating directions for the future. Collegian 18(2):55–60

Grzybowski S, Stoll K, Kornelsen J 2011 Distance matters: a population based study examining access to maternity services for rural women. BMC Health Service Research 11:147

Haines H M, Critchley J 2009 Developing the Nurse Practitioner role in a rural Australian hospital – a Delphi study of practice opportunities, barriers and enablers. Australian Journal of Advanced Nursing 27(1):30–36

Harvey C 2011 Legislative hegemony and nurse practitioner practice in rural and remote Australia. Health Sociology Review 20(3):269–280

Health Workforce Australia 2011 National health workforce innovation and reform strategic framework for action 2011–2015, Health Workforce Australia, Canberra, Australia

Health Workforce New Zealand 2011 Health Workforce New Zealand: retention initiatives, Wellington

Hegney D, McCarthy A, Rogers-Clarke C, Gorman D B 2002 Why nurses are resigning from rural and remote Queensland health facilities. Collegian 9(2):33–39

Holt B 2010 On being rural: identity claims, higher education and the global citizen, Australian Association for Research in Education (AARE). AARE, Deakin, Australian Capital Territory, p 20

Howie L 2008 Contextualised nursing practice. In: Ross J (ed) Rural nursing: aspects of practice. Rural Health Opportunities, Dunedin, pp 33–49

Humphreys J S, Wakerman J, Wells R, Kuipers P, Jones J, Entwistle P 2008 Beyond workforce: a systemic solution for health service provision in small rural and remote communities. Medical Journal of Australia 188(8 suppl):S77–S80

Judd F, Jackson H, Komiti A et al 2006 Help-seeking by rural residents for mental health problems: the importance of agrarian values. Australian and New Zealand Journal of Psychiatry 40:769–776

Kenny A, Allenby A 2011 Implementing clinical supervision for Australian rural nurses. Nurse Education in Practice. Online early view. Available: http://dx.doi. org/10.1016/j.nepr.2012.08.009

Kulig J C, Andrews M E, Stewart N L et al 2008. How do registered nurses define rurality? Australian Journal of Rural Health 16:28–32

Lenthall S, Wakerman J, Opie T et al 2011 Nursing workforce in very remote Australia, characteristics and key issues. The Australian Journal of Rural Health 19:32–37

Liu L, Hader J, Brossart B et al 2001 Impact of rural hospital closures in Saskatchewan, Canada. Social Science & Medicine 52(12):1793–1804

Mahnken J E 2001 Rural nursing and health care reforms: building a social model of health. Rural and Remote Health 1:104

Mills J, Francis K, Bonner A 2007 Live my work: rural nurses and their multiple perspectives of self. Journal of Advanced Nursing 59(6):583–590

Mills J, Birks M, Hegney D 2010a The status of rural nursing in Australia: 12 years on. Collegian 17(1):30–37

Mills J E, Francis K, Birks M et al 2010b Registered nurses as members of interprofessional primary health care teams in remote or isolated areas of Queensland: Collaboration, communication and partnerships in practice. Journal of Interprofessional Care 24(5):587–596

Ministry of Health 2012. Mātātuhi Tuawhenua: health of rural Māori 2012. Wellington

O'Brien L M, Jackson D 2007 It's a long way from the office to the creek bed: remote area mental health nursing in Australia. Journal of Transcultural Nursing 18(2):135–141

Opie T, Dollard M, Lenthall S et al 2010 Levels of occupational stress in the remote area nursing workforce. Australian Journal of Rural Health 18(6):235–241

Ostini F, Bonner A 2012 Australian new graduate experiences during their transition program in a rural/regional acute care setting. Contemporary Nurse 41(2):242–252

Pearson A 2008 Claims, contradictions and country life in Australia: the evidence on rural nursing and midwifery. International Journal of Nursing Practice 14(6): 409–410

Place J, MacLeod M, John N et al 2012 'Finding my own time': Examining the spatially produced experiences of rural RNs in the rural nursing certificate program. Nurse Education Today 32(5):581–587

Playford D, Larson A, Wheatland B 2006 Going country: rural student placement factors associated with future rural employment in nursing and allied health. Australian Journal of Rural Health 14(1):14–19

Pront L, Kelton M, Munt R, Hutton A 2012 Living and learning in a rural environment: a nursing student perspective. Nurse Education Today. Online. Available: http://www.nurseeducationtoday.com/article/S0260-6917(12)00180-3/abstract

Scott-Jones J, Lawrenson R, Maxwell N 2008 Sharing after hours care in a rural New Zealand community – a service utilization survey. Rural and Remote Health 8:1024

Statistics New Zealand 2007 New Zealand: an urban/rural profile. New Zealand Government

The Human Rights Commission 2000 Rural health: healthy community projects. Australia

Townsend R 2008 Public health policy, legal uncertainty and the standard of care in rural and remote communities. Journal of Law and Medicine 15(5):693–703

Wakerman J, Humphreys J S, Wells R W et al 2007 Improving rural and remote health. Medical Journal of Australia 186(9):486

Webster S, Lopez V, Allnut J et al 2010 Undergraduate nursing students' experiences in a rural clinical placement. Australian Journal of Rural Health 18(5):194–198

Yates K, Kelly J, Lindsay D, Usher K 2012 The experience of rural midwives in dual roles as nurse and midwife: 'I'd prefer midwifery but I chose to live here': women and birth. Online. Available: http://download.journals.elsevierhealth.com/pdfs/journals/1871-5192/PIIS1871519212000200.pdf

Diversity in the context of multicultural communities: implications for nursing and midwifery practice

Kim Usher, Jane Mills and Roianne West

LEARNING OBJECTIVES

Upon completion of this chapter, the student should be able to:

- explain the concept of culture and its relationship to nursing and midwifery practice
- define the terms *cultural safety* and *cultural competence*
- trace relevant government policy changes related to immigration and multiculturalism
- examine the impact of diverse cultural influences on access to healthcare services
- identify considerations for the provision of nursing and midwifery care in multicultural communities.

KEY WORDS

Multiculturalism, cultural diversity, culturally competent, cultural safety

THE CONCEPT OF CULTURE AND ITS RELATIONSHIP TO NURSING AND MIDWIFERY PRACTICE

Australia and New Zealand are multicultural societies with a history of colonisation. The health of Indigenous peoples in colonised countries is less than acceptable with life expectancies well below their non-indigenous counterparts. Popular understandings of the concept of culture differ, so before beginning this chapter addressing diversity in multicultural Australia and New Zealand, we ask you, the reader, to take a moment to reflect on your own understanding of 'culture' and how this impacts on the provision of nursing and midwifery care.

Activity 1: What is culture?

Allocate ten minutes to this free writing activity. Firstly, open a blank document on your computer, or find a piece of paper and a pen. Take a moment to think back on your clinical experience to date. Has there been a moment that caused you to reflect on 'culture' as something that determines a person's actions and behaviours? Describe the episode of care that has influenced your ideas about culture. Write down a definition of culture—what do you think it means? How do you think culture influences nursing and midwifery practices?

Much has been written about the importance of cultural safety in nursing and midwifery practice (Fredericks & Thompson 2012, Phiri et al 2010), particularly in countries such as New Zealand, which has led the way in the notion of cultural safety (Ramsden 2002), and Australia, which prides itself on being a nation that embraces multiculturalism and diversity. In the foreword to *The People of Australia: Australia's multicultural policy*, the Prime Minister, the Honourable Julia Gillard MP, says, 'We sing "Australians all" because we are. Our country's story is the story of our people in this place. Australia has provided a new home and a chance at a better life for millions of people' (Australian Government 2011b:iv). The term *cultural safety* originates in New Zealand from the work of Indigenous (Māori) nursing scholar Irihapeti Ramsden (2002) and provides a framework for nursing and midwifery practice that recognises the importance of individuals, families and communities being able to judge the quality and appropriateness of nursing and midwifery care provided to them (Wilson & Grant 2008). The Nursing Council of New Zealand (2009) defines cultural safety as:

> The effective nursing practice of a person or family from another culture, and is determined by that person or family. Culture includes, but is not restricted to, age or generation; gender; sexual orientation; occupation and socioeconomic status; ethnic origin or migrant experience; religious or spiritual belief; and disability.
>
> The nurse delivering the nursing service will have undertaken a process of reflection on his or her own cultural identity and will recognise the impact that his or her personal culture has on his or her professional practice. Unsafe cultural practice comprises any action which diminishes, demeans or disempowers the cultural identity and wellbeing of an individual.

You will notice in this definition that the New Zealand Nursing Council also defines the concept of culture, using the notion of difference from the nurse or midwife providing care under the broad categories of: age, generation, gender, sexual orientation, occupation and socioeconomic status, ethnic origin or migrant experience, religious or spiritual belief and disability. A number of authors argue that this is an essentialist view of culture (Gray & Thomas 2006, Gregory et al 2010)—assigning a set of differences to each of the categories that people other than the dominant cultural group can use as a method of identification or signification, and which can work to marginalise individuals in the context of mainstream healthcare services. Using an essentialist definition of culture leads to the understanding that different cultures are static—that there are a set of characteristics and issues that members of each cultural group face regardless of context and that these cultural norms are handed down from generation to generation (Gregory et al 2010). This notion of culture is problematic. It is important to understand that just because people come from the same culture, it does not mean they will all believe the same things and act in the same way. For example, consider Australian Aboriginals; there are hundreds of different groups who speak many different languages, so assuming all Aboriginal Australians can be understood as a group with exactly the same beliefs or qualities is misleading or even dangerous. Unfortunately this view of culture leads to the situation where clinicians develop stereotypes and use a blueprint approach to try to explain peoples' actions (Gregory et al 2010), including their experiences of health and illness.

Reformulating the concept of culture to a dynamic process, as opposed to a static entity, leads to the concept of cultural constructivism (Gray & Thomas 2006) whereby nurses and midwives begin with the individuals with whom they practise, and seek to understand their worldviews and ways of being and knowing. From this approach, people of a different culture are not seen as a member of a group with similar beliefs and qualities. Rather, clinicians will work with people from different cultures by seeking to understand each individual as a unique person with qualities and beliefs, and taking their social context into account (Gregory et al 2010).

In many ways, the definition of cultural safety cited previously is a mix of cultural essentialism and cultural constructivism given the emphasis on a consumer's self-determination of identity and wellbeing. Advocates of cultural constructivism argue that 'students' abilities to critically examine and question ways in which culture is constructed and the consequences of those constructions for both individuals (self and others) and society at large' (Gray & Thomas 2006:81) are at the heart of what makes a culturally competent clinician, as opposed to learning a set of facts about different cultural groups. While we offer this argument as a stimulus to debate, it is also important to discuss mainstream definitions and understandings of cultural competence in nursing and midwifery practice in order to understand the wider social and political context in which we work. Before we move on to the next section, take a moment to reflect on your own definition of culture and decide if your initial ideas have most in common with either an essentialist or constructivist view of culture and think about what has influenced your understanding of 'culture'. Also think about the issues that can arise if culture is conceived as a static rather than dynamic concept.

Cultural competence

Cultural competence is defined as a set of congruent behaviours, practices, attitudes and policies related to embracing cultural differences that are integrated into a system or agency or among professionals (Mays et al 2002). Andrews and Boyle (2008) identify two major categories of cultural competence: organisational cultural competence and individual cultural competence. Organisational competence requires:

... a defined set of values and principles and demonstration of behaviours, attitudes, policies and structures that enable people to work effectively cross-culturally. Individual cultural competence refers to a complex integration of knowledge, attitudes, beliefs, and encounters with those from cultures different from one's own.
(*Andrews & Boyle* 2008:16)

Cultural competence in nursing has been defined as a process, as opposed to an end point, in which nurses continuously strive to work effectively within the cultural context of an individual, a family or community with diverse backgrounds (Andrews & Boyle 2008, Campinha-Bacote 2008). Campinha-Bacote suggests that 'the process involves the integration of cultural desire, cultural awareness, cultural knowledge, cultural skill and cultural encounter' (2008:14).

Assuring culturally competent nursing and healthcare is the responsibility of systems, agencies and institutions (Omeri 2003). There is a growing understanding revealed in the literature that organisations providing culturally and linguistically appropriate services (i.e. culturally competent services) have the potential to reduce cultural and ethnic health disparities (Anderson et al 2003). The nursing profession is responsible for developing cultural competence in its practitioners, not only in its novitiates, but also on a continuing basis as measured by the demonstration of requisite skills, knowledge and attitudes. However, there is no agreement as to how continuing competence should be monitored, nor is there any provision for continuing education in transcultural nursing for faculty and nurse administrators. The purpose of this chapter is to develop the reader's awareness of Australia's cultural diversity, in order to promote self-reflection on their own cultural identity and how this influences their way of being in the world—including how they develop interpersonal connections and respectful ways of communication in their professional life.

AUSTRALIA'S DIVERSE POPULATION

The Australian people represent a wealth of diversity. Recent census data (Australian Bureau of Statistics 2012a) reports that of the total population of 21,507,717 there are 548,370 self-identified Aboriginal or Torres Strait Islander people (2.5%) (Australian Bureau of Statistics 2012b). Australia has one of the largest proportions of immigrant populations in the world, with an estimated 26% of the total population born overseas and a further 20% having at least one parent born overseas. Interestingly, 81% of Australians aged 5 years and over speak only English at home, with only 2% of the population not speaking English at all (Australian Bureau of Statistics 2012c).

The Australian Government (2011b) describes multiculturalism as being:

in Australia's national interest and speaks to fairness and inclusion. It enhances respect and support for cultural, religious and linguistic diversity. It is about Australia's shared experience and the composition of neighbourhoods. It acknowledges the benefits and potential that cultural diversity brings.
(2011b:iv)

From an historical perspective, Australia's policies on immigration have evolved in response to social changes and a commitment to the development of society as a whole (see Table 20.1). Since 1947, Australia's immigration policies have shifted between phases of assimilation, integration, multiculturalism and mainstreaming, to inclusiveness and being united in diversity.

Table 20.1
Periods in immigration policy development

Years	Policy	Features	Health policy implication
1945–70	Assimilation	Predominantly White Australian Anglo-Saxon policies.	Absence of government assistance.
1970–80	Integration	White Australia policy relaxed and gradually abandoned. Some cultural characteristics tolerated.	Relevant services provided. Welfare needs of migrants being addressed.
1980–89	Multi-culturalism	Pluralistic approach to immigration. Policies to limit discrimination on racial and ethnic grounds. Cultural and ethnic diversity becoming more accepted in Australian society. Cultural identity, social justice and economic efficiency were adopted.	Provision of various health services. Equality of access to culturally appropriate services.
1983	Mainstreaming	Redirecting service delivery from marginal to a central base. Concern of government institutions based on social equity and access; economic efficiency and cultural identity.	Promotion of culturally sensitive health services. Equality of access to health services by immigrants.
1999	Inclusiveness	Diversity. Multicultural policies built upon civic duty, cultural respect, social equity and productive diversity. The term *multiculturalism* to remain. Inclusiveness.	Promotion of culturally sensitive health services. Equality of access to health services by immigrants.
2000–08	United in diversity	National agenda for a multicultural Australia. Policy framework including: all Australians are expected to have a 'loyalty to Australia and its people, and to respect the basic structures and principles underpinning our democratic Society. These are: Constitution, Parliamentary democracy, freedom of speech and religion, English as the National language, the rule of law, acceptance and equality' (Commonwealth of Australia 2003:6).	Main components of 'Multicultural Australia: united in diversity policy 2003–06': responsibility, respect, fairness and benefits for all.
2008–12	Benefits of cultural diversity	Celebrate and value the benefits of cultural diversity. Emphasis on justice, inclusivity, trade, racism and discrimination.	*The People of Australia: Australia's multicultural policy* launched in 2011.

Source: Commonwealth of Australia (1999, 2003, 2007, 2008)

Australia's current multicultural policy document (Australian Government 2011b) is underpinned by four principles. The policy is intended for all Australians, not just for those people from non-English-speaking backgrounds.

1. The Australian Government celebrates and values the benefits of cultural diversity for all Australians, within the broader aims of national unity, community harmony and maintenance of our democratic values.

2. The Australian Government is committed to a just, inclusive and socially cohesive society where everyone can participate in the opportunities that Australia offers and where government services are responsive to the needs of Australians from culturally and linguistically diverse backgrounds.

3. The Australian Government welcomes the economic, trade and investment benefits which arise from our successful multicultural nation.

4. The Australian Government will act to promote understanding and acceptance while responding to expressions of intolerance and discrimination with strength and, where necessary, with the force of the law.

NEW ZEALAND'S DIVERSE POPULATION

New Zealand has a diverse multicultural population of over 4 million people, with New Zealand's Indigenous Māori making up about 15% of the population. While British migrants predominated during the first half of the twentieth century, the 1950s saw an increasing number of migrants come from the Pacific Island countries. However, since the 1990s there has been a rapid diversification of migrants arriving in New Zealand with increasing numbers of migrants arriving from Asia and Africa (Lawrence & Kearns 2005).

Characteristics of diversity

The Treaty of Waitangi, signed in 1840, is the founding document of New Zealand. The Treaty is the basis for all legislation, and its principles are incorporated into all health service initiatives in New Zealand (Crawford et al 2008, Health Practitioners Competency Assurance (HPCA) Act 2003, Nursing Council of New Zealand (NCNZ) 2004). The Treaty contains three Articles: Article 1 (Kāwanatanga) refers to self-governance, Article 2 (Tino Rangatiratanga) to Māori self-determination and Article 3 to the rights and protection of Māori (Orange 1989). The Treaty is simplified into three guiding principles: partnership, participation and protection. Together, these form the basis of cultural safety within the New Zealand health services (NCNZ 2002, Wepa 2005) and are used to guide health service delivery.

Māori have poorer health and social outcomes than other New Zealanders. While non-Māori life expectancy has continued to improve since the 1980s, there has been little change in the life expectancy of Māori. Access to affordable, quality care is one reason for this disparity (Anderson et al 2006).

CULTURAL INFLUENCES ON ACCESS TO HEALTHCARE SERVICES

Language diversity

Culture is a shared experience that is mediated through language and other symbols. Spradley (1979) states that language is an important cultural expression and the major means for humans to share, construct and understand the world around them. He goes

Box 20.1

Some key dates in New Zealand's history

1300	East Polynesian people arrive—now known as Māori
1642	Abel Tasman visits
1769	James Cook arrives and claims New Zealand for Great Britain
1835	Declaration of Independence signed by 34 Māori chiefs
1840	Treaty of Waitangi
1865	Wellington declared capital in place of Auckland
1893	New Zealand becomes the first country to give all women the right to vote
1907	New Zealand becomes a dominion
1908	Population reaches 1 million
1933	Adopts own currency
1947	Adopts the Statute of Westminster (1931) and becomes independent of Great Britain
1952	Population reaches 2 million
1967	Decimalisation of currency
1973	Population reaches 3 million
1983	Closer Economic Relations (CER) agreement signed with Australia
1985	Waitangi Tribunal given power to hear Māori land grievances going back to 1840
2003	Population reaches 4 million

on to say that the decoding of cultural symbols and identification of meaning involves the discovery of relationships between the symbols, their usage and the cultural context in which they are expressed. Accordingly, language needs to be understood in relation to the cultural and social structures that influence the development of an individual's beliefs, values and behaviour patterns.

In response to the diversity of languages that exist in Australia and New Zealand, a number of both government and non-government interpreter and translator language support services and resources are currently available for both healthcare workers and clients of healthcare services. There are benefits to accrue from a healthcare workforce that is either bilingual or multilingual, particularly one that reflects the demographic language characteristics of the population as a whole (Australian Bureau of Statistics 2012c).

Religion

The religious, spiritual and philosophical beliefs adopted by people influence the way that individuals, families and community groups respond to significant life events such as birth, illness, death and dying, as well as their behaviours to maintain health and wellbeing.

There is diversity in the religious affiliations of Australians (Australian Bureau of Statistics 2012c). They comprise 25.3% Catholic, 17.1% Anglican and 36.9% other Christian denominations. Major non-Christian religions comprise 7.2% and include Buddhism (2.5%), Hinduism (1.3%), Islam (2.2%) and Judaism (0.5%). In New Zealand, the religious denomination of the country is similarly diverse. In 2006, 55% of New Zealanders affiliated with a Christian religion (Anglican, Catholic, Presbyterian Christian not defined and Methodist in that order), while a significant number indicated they followed other religions such as Hinduism (64,392), Islam (23,631) and Sikh (9,507) or followed no religion (34.7%) (Statistics New Zealand 2011).

Religious diversity has enormous implications for the planning, development and delivery of mainstream health services. Religious ceremonies may involve family members, requests for religious representatives or prayer sessions during hospitalisation or procedures. In compliance with the codes of ethics and professional conduct (Australian Nursing & Midwifery Council 2008a, 2008b) and competency standards for nurses (Australian Nursing and Midwifery Council 2006), nurses are required to demonstrate respect for the beliefs and values of diverse cultural groups in their care. Knowledge of different cultural rites and ceremonies and accommodation of such requests is one example of how a nurse can demonstrate respect for diverse beliefs, values and life ways.

Health and wellbeing

The World Health Organization (WHO) defines health as a state of complete physical, mental and social wellbeing, not merely the absence of disease or infirmity (McMurray 2007). The degree to which a society experiences health and wellbeing is largely dependent upon the social and cultural structures in place to support the nation's most vulnerable population groups (Australian Institute of Health and Welfare 2012).

Groups such as the very young, the very old and the very poor, newly arrived refugees and people living with a disability are undeniably a nation's most vulnerable, and in need of support at a far greater level than other population groups. Compared with those who have social and economic advantages, disadvantaged Australians are more likely to have shorter lives, higher levels of disease risk factors and lower use of preventive health services. Despite their right to equal health status, Indigenous people from countries such as Australia and New Zealand suffer health disparities when compared with non-indigenous populations within their countries (United Nations 2007). For example, while the life expectancy of Australians is high when compared with that of the rest of the world, the life expectancy of Indigenous Australians is among the lowest worldwide and Indigenous Australians continue to experience poorer health and higher death rates than non-Indigenous Australians (Australian Institute of Health and Welfare 2008). In addition, many Indigenous Australians and New Zealanders are reluctant to access health services because of their reliance on Westernised biomedical models of service delivery that fail to accommodate Indigenous notions of health (Sherwood 2009). For example, Indigenous people prefer to use the term 'social and emotional wellbeing' rather than 'mental illness' because it is more positive and holistic which fits better with Indigenous beliefs about health (Usher & West 2011). The following box (20.2) identifies some key points to consider when working with Indigenous Australians.

Box 20.2
Working with Indigenous Australians

Things to be aware of when working with Australian Indigenous people include:

- Indigenous people perceive health and illness differently to the Western biomedical model.

- It may not be appropriate for a nurse to care for an Indigenous consumer of a different gender.

- Indigenous consumers must be consulted and included in all decisions about their care.

- Indigenous consumers often have an extended family and group of carers who should all be consulted about their care.

- Avoid asking questions about ceremonial business, bereavement, sexuality, fertility, domestic habits and other similar sensitive issues.

Source: (Haswell et al 2009, Westerman 2004)

Research has also found that most immigrants enjoy health that is at least as good as, if not better than, that of the Australian-born population and that they often have lower death and hospitalisation rates, as well as lower rates of disability and lifestyle-related risk factors (AIHW 2012). A similar situation occurs in New Zealand where Pacific Islanders and other migrants have health outcomes better than Māori even though they remain less than that of the other non-Indigenous New Zealanders (Lawrence & Kearns 2005). This 'healthy migrant' effect is believed to result from two main factors. First, a self-selection process includes those who are willing and economically able to migrate, and excludes those who are sick or disabled. Second, the government selection process involves certain eligibility criteria based on health, education, language and job skills.

Refugees and asylum seekers

The Australian Government's Humanitarian Program aims to protect refugees who have been forced to leave their country due to a dereliction of human rights and warfare. The quota resettled in the Humanitarian Program in 2010–11 was 13,799. Nearly 6000 of these places were provided to refugees of which 12.7% were awarded to women at risk. In 2010–11 the top five countries of origin of offshore refugee and Special Humanitarian Program entrants were Iraq, Burma, Afghanistan, Bhutan and Congo (Australian Government 2011a).

Refugees may have experienced severe deprivation, trauma and torture that can lead to post-traumatic stress disorder (PTSD), a condition that can profoundly affect a person's health and capacity to resettle. There is a body of literature on the medical and psychological responses of people to war and conflict that includes Afghan refugees in Australia (Harris & Telfer 2001, Omeri et al 2004, 2006, Proctor 2004a, 2004b, Steel & Sil 2001, Sultan & K 2001). The specific factors that impact on resettlement of refugees are poorly understood outside of relief agencies (Summerfield 2000). In their study of

Afghan refugees in New South Wales, Omeri et al (2006) identify a number of issues of central concern to this group, including: emotional responses to trauma; migration and resettlement experiences; culture-specific health maintenance strategies; and barriers impeding access to and appropriateness of Australian healthcare services. The findings have relevance for improving the quality of culture-specific healthcare for the Afghan community in Australia. A New Zealand study found that the delivery of healthcare to migrants is plagued by issues such as the poor physical and mental health of refugees, their expectations of health services, lack of cultural awareness among health workers, the lack of English-speaking translators, the resources required to provide affordable and accessible care and retention of health workers (Lawrence & Kearns 2005).

The Australian Government's 'Review of settlement services for migrants and humanitarian entrants report' (Commonwealth of Australia 2003) outlined in recommendation 29 a proposal that the department seek further opportunities to settle humanitarian entrants in regional Australia. The report also highlighted the need for the department to liaise more closely with stakeholders regarding regional locations where employment opportunities exist and where appropriate community services and support currently exists or may be developed. As a result of this recommendation, many newly arrived immigrants and refugees now transfer to country locations for employment and affordable housing (Australian Government 2007). However, social support networks and access to culturally appropriate services are reduced in regional areas, in comparison with urban and metropolitan regions in Australia.

CONSIDERATIONS FOR NURSING AND MIDWIFERY CARE IN MULTICULTURAL COMMUNITIES

Irihapeti Ramsden has had significant influence in New Zealand and internationally through her contribution to the notion of *cultural safety*. Originally proposed as a political response to the long-term effects of colonisation on the Māori people, cultural safety is situated within a framework of biculturalism between the Māori and non-Māori (immigrant others to New Zealand) with the goal of better healthcare for all (Ramsden 2002, Wepa 2005). Importantly, the notion rests on the principle that culturally safe healthcare is determined by the end users rather than the healthcare providers (Clarke 2005). Therefore, it is an expectation that the notion of cultural safety will guide all healthcare delivery. Cultural safety is therefore a pivotal component of all nursing and midwifery curricula and nursing and midwifery registration (Nursing Council of New Zealand 2009).

Skills are needed to deliver culturally competent care, and the following description includes a summary of those skills needed for the planning, development and delivery of culturally competent nursing care. These guidelines have been adapted from Andrews and Boyle (2008). They are:

- **Cultural self-assessment.** This enables nurses to develop an awareness of their own cultural values, attitudes, beliefs and practices. These insights enable one to overcome ethnocentric tendencies and cultural stereotypes, which are often vehicles for perpetuating prejudice and discrimination. Cultural self-assessment is the foundation for culturally competent and culturally congruent nursing care.

- **Cross-cultural communication.** This is identified as one of the most important landmarks in cultural assessment in establishing a culturally congruent care plan. Therefore, it is necessary to examine the ways in which people from various cultural backgrounds communicate with one another. In addition to oral and verbal communication, messages are conveyed non-verbally through gestures, body movements, posture, tone of voice and facial expressions.

- **Non-verbal communication.** Non-verbal communication patterns vary widely across cultures. Therefore, nurses must be alert for cues that convey cultural differences in the use of silence, eye contact, touch, space, distance and facial expressions. Cultural influences on appropriate communication between individuals of different genders also need to be considered. Non-verbal behaviours are culturally significant and failure to adhere to cultural norms of behaviour may be viewed as a serious transgression. Violating norms that relate to appropriate male–female relationships among various cultural groups may jeopardise nurses' therapeutic relationship with patients and their families.

- **Touch.** This deserves careful consideration. While we recognise the often-reported benefits in establishing rapport with clients through touch, including the promotion of healing through therapeutic touch, physical contact with clients conveys various meanings cross-culturally.

- **Space and distance.** These are significant in cross-cultural communication. The perception of appropriate distance zones varies widely among cultural groups. In the early 1960s, Edward Hall pioneered the study of proxemics, which focuses on how people in various cultures relate to their physical space. Although there are intercultural variations, the intimate distance in interpersonal interactions ranges from 0–0.5 metres. At this distance, people experience visual detail and each other's odour, health and touch. Personal distance varies from 0.4–1.2 metres, the usual space within which communication between friends and acquaintances occurs. Nurses frequently interact with clients in the intimate or personal distance zones. Socially acceptable personal distance between people refers to approximately 1 metre, whereas anything greater than 1.5 metres is considered public space (Hall 1963, cited in Andrews & Boyle 2008:26).

CONCLUDING REMARKS

Meeting the healthcare needs of individuals living in a multicultural country such as Australia requires careful reflection and consideration on behalf of nurses and midwives. This chapter has provided an overview of Australia's population and the ways this composition impacts on the role and function of nurses and midwives. The importance of understanding culture as a dynamic process was also addressed. A number of strategies to promote critical thinking and reflective practice around particular issues that impact on nursing and midwifery care are provided.

REFLECTIVE QUESTIONS

1. What are some of the factors influencing healthcare for diverse populations in Australia? Reflect upon those discussed in this chapter.

2. How are social context and cultural beliefs linked to health and wellbeing outcomes?

3. Take some time to think about your own cultural beliefs in relation to health and healthcare. How might your own beliefs be similar or different from that of someone from another culture?

4. Why is it important to change the existing view of culture from a static to a dynamic process?

RECOMMENDED READINGS

Australian Government 2011 The people of Australia: Australia's multicultural policy. Australian Government, Canberra. Online. Available: http://www.immi.gov.au/living-in-australia/a-multicultural-australia/multicultural-policy/

Fredericks B, Thompson M 2012 Collaborative voices: ongoing reflections on cultural competency and the health care of Australian Indigenous people. Journal of Australian Indigenous Issues 13(3):10–20

Gregory D, Harrowing J, Lee B et al 2010 Pedagogy as influencing nursing students' essentialized understanding of culture. International Journal of Nursing Education Scholarship 7(1):Article 30

Nursing Council of New Zealand 2009 Guidelines for cultural safety, the Treaty of Waitangi and Māori health in nursing education and practice. Nursing Council of New Zealand, Wellington

REFERENCES

Anderson I F, Crengle S, Kamaka M et al 2006 Indigenous health 1 – indigenous health in Australia, New Zealand, and the Pacific. Lancet 367:1775–1785

Anderson L, Scrimshaw S, Fullilove M et al 2003 Culturally competent healthcare systems: a systematic review. American Journal of Preventative Medicine 24(3S):238–246

Andrews M, Boyle J 2008 Transcultural concepts in nursing care, 5th edn. Kluwer/Lippincott, Williams & Wilkins, Philadelphia

Australian Bureau of Statistics 2012a Census home – data & analysis. Online. Available: http://www.abs.gov.au/websitedbs/censushome.nsf/home/data?opendocument&navpos=200 25 July 2012

Australian Bureau of Statistics 2012b Census of population and housing – counts of Aboriginal and Torres Strait Islander Australians, 2011. Online. Available: http://www.abs.gov.au/ausstats/abs@.nsf/Lookup/2075.0main+features32011 25 July 2012

Australian Bureau of Statistics 2012c Reflecting a nation: stories from the 2011 census, 2012–2013. Online. Available: http://www.abs.gov.au/ausstats/abs@.nsf/Lookup/2071.0main+features902012-2013 25 July 2012

Australian Government 2007 Fact sheet 66: integrated humanitarian settlement strategy. Online. Available: http://www.immi.gov.au/media/fact-sheets/66hss.htm 26 July 2013

Australian Government 2011a Fact Sheet 60 – Australia's Refugee and Humanitarian Program. Online. Available: http://www.immi.gov.au/media/fact-sheets/60refugee.htm 26 July 2012

Australian Government 2011b The people of Australia: Australia's multicultural policy. Canberra: Australian Government. Online. Available: http://www.immi.gov.au/living-in-australia/a-multicultural-australia/multicultural-policy/

Australian Institute of Health and Welfare (AIHW) 2008 The health and welfare of Australia's Aboriginal and Torres Strait Island peoples. AIHW, Canberra, p 283

Australian Institute of Health and Welfare (AIHW) 2012 Australia's health 2012. AIHW, Canberra, p 580

Australian Nursing and Midwifery Council 2006 RN competency standards. Online. Available: http://www.nursingmidwiferyboard.gov.au/Codes-Guidelines-Statements/Codes-Guidelines.aspx#codeofethics 22 August 2008

Australian Nursing and Midwifery Council 2008a Code of ethics for nurses in Australia. Online. Available: http://www.nursingmidwiferyboard.gov.au/Codes-Guidelines-Statements/Codes-Guidelines.aspx#codeofethics 26 July 2012

Australian Nursing and Midwifery Council 2008b Code of professional conduct for nurses in Australia. Online. Available: http://www.nursingmidwiferyboard.gov.au/Codes-Guidelines-Statements/Codes-Guidelines.aspx#codeofethics 26th July 2012

Campinha-Bacote J 2008 Cultural desire 'caught' or 'taught'. Contemporary Nurse 28(1–2):141–148

Clarke M 2005 Preface. In: Wepa D (ed), Cultural Safety in Aotearoa New Zealand. Pearson Education New Zealand, Auckland, pp v–vii

Commonwealth of Australia 1999 Australian multiculturalism for a new century: towards inclusiveness. Online. Available: www.immi.gov.au/fact-sheets/06evolution.html 23 Aug 2008

Commonwealth of Australia 2003 Multicultural Australia: united in diversity. Updating the 1999 new agenda for multicultural Australia: strategic directions for 2003–06. Online. Available: www.immi.gov.au/media/fact-sheets/06evolution.htm 23 Aug 2006

Commonwealth of Australia 2007 Fact sheet 66: integrated humanitarian settlement strategy. Department of Immigration and Citizenship. Online. Available: www.immi.gov.au/media/fact-sheets/66ihss.htm 25 Aug 2008

Commonwealth of Australia 2008b A new lease of life for multicultural Australia. Online. Available: www.minister.immi.gov.au/parlsec/media/media-releases/2008/lf08004.htm 23 Aug 2008

Crawford B, Lilo S, Stone S, Yates A 2008 Review of the quality, safety and management of maternity services in the Wellington area. Ministry of Health, Wellington

Fredericks B, Thompson, M 2012 Collaborative voices: ongoing reflections on cultural competency and the health care of Australian Indigenous people. Journal of Australian Indigenous Issues 13(3):10–20

Gray P, Thomas D 2006 Critical reflections on culture in nursing. Journal of Cultural Diversity 13(2):76–82

Gregory D, Harrowing J, Lee B et al 2010 Pedagogy as influencing nursing students' essentialized understanding of culture. International Journal of Nursing Education Scholarship 7(1):Article 30

Harris M, Telfer B 2001 The health needs of asylum seekers living in the community. Medical Journal of Australia 175:589–592

Haswell M, Hunter E, Wargent R et al 2009 Protocols for the delivery of social and emotional wellbeing and mental health services in Indigenous communities: guidelines for health workers, clinicians, consumers and carers. University of Queensland and Queensland Health, Cairns

Health Practitioners Competence Assurance Act 2003. Online. Available: www. legislation.govt.nz (statutes)

Lawrence J, Kearns R 2005 Exploring the 'fit' between people and providers: refugee health needs and health care services in Mt Roskill, Auckland, New Zealand. Health and Social Care in the Community 13(5):451–461

McMurray A 2007 Community health and wellness: a socio-ecological approach, 3rd edn. Mosby Elsevier, Sydney

Mays R, De Leon Siantz M, Viehweg S 2002 Accessing cultural competence of policy organisations. Journal of Transcultural Nursing 13(2):139–144

Nursing Council of New Zealand 2002 Guidelines for cultural safety, the treaty of Waitangi, and Māori health in nursing and midwifery education and practice. Nursing Council of New Zealand, Wellington

Nursing Council of New Zealand 2004 Report of the Nursing Council of New Zealand for the year ending 31 March 2004. Nursing Council of New Zealand, Wellington

Nursing Council of New Zealand 2009 Guidelines for cultural safety, the Treaty of Waitangi and Māori health in nursing education and practice. Nursing Council of New Zealand, Wellington

Omeri A 2003 Meeting diversity challenges: pathways of advanced transcultural nursing practice in Australia. Contemporary Nurse 15(3):175–187

Omeri A, Lennings C, Raymond L 2004 Hardiness and transformational coping in asylum seekers: the Afghan experience. Diversity in Health and Social Care 1(1):21–30

Omeri A, Lennings C, Raymond, L 2006 Beyond asylum: implications for nursing and health care delivery for Afghan refugees in Australia. Journal of Transcultural Nursing 17(1):30–39

Phiri J, Dietsch E, Bonner A 2010 Cultural safety and its importance for Australian midwifery practice. Collegian 17:105–111

Proctor N 2004a Beyond asylum: the significance of supportive counselling in the process of seeking asylum. Nursing Review March:5

Proctor N 2004b Retraumatization, fear and suicidal thinking: a case study of 'boat people' to Australia. Migration Letters: An International Journal of Migration 1(1):42–49

Ramsden I 2002 Cultural safety and nursing education in Aotearoa and Te Waipounamu. Victoria University of Wellington, Wellington

Sherwood J 2009 Who is not coping with colonization? Laying out the map for decolonization. The Royal Australian and New Zealand College of Psychiatrists 17(1)

Spradley J 1979 The ethnographic interview. Harcourt Brace Jovanovich, Fort Worth

Statistics New Zealand 2011 New Zealand in Profile 2011. New Zealand Ministry of Foreign Affairs and Trade, Manatu Aorere, New Zealand

Steel Z, Sil D 2001 The mental health implications for detaining asylum seekers. Medical Journal of Australia 175:596–604

Sultan A, K O S 2001 Psychological disturbances in asylum seekers. Medical Journal of Australia 175:593–596

Summerfield D 2000 Childhood war refugeedom and trauma: three core questions for mental health professionals. Transcultural Psychiatry 37:417–433

United Nations 2007 United Nations Declaration on the rights of Indigenous peoples. United Nations, New York

Usher K, West R 2011 Indigenous mental health. In: Edwards K, Munro I, Robins A, Welch A (eds), Mental health nursing: dimensions of praxis. Oxford, Melbourne, pp 397–408

Wepa D (ed), Cultural Safety in Aotearoa New Zealand. Pearson Education New Zealand, Auckland

Westerman T 2004 Engagement of Indigenous clients in mental health services: what role do cultural differences play? Australian e-Journal for the Advancement of Mental health (AeJAMH) 3(3)

Wilson D, Grant J 2008 Culturally competent partnerships with communities. In: Francis K, Chapman Y, Hoare K, Mills J (eds) Australia and New Zealand community as partner: theory and practice in nursing. Lippincott, Williams & Wilkins, Broadway, Australia

CHAPTER 21

Cultural awareness: nurses working with Indigenous Australian people

Isabelle Ellis, Christine Davey and Vicki Holliday

LEARNING OBJECTIVES

After completing this chapter, readers will be able to:

- outline the cultural diversity of Australia and identify where Indigenous people live
- recognise the effect of racism and social class on the health of Indigenous people
- differentiate between the terms *cultural awareness*, *cultural safety* and *cultural competence*
- assess the healthcare environment through the lens of cultural competence
- develop a plan to increase personal cultural competence, particularly in relation to working with Indigenous people.

KEY WORDS

Indigenous health, Aboriginal health, cultural competence, racism, social class

INTRODUCTION

Indigenous Australians are made up of two distinct groups—Aboriginal people and Torres Strait Islander people. Aboriginal culture is said to be the oldest living culture in the world, spanning more than 40,000 years. Prior to colonisation of Australia by the Europeans, it is thought that there were more than 500 Aboriginal clans living in Australia. It is estimated that there were 200 distinct languages spoken and many more dialects (Aboriginal and Torres Strait Islander Commission 1998:8). The Torres Strait is located between the tip of Queensland and Papua New Guinea. This Strait was named by a Spanish explorer, Luis Baez de Torres, in the early 1600s. There are approximately 100 islands of the Strait, of which 15 are inhabited. People originating from these islands are called Torres Strait Islanders (Dudgeon et al 2000).

Since colonisation, Australia has developed into a multicultural society with 23.8% of its population born overseas. However, of those, almost half, 43%, come from just four countries: the United Kingdom, New Zealand, Italy and Vietnam (Australian Bureau of Statistics (ABS) 2005b). Thomson et al (2010) report that there is very little information available about each of the distinct groups of Indigenous Australians. In general, Aboriginal and Torres Strait Islander peoples are counted together; additionally, despite improvements in reporting, there remains a persistent problem of under-reporting in the health-related data collections, which is why you often see an estimate of Indigenous figures.

Aboriginal and Torres Strait Islander people make up approximately 2.6% of the Australian population (ABS 2009a), Anglo-celtic 74%, other European 19% and Asians 4.5% (ABS 2005a). So although Australia considers itself multicultural, Australians are predominantly from an English-speaking background and of the dominant coloniser culture.

Australians generally enjoy longevity, which can be used as a proxy for an effective healthcare system. However, there is a disparity between groups. It is difficult to categorically state the differences, owing to the changes recently introduced by the Australian Bureau of Statistics in calculating Indigenous mortality rates. In fact, in the last few years, the press has reported the disparity in life expectancy is declining despite the Australian Bureau of Statistics highlighting that the decline is due to changes in statistical processes and may not reflect an actual decline. The ABS estimates that Australian girls born between 2005 and 2007 can expect to live to 82.6 years but an Indigenous girl's life expectancy is reduced to 72.9 years. Australian boys born in the same year period have a lower life expectancy and can expect to live to 78.7 years. Indigenous boys, though, can only expect to live to 67.2 years (ABS 2009b).

In this chapter we will explore some of the issues involved in working with Indigenous people as consumers, clients, patients, families and communities. We will identify why cultural competence is equally as important as clinical competence in improving the health of Aboriginal and Torres Strait Islander people for whom we care. We will also touch on some of the rewards and challenges of working cross-culturally with Aboriginal and Torres Strait Islander people.

WHAT DOES IT MEAN TO BE INDIGENOUS IN AUSTRALIA?

Being an Indigenous person means that a person identifies as an Indigenous person and acknowledges their Indigenous heritage. The United Nations has rejected the need for a definition for Indigenous people; however, it endorses the notion of a description of the concept of Indigenous, particularly the one put forward by José R Martínez Cobo in his famous study on the problem of discrimination against Indigenous populations.

> Indigenous communities, peoples and nations are those which, having a historical continuity with pre-invasion and pre-colonial societies ... consider themselves distinct from other sectors of the societies now prevailing in those territories ... They form at present non-dominant sectors of society and are determined to preserve, develop and transmit to future generations their ancestral territories, and their ethnic identity, as the basis of their continued existence as peoples, in accordance with their own cultural patterns, social institutions and legal systems.
> (*Cobo* 1983:379–382)

The Department of Aboriginal Affairs published a report in 1981 with the working definition of Aboriginal and Torres Strait Islander, which has been tested in the courts in relation to Indigenous land claims, the jurisdiction of the Royal Commission into Aboriginal Deaths in Custody and clarifying elements of the Constitution (Gardiner-Garden 2000).

> An Aboriginal or Torres Strait Islander is a person of Aboriginal or Torres Strait Islander descent who identifies as an Aboriginal or Torres Strait Islander and is accepted as such by the community in which he (she) lives.

This working definition has been adopted by government departments and organisations to determine eligibility for some programs and services. Although this three-part working definition, which comprises descent, self-identification and community recognition and acceptance, is in line with the concept of Indigenous accepted by the United Nations, it has been criticised as not originating from Indigenous people. However, it should be noted that many Indigenous people prefer to be referred to as being Aboriginal or Torres Strait Islander people rather than by the term *Indigenous*.

The history of recognition as an Indigenous person or community has not been straightforward in Australia. Early definitions used family tree mapping as a way of defining people's Aboriginality and alluded to notions of dilution of Aboriginality through mixing of blood with the colonisers. These definitions were regularly used by the government to develop and implement policies from 1788 to the 1960s, and led to descriptions of people as full blood, half caste or quarter caste, based mainly on the description of skin colour by those wishing to describe, exclude or implicate the Aboriginal person in question (Eckermann et al 2010). The 1936 Native Administration Bill, introduced in Western Australia, highlights this clearly, as Collard (in Dudgeon et al 2000) points out. 'People of less than "quadroon" (one fourth) descent were not allowed to live with people who were classified as "natives" even if they were related'. These terms are no longer used and it is inappropriate to do so; as described by Eckermann et al (2010), it is considered to be a form of scientific racism.

THE EFFECT OF CULTURE, RACE AND CLASS ON HEALTH

Stratification of society exists in all countries. In Australia, the strata are not only between rich and poor suburbs in our major cities, but also between urban and remote areas and between non-Indigenous and Indigenous Australians. Social class, according to Walter and Saggers (2007:88), is a 'broad concept which encapsulates both objective material position and subjective understandings and incorporates the important notion of differential access to power'. Social class also relates to social mobility, which refers to an individual's opportunity to move up or down the social class structure. This is often leveraged through access to education, employment and health services, resulting in a sustainable standard of living. Generally speaking, the further from the major capital cities you go, the poorer you are likely to be; and being Indigenous also makes you more likely to be poor. The key measures of Indigenous social disadvantage nationally include education, employment and income. The Australian Bureau of Statistics School Report (2009c) revealed that school retention from years 7/8 amongst non-Indigenous school children was 100% but for Indigenous school children it was 89%, dropping to 46% for children completing year 12, compared to a drop to 76% for non-Indigenous children. The 2006 Census reported the commonest employment classification for an Indigenous person was 'labourer' (24%) and for non-Indigenous person 'professional' (20%) and the average equalised weekly household income for Indigenous people was 62% less than for non-Indigenous people (ABS 2008a).

Social class structures are maintained or strengthened by the process of 'othering' (Cahoone 2003), whereby the dominant culture, structure or class maintains its hierarchy by creating a duality and then actively excluding or opposing the other. Difference is highlighted and accentuated. The classic Dr Seuss story about the Sneetches on the beaches is a wonderful example of othering; the only difference between the two groups is whether they have a star on their belly or not. The star-bellied Sneetches create and maintain their privileged position by highlighting this difference. Othering can be expressed as bullying, social exclusion and excessive vigilance by authority figures, such as when young people are followed in shops in case they shoplift. When expressed as racism, the effects on the health of individuals and communities can be profoundly negative (Larson et al 2007).

Defining racism is not easy. In his 2006 systematic review on self-reported racism, Paradies found that of the 138 studies included in the review, only 34 gave a definition of racism. Paradies proposes that racism is a form of:

> ... oppression/privilege which exists in a dialectical relationship with antiracism ... a societal system in which people are divided into races, with power unevenly distributed, or produced based on their racial classifications.
> (Paradies 2006:68)

Interpersonal racism is experienced as emotional upset (anger, sadness or frustration)—when a person perceives that they have been treated unfairly or have been demeaned in some way on the basis of their race. It can also be experienced as physical upset (headaches, an upset stomach, tensing of the muscles or a pounding heart). The study by Larson et al (2007) that examined the experiences of 639 residents of a town, of whom 138 identified as Aboriginal, found that Aboriginal people reported that they had received 3.6 times more negative racially-based treatment than non-Aboriginal people. They were more than twice as likely to report their health as fair to poor.

The experience or perception of racism has a negative impact on mental and physical health (Coffin 2007, Eades 2000, Karlsen & Nazroo 2002, Paradies 2006). The research by Larson et al (2007) concluded that racially-based negative treatment was so common in their study population that 40% of their Aboriginal respondents reported it. The research found no association of negatively racially-based treatment for the variables of gender, education or employment status and they concluded that all Aboriginal people in this town may equally experience or perceive racism as part of their daily lives. Durey (2010) highlights that Aboriginal people may be internalising and accepting the privileged position of non-Aboriginal people owing to their historical, long-standing oppression. She challenges non-Aboriginal people to turn the lens on themselves and reflect on the advantages of being white, when considering health, education, training and employment. She refers to McIntosh (1990) when she argues that the beliefs and practices that entrench 'white privilege' are an 'invisible package of unearned assets'.

Interpersonal racism can be overt or covert. Covert racism may be unintentional, hidden or less obvious than overt racism. The perpetrator may not even be aware that they are making a racist comment (Henry et al 2004). An example of this is to claim Indigeneity having been born in a particular country without having Indigenous heritage. This comment would be hurtful to Indigenous people, and it demonstrates lack of information or insight. Overt racism is intentional and can be perpetrated in many ways, such as: commenting on the dress or smell of a person and linking it to race; treating people in unequal ways based on race, such as making people wait while others are attended to straight away based on their race; speaking to adults as if they are children by simplifying explanations and using a tone of voice that sounds scolding or patronising.

Organisations are also able to create an atmosphere of 'othering'. When service organisations do not recognise the need for and provide culturally safe services, they can be accused of institutional racism (Henry et al 2004). Australia recently ratified the 2007 United Nations Declaration on the Rights of Indigenous Peoples. Article 24 states that individuals have the right 'to access, without any discrimination all social and health services, and to have an equal right to the enjoyment of the highest attainable standard of physical and mental health' (Durey 2010). Henry et al provide several examples of institutional racism within the healthcare system, such as cultural barriers, insufficient funding and the inequities in addressing overspending (e.g. an Aboriginal Medical Service had funding cut for overspending, while a government service was given an additional $100 million to address the overspend).

Institutional racism occurs when the policies of an organisation or institution result in Aboriginal or Torres Strait Islander people receiving less benefit from the same policies. This can occur in intentional or non-intentional ways (e.g. when the visiting times of a hospital do not coincide with the public transport schedules, or when the policy of the hospital states only immediate family members are able to visit an inpatient (Coffin 2007)).

Where do Aboriginal and Torres Strait Islander people live?

Indigenous people make up 2.6% of the total Australian population, with 32% living in major cities, 43% in regional areas and 25% in remote areas (ABS Australian Institute of Health and Welfare 2008:xxi). According to the Australian Bureau of Statistics (2007), more than half of all Indigenous people live in nine of the former 37 Aboriginal and Torres Strait Islander Commission (ATSIC) regions, namely Sydney, Brisbane, Coffs Harbour, Perth, Townsville, Cairns, Adelaide, Tasmania and Wagga Wagga. The population of the Torres Straits is approximately 8,000. Most outer island populations range from 100 to 500. The remainder of the approximately 33,000 Torres Strait Islanders and the 20,000 people of both Aboriginal and Torres Strait Islander descent live mostly in Queensland with New South Wales being the only other state with large numbers of Torres Strait Islanders (ABS 2007). Indigenous and non-Indigenous people are not distributed across the country in similar proportions. The percentage of the total population who live in very remote areas of Australia is 1%, as classified by the Australian Standard Geographical Classification (ASGC). Of those, Indigenous people make up approximately 45%. In contrast, 89% of non-Indigenous people live in the major capital cities and regional areas of Australia and only 3% live in remote or very remote areas.

Larson's analysis of the migration patterns and fertility trends for remote Australia point to a continuing increase in the remote Indigenous population, as a result of both a higher fertility rate and an increase in total numbers of Indigenous people due to a lower out-migration trend. This is in contrast to a higher out-migration of non-Indigenous people. She proposes that these factors will lead to increasing Indigenisation of remote Australia (Larson 2006).

The health of Aboriginal and Torres Strait Islander people

The story of disadvantage and disparity in health outcomes for Indigenous Australians should be alarming to all healthcare professionals. As previously stated, the Australian Bureau of Statistics and the Australian Institute of Health and Welfare acknowledge there has been difficulty in giving accurate statistical information in relation to Aboriginal and Torres Strait Islander people; however, the degree of disadvantage makes the small margins of error in statistical accuracy immaterial. We know that the Indigenous population is significantly younger overall than the non-Indigenous population. According to the 2006 Census, 37% of Indigenous people were under 15 years compared with 19% of non-Indigenous people. That contrasts starkly with the percentage of people over 65 years. The Indigenous rate is 3% compared with 13% for the non-Indigenous rate. Aboriginal and Torres Strait Islander people were twice as likely to report their health as fair to poor (ABS 2007).

Cardiovascular disease, which includes heart disease and stroke, were the major cause of death for both Indigenous men and women. The number of deaths after age-cause-specific statistical adjustment was more than 3 times the number expected for non-Indigenous men and 2.7 times the number expected for non-Indigenous women. The next most frequent cause of death for Indigenous men was injury, including transport accidents, self-harm and assault. Diabetes is a major cause of morbidity and although there are real problems with the reporting of diabetes numbers, we do know that the prevalence of diabetes increases with age and Aboriginal and Torres Strait Islander people experience it at younger ages than expected for non-Indigenous people. The prevalence of diabetes reported at the 2006 Census for Indigenous people aged between 35 and 44 years was five times that reported by non-Indigenous people (ABS 2006). Renal disease is more prevalent among Indigenous people than non-Indigenous people. Data from the Australian and New Zealand Dialysis and Transplant Registry reveal that a total of 846 Indigenous people were newly identified with End Stage Renal Disease in the period 2004–2007. Indigenous people from the Northern Territory had a rate more than 20 times the rate of non-Indigenous people and three times the rate of other Indigenous people. The story of Indigenous disadvantage does not just relate to chronic diseases. The National Aboriginal and Torres Strait Islander Social Survey (ABS 2008a) collected data on ear and hearing problems. It concluded that there was no significant difference between children living in urban or remote areas; 1 in 10 Indigenous children aged 4–14 had experienced ear or hearing problems. The Western Australian Child Health Survey identified that Western Australian Aboriginal children suffer significantly more from skin, ear and respiratory infections than non-Aboriginal children (Zubrick et al 2004).

The statistics paint a bleak picture of the physical health of Indigenous Australians. They paint a picture of many people suffering increasing disadvantage, starting from birth, that spirals through a childhood marred by acute infections and illness, to the early onset of chronic disease and deterioration in health status and early death. Identifying the causes of poor health is the first step in trying to address poor outcomes. We are constantly reminded in the media that if we eat less, drink less alcohol, exercise more and do not smoke we will be less likely to suffer chronic disease, and we will become healthier and live longer. This puts responsibility for improving health status squarely at the feet of individuals. However, there are other opinions that suggest that individuals do not have total control or autonomy over various aspects of their lives; that, in reality, their lives and decisions are governed by social obligations and norms and the assumption of control when it comes to chronic disease self-management is flawed, thereby undermining the usefulness of the current chronic disease self-management models (Skinner & Ellis 2009).

There is a growing body of research that has looked at the social determinants of health and tried to identify their impact on health outcomes (Marmot & Wilkinson 1999, Saggers & Gray 2007, Turrell & Mathers 2000). It is clear that income, environmental issues and education have a profound impact on health across the lifespan for all people, but the stories of Indigenous people describe a specific group of social determinants that impact on their health. Indigenous people describe their health in terms of culture, community, access to land and sacred sites, access to resources and key services and involvement in the political, economic and social life of post-colonised Australia (Hunter 1993).

USE OF HEALTH SERVICES BY ABORIGINAL AND TORRES STRAIT ISLANDER PEOPLE

Indigenous Australians visit their general practitioner (GP) and are hospitalised for circulatory diseases, diabetes, respiratory diseases, musculoskeletal conditions, kidney disease, eye and ear problems and mental and behavioural disorders (Australian Institute of Health and Welfare 2009). However, they are less likely to visit their GP, use private health services or residential aged care than non-Indigenous Australians. They are more likely to use public hospitals for a range of care needs and are twice as likely to be hospitalised (Australian Bureau of Statistics 2006).

In his 2005 Social Justice report, Tom Calma, Aboriginal and Torres Strait Islander Social Justice Commissioner, made recommendations for equity in health within a generation culminating in the Close the Gap Campaign in March 2006 (Aboriginal and Torres Strait Islander Social Justice Commissioner and the Steering Committee for Indigenous Health Equality 2008). As a result of this, the Steering Committee for Indigenous Health Equality was formed and has worked tirelessly since to gain a commitment from government and non-government stakeholders to work collaboratively to 'close the gap'. On 13 February 2008, the Prime Minister, Kevin Rudd, apologised to Aboriginal and Torres Strait Islander peoples for the wrongdoings by governments of the past. In his speech, not only did the Prime Minister apologise, but he also committed to developing partnerships with Indigenous people to close the gap in life expectancy, employment and educational opportunities (Aboriginal and Torres Strait Islander Social Justice Commissioner and the Steering Committee for Indigenous Health Equality 2008).

In March 2008, a Close the Gap Indigenous Health Equality summit was held in Canberra. On the final day of the summit, a Statement of Intent to work in partnership to reduce the gap in life expectancy of Indigenous people within a generation was produced. The statement was signed by the Prime Minister, Minister of Health, Minister of Indigenous Affairs, Leader of the opposition, the Aboriginal and Torres Strait Islander Social Justice Commissioner, Leaders of National Aboriginal Community Controlled Health Organisation (NACCHO), Congress of Aboriginal and Torres Strait Islander Nurses (CATSIN), Australian Indigenous Doctors Association (AIDA) and the Indigenous Dentists Association of Australia. During the three-day summit, targets were developed to address disparities in the morbidity and mortality of Indigenous people.

The targets are addressed under five broad categories:

1. partnerships
2. health status
3. primary healthcare and other health services
4. infrastructure, and
5. social determinants.

In his speech on 20 March 2008, Tom Calma highlighted the importance of working together to achieve the health targets; this has been further supported more recently with the Australian government allocation of funds to address inequities (Aboriginal and Torres Strait Islander Social Justice Commissioner and the Steering Committee for Indigenous Health Equality 2008).

In response to the Close the Gap campaign and the signing of the 'Statement of Intent', the Australian Government established the Closing the Gap Strategy to address Aboriginal and Torres Strait Islander disadvantage; the Strategy is monitored by the Council of Australian Governments (COAG). The National Partnership Agreement on Closing the Gap in Indigenous Health Outcomes National Healthcare Agreement was signed in December 2008 by the prime minister and the state and territories' leaders. This agreement outlines how governments will work together to address the disparities in life expectancy of Aboriginal and Torres Strait Islander peoples (Australian Government 2008).

The Agreement has 6 targets:

1. to close the gap in life expectancy within a generation;
2. to halve the gap in mortality rates for Indigenous children under five within a decade;
3. to ensure all Indigenous four-year-olds in remote communities have access to early childhood education within five years;
4. to halve the gap in reading, writing and numeracy achievements for Indigenous children within a decade;
5. to halve the gap for Indigenous students in year 12 attainment or equivalent attainment rates by 2020; and
6. to halve the gap in employment outcomes between Indigenous and non-Indigenous Australians within a decade (Australian Government 2008).

Since its inception, each year in March the prime minister tables a report in Parliament outlining the progress of the Agreement in closing the gap. At the same time, the Close the Gap Committee develops a 'Shadow report on the Australian Government's progress to close the gap'. The Close the Gap Committee continues to lobby government for equality in health for Aboriginal and Torres Strait Islander people with National Close the Gap day being held in March each year.

In 2011 the peak Indigenous health organisations joined with the Congress of Australia's First People to take the lead in lobbying and informing the Australian Government. This committee, led by the Congress of Australia's First People, enables links with governments and the Close the Gap Committee. It will be monitored and measured through existing frameworks, the Overcoming Indigenous Disadvantage and Aboriginal & Torres Strait Islander Health Performance Framework (Congress of Australia's First People 2011).

The Australian Institute of Health and Welfare (2011) reports some recent health gains such as an increase in the life expectancy for Aboriginal and Torres Strait Islander people of 11.5 years for females and 9.7 years for males and a decrease in infant mortality, although it remains two times higher than for non-Indigenous infants. Whilst there are gains, there are also some areas where there is little or no improvement, such as the prevalence of trachoma, mental ill health, cardiovascular disease and renal disease to name a few.

Access to health services

Accessibility to health services is widely acknowledged as a factor determining their use. Access is one of the pillars of Primary Health Care and has been further described by the World Health Organization declarations since the first Alma Ata declaration in 1978. The Australian Institute of Health and Welfare (2012) website notes:

> Overall, Indigenous Australians experience lower levels of access to health services than the general population, attributed to factors such as proximity, availability and cultural appropriateness of health services, transport availability, health insurance and health services affordability and proficiency in English.

The availability of transport and the distance to the nearest health service is a factor in accessibility of health services. The 2006 Social Health Survey found that 84% of Australians found it relatively easy to get to places they needed to go to, including health services. Only 4% found it difficult to get to places they needed to visit (ABS 2006). Indigenous people, on the other hand, found it much more difficult to get to places they needed to go to. Twenty-six per cent nationally had no access to a motor vehicle when needed, with 18% having no access to public transport (ABS 2010). The situation is worse in remote areas: the Australian Bureau of Statistics reported that in 2008 71% of Indigenous adults living in remote areas had no access to public transport. It needs to be noted that in rural and remote areas, 78% of discrete Indigenous communities are located more than 50 kilometres from the nearest hospital and 50% are located more than 25 kilometres from the nearest community health service (ABS 2006).

Although English is the official language of Australia, many Indigenous people do not speak it as their primary language. State hospitals and health services do have interpreter services available for a range of languages, but there are very few trained interpreters for Indigenous languages and there is very little written material that has been translated into Indigenous languages. Aboriginal and Torres Strait Islander health workers, liaison officers or extended family members are the key resources for providing translation services.

Aboriginal and Torres Strait Islander health services

Aboriginal Community Controlled Health Services (ACCHS) were established in the 1970s to provide Aboriginal people with choice relating to their medical care provider. These services can be found in urban, rural and remote areas and are governed by an elected Board of Directors. Services are funded by the Australian Government through the Office of Aboriginal and Torres Strait Islander Health (OATSIH). These comprehensive primary healthcare services can be general practice medical services, or offer a range of services to include the social and emotional wellbeing needs of the community they serve. The services can be exclusively for Aboriginal people in the local community or can cater to the general public, depending on the decisions of the Aboriginal Board of Directors. ACCHS often work in partnership with government and non-government organisations to streamline services for their community members. Many of these services work very hard to address accessibility by providing transport services and training local Aboriginal and Torres Strait Islander people for health careers. They also place a high value on the cultural competence of their employees as a strategy to address the lack of cultural safety experienced by Aboriginal and Torres Strait Islander people when accessing mainstream services.

CULTURALLY COMPETENT NURSING PRACTICE

Nursing competency standards have developed over the last two decades to better inform the public and the profession of what can be expected from nurses in a range of practice settings. The Australian Nursing and Midwifery Council competency standards have been adopted by the new accrediting body, the Australian Nursing and Midwifery Accreditation Council (ANMAC), and are the basis for all nursing education in Australia leading to registration with the Australian Health Practitioners Regulation Agency (AHPRA). In addition to competency standards, nursing practice is governed by a code of ethics and a code of professional conduct. The most recent code of ethics was revised in 2008; it clearly recognises that nurses have a responsibility to consider human rights in their care of individuals and communities.

The code of ethics outlines the profession's view of the 'critical relationship between health and human rights' and the importance of reconciliation between Aboriginal and Torres Strait Islander peoples and non-Indigenous Australians. It also states that the model of care for Aboriginal and Torres Strait Islander peoples must include physical, spiritual and cultural wellbeing as an 'expected whole'. The code of ethics explicitly states that nurses have a responsibility to provide 'just, compassionate, culturally competent and culturally responsive care to every person requiring or receiving nursing care' (Australian Nursing and Midwifery Council 2008). Cultural competence has been defined as a set of 'congruent behaviours, attitudes and policies that come together in a system, agency or among professionals to enable that system, agency or that group of professionals to work effectively in cross cultural situations' (National Health and Medical Research Council 2005). Betancourt (2006:183) expands on that definition to include:

knowledge and information from and about individuals and groups that is integrated and transformed into clinical standards, skills, service approaches, techniques ... that match the cultural experiences and traditions of clients and that increase both the quality and appropriateness of health care services and health outcomes.

How nurses develop cultural competence has been variously studied; particularly looking at knowledge acquisition immediately after a period of training. Long-term evaluations that assess the impact on patient outcomes of cultural competence training are yet to be conducted (Durey 2010).

CULTURAL SAFETY

Cultural safety is a term that originated in New Zealand in the 1980s (Ramsden 1992, 2002). It supports a social justice approach to healthcare and, unlike cultural competence which is generic, pertains to all cross-cultural situations. Cultural safety is specific to working in a cross-cultural context with Indigenous peoples. The Congress of Aboriginal and Torres Strait Islander Nurses (CATSIN) endorse cultural safety as a model for providing healthcare to Aboriginal and Torres Strait Islander peoples (Indigenous Nurse Education Working Group 2002). It is a philosophy of healthcare that 'aims to improve the health of all Indigenous peoples in First World Colonised Countries, by providing culturally appropriate healthcare services' (Edwards et al 2007:62). The development of culturally safe practice requires openness, honesty, commitment and respect. It is achieved by personal reflection and understanding your own culture and values before you can meaningfully interact with Indigenous people (Ramsden 2002). There are three principles that underpin cultural safety: partnership, participation and protection.

Partnership and participation require the development of responsive service delivery models in partnership with the Indigenous people who are expected to use the service. This may be a service designed specifically for Indigenous people to reduce inequity or it may be a mainstream service. Protection is against individual, structural and institutional racism. There needs to be a recognition that Indigenous people may have had past negative experiences with the system, either personally as a recipient of care or as an observer watching others receive care. There needs to be acknowledgement that language and cultural barriers may prevent meaningful exchanges and that there are variances between the concepts of health and wellness between cultures (Edwards et al 2007). When a health service institutes policies and protocols to ensure that consumers receive a culturally safe service, then the service is said to be culturally secure (Coffin 2007).

Cultural awareness

Cultural awareness is about acknowledging that we do not all have a shared history— nor a shared understanding of the present. The culturally aware nurse is able to question the source of information and recognise the filter through which information is presented. It may be information in the news or popular press. It may be organisational or policy documents. The culturally aware nurse recognises the importance of listening. Most health services in rural and remote Australia and some government and non-government health services in urban areas have a requirement for health professionals to attend cultural awareness training on commencement of employment. This needs to be meaningful and presented by Aboriginal or Torres Strait Islander people, preferably people who are Indigenous to the area in which the health service is provided.

Cultural awareness does not develop from a generalised summary about Aboriginal and Torres Strait Islander cultures, which often serves no greater function than to reinforce stereotypes. Where health services have engaged the services of an appropriate Aboriginal or Torres Strait Islander facilitator, you will find you learn most by listening. Edwards et al (2007) suggest that the first principle for working effectively with Australian Indigenous people is to 'stand back, be quiet, listen, hear and wait'. If you adopt this from your first encounter, you will find that you will learn much more than by asking.

Cultural sensitivity

Cultural sensitivity is a process—a dawning. By reflecting on what you have learnt about the local Aboriginal or Torres Strait Islander community and about how your own life experiences impact on others and therefore your practice as a health professional, you gradually come to the realisation that your actions and interactions have an effect on the health of the people for whom you are caring. The culturally sensitive nurse will work to get to know the community and be respectful at all times, being open to different understandings, beliefs, values, practices and norms. In time, you may even enjoy a joke at your own expense, particularly as you realise how you have been and are perceived by others (Eckermann et al 2010, Edwards et al 2007).

PLANNING YOUR OWN JOURNEY TOWARDS CULTURAL COMPETENCE AND SAFETY

Developing into a culturally safe practitioner requires leadership on your part. It requires you to reflect on your own values and culture. It requires you never to participate in racist behaviour. It requires you to work with others to build a culturally secure health service which is participative, and works in partnership with the Aboriginal and Torres Strait Islander people it is set up to serve. It requires you to actively engage with the social justice agenda.

The exercise in the box on the next page is a cultural competence self-reflection tool. You can use it to help you on your journey towards cultural competence. It is a practical tool that can be used at any time and can be used periodically to gauge how you are progressing, or as a reminder when you commence a new role or you move to a new location, of the kinds of information you need to discover and the people you might find useful to talk with.

It has been adapted from the Multicultural Disability Advocacy Association of New South Wales (MDAA) http://www.mdaa.org.au/.

CONCLUDING REMARKS

Providing appropriate holistic nursing care to Aboriginal and Torres Strait Islander people needs to be a priority for all nurses. The health of Australia's Indigenous people is negatively impacted by interpersonal and institutional racism. Aboriginal and Torres Strait Islander people may have internalised structural racism and may be suspicious of changing attitudes. Developing your own cultural competence and working to provide culturally safe care in a culturally secure health service will have a positive impact on health outcomes for the people you are caring for.

In this chapter, we have provided a snapshot of what it means to identify as an Aboriginal or Torres Strait Islander and where Indigenous people live. We have highlighted some of the health inequities and provided insight into the complexity of the causes. We recognise that it would be preferable to have a 'quick fix' to some of the worst problems faced by Aboriginal people living in very remote areas, and to be able to address some of the social and emotional wellbeing issues caused by racism, but in our experience there is no recipe book or instant solution. We hope you see this personal leadership journey of becoming culturally safe as a way that you can impact positively on the health of all of the Aboriginal and Torres Strait Islander people that you come across in both your personal and your professional life.

REFLECTIVE QUESTIONS

1. Reflect on the number of Aboriginal or Torres Strait Islander people you know. Where would you find out who are the traditional owners of the land where you live?
2. Take time to consider your own family history. How might you learn about the history of colonisation and the impact of past government policies on the Indigenous peoples in the state or territory in which you live?
3. Find one dreamtime story and reflect on its place in Aboriginal or Torres Strait Islander culture.

Cultural competence self-test

Read each statement and record a number from 1 to 3 that most closely reflects what you do, or would do, when caring for someone from a culturally or linguistically different background from your own.

1 I frequently do this.

2 I occasionally do this.

3 I rarely or never do this.

My communication			
When speaking with people who speak languages other than my language; I attempt to learn basic greetings.	1	2	3
I am competent and confident in determining the language used by the users of my service. I am competent in using accredited interpreters.	1	2	3
When interacting with people who have limited proficiency in my language, I always keep in mind that: limited language skill does not equate to limited intellectual capacity.	1	2	3
Limited second or subsequent language skills have no bearing on a person's ability to express themselves in their first language.	1	2	3

Our workplace			
I seek information from clients/patients and other community contacts to assist me in adapting my practice to the diverse needs and preferences of users of our service.	1	2	3
I attend training sessions that enhance my cultural competence.	1	2	3
The workplace reflects the cultural diversity of the community my agency serves. There are relevant images, objects or art works and education materials for these different cultural groups.	1	2	3
My values			
I explore my own values, beliefs, assumptions and attitudes about cultural diversity and reflect on how they impact on how I work with people using our service.	1	2	3
I avoid imposing my values.	1	2	3
In every situation I discourage colleagues, service users and others from using racial and ethnic slurs by helping them understand the impact their language can have on others.	1	2	3

If you frequently responded with a 1, you are engaged in practices that demonstrate cultural awareness and you aim to deliver a culturally competent service. If you found you frequently responded with a 2, you may need to reflect on your practices to respond more effectively to the needs of people from culturally or linguistically different backgrounds from your own. If you responded with a 3 to any statement, you may need to learn more about the people who use your service.

RECOMMENDED READINGS

Eckermann A-K, Dowd T, Chang E et al 2010 Binan Goonj: bridging cultures in Aboriginal health, 3rd edn. Elsevier Australia, Sydney

Edwards T, Dade Smith J, Smith R et al 2007 Cultural perspectives. In: Dade Smith J (ed) Australia's rural and remote health: a social justice perspective, 2nd edn. Tertiary Press, Melbourne

Larson A, Gilles M, Howard P J, Coffin J 2007 It's enough to make you sick: the impact of racism on the health of Aboriginal Australians. Australian and New Zealand Journal of Public Health 31(4):322–329

Walter M, Saggers S 2007 Poverty and social class. In: Carson B, Dunbar T, Chenhall R, Baillie R (eds) Social determinants of Indigenous health. Allen & Unwin, Sydney, pp 87–94

REFERENCES

Australian Government (2008) National partnership agreement on closing the gap in Indigenous health outcomes: an agreement between the Commonwealth of Australia: the State of New South Wales; the State of Victoria; the State of Queensland; the State of Western Australia; the State of South Australia; the Australia Capital Territory and the Northern Territory. Online. Available: www.health.gov.au/internet/main/Publishing.nsf/Content/closinggap-tacklingchronicdisease/$File/commonwealth_implementation_plan.pdf

Aboriginal and Torres Strait Islander Commission (ATSIC) 1998 As a matter of fact: answering the myths and misconceptions about Indigenous Australians. ATSIC, Canberra

Aboriginal and Torres Strait Islander Health and Welfare Unit 2012 Access to health services. AIHW, Canberra. Online. Available: www.aihw.gov.au/indigenous/health/access.cfm

Aboriginal and Torres Strait Islander Social Justice Commissioner 2005 Social Justice Report, 3/2005. HREOC, Canberra

Aboriginal and Torres Strait Islander Social Justice Commissioner and the Steering Committee for Indigenous Health Equality 2008 Close the gap: national Indigenous health equality targets. HREOC, Sydney

Australian Bureau of Statistics (ABS) 2003 The health and welfare of Australia's Aboriginal and Torres and Strait Islander peoples. AIHW, Canberra

Australian Bureau of Statistics (ABS) 2005a The health and welfare of Australia's Aboriginal and Torres Strait Islander peoples. ABS, Canberra

Australian Bureau of Statistics (ABS) 2005b Year book Australia 2005. 1301.0. ABS, Canberra

Australian Bureau of Statistics (ABS) 2006 National Aboriginal and Torres Strait Islander health survey 2004–05. ABS, Canberra

Australian Bureau of Statistics (ABS) 2007 Population distribution Aboriginal and Torres Strait Islander Australians 4705.0 ABS, Canberra

Australian Bureau of Statistics (ABS) 2008a National Aboriginal and Torres Strait Islander social survey ABS, Canberra

Australian Bureau of Statistics (ABS) 2008b Population characteristics Aboriginal and Torres Strait Islander Australians 4713.0 ABS, Canberra

Australian Bureau of Statistics (ABS) 2009a Experimental estimates and projections, Aboriginal and Torres Strait Islander Australians 1991 to 2021 3238.0 ABS, Canberra

Australian Bureau of Statistics (ABS) 2009b Experimental life tables for Aboriginal and Torres Strait Islander Australians 2005 to 2007 3302.0.55.003 ABS, Canberra

Australian Bureau of Statistics (ABS) 2009c Schools Australia 2008 4221.0 ABS, Canberra

Australian Bureau of Statistics (ABS) 2010 The health and welfare of Australia's Aboriginal and Torres Strait Islander peoples 4704.0 ABS, Canberra

Australian Bureau of Statistics (ABS) Australian Institute of Health and Welfare (AIHW) 2008 The health and welfare of Australia's Aboriginal and Torres Strait Islander peoples 2008. AIHW, Canberra

Australian Institute of Health and Welfare 2009 Australian hospital statistics 2007–08 Health Service Series 33 HSE71. AIHW, Canberra

Australian Institute of Health and Welfare 2011 The health and welfare of Australian Aboriginal and Torres Strait Islander people, an overview 42 AIHW, Canberra

Australian Institute of Health and Welfare 2012. Online. Available: http://www.aihw.gov.au/indigenous-health/

Australian Nursing and Midwifery Council (ANMC), Royal College of Nursing Australia (RCN), Australian Nursing Federation (ANF) 2008 Code of ethics for nurses in Australia. ANMC, RCN and ANF, Canberra

Betancourt J 2006 Cultural competence and medical education: many names, many perspectives, one goal. Academic Medicine 81(6):182–191

Cahoone L 2003 From modernism to postmodernism: an anthology, expanded 2nd edn. Blackwell, Cambridge

Cobo J R M 1983 Study of the problem of discrimination against Indigenous populations. United Nations, Geneva

Coffin J 2007 Rising to the challenge of Aboriginal health by creating cultural security. Aboriginal and Islander Health Worker Journal 31(3):22–24

Congress of Australia's First Peoples 2011 Congress joins with health groups to lead on Aboriginal health media release. Online. Available: http://nationalcongress.com.au/news-pics/

Dudgeon P, Garvey D, Pickett H 2000 Working with Indigenous Australians: a handbook for psychologists. Gunada Press, Perth

Durey A 2010 Reducing racism in Aboriginal health care in Australia: where does cultural education fit in? Australian and New Zealand Journal of Public Health 34:S87–S92

Eades S J 2000 Reconciliation, social equity and Indigenous health. Medical Journal of Australia 172:468–469

Eckermann A-K, Dowd T, Chang E et al 2010 Binan Goonj: bridging the cultures in Aboriginal health, 3rd edn. Elsevier, Sydney

Edwards T, Dade Smith J, Smith R, Elston J 2007 Cultural perspectives. In: Dade Smith J (ed) Australia's rural and remote health: a social justice perspective, 2nd edn. Tertiary Press, Melbourne

Gardiner-Garden J 2000 Research policy note 18: 2000–01. The definition of Aboriginality. Social Policy Group, Canberra

Henry B, Houston S, Mooney G 2004 Institutional racism in Australian health care: a plea for decency. Medical Journal of Australia 180(10):517–520

Human Rights and Equal Opportunities Commission (2008–2012). Close the Gap: Campaign for Indigenous Health Equality. http://www.hreoc.gov.au/social_justice/health/index.html#what

Hunter E 1993 Aboriginal health and history. Cambridge University Press, Melbourne

Indigenous Nurse Education Working Group (INEWG) 2002 Getting 'em 'n' keepin' 'em: report of the Indigenous Nursing Education Working Group to the Commonwealth Department of Health and Ageing Office for Aboriginal and Torres Strait Islander Health, September 2002 INEWG, Canberra

Karlsen S, Nazroo J 2002 Relation between racial discrimination, social class and health among ethnic minority groups. American Journal of Public Health 92(4):624–631

Larson A 2006 Rural health's demographic destiny. Rural and Remote Health 6(551):1–8

Larson A, Gilles M, Howard P et al 2007 It's enough to make you sick: the impact of racism on the health of Aboriginal Australians. Australian and New Zealand Journal of Public Health 31(4):322–329

Marmot M, Wilkinson R G 1999 Social determinants of health. Oxford University Press, New York

National Health and Medical Research Council (NHMRC) 2005 Cultural competency in health: a guide for policy, partnership and participation. NHMRC, Canberra

Oxfam: Close the Gap. Available: www.oxfam.org.au/explore/indigenous-australia/close-the-gap/

Paradies Y 2006 A systematic review of empirical research on self-reported racism. International Journal of Epidemiology 35(4):888–901

Ramsden I 1992 Kawa Whakaruruhau: guidelines for nursing and midwifery education. Nursing Council of New Zealand, Wellington

Ramsden I 2002 Cultural safety and nursing education in Aotearoa and Te Waipounamu. Victoria University, Wellington

Saggers S, Gray D 2007 Defining what we mean. In: Carson B, Dunbar T, Chenhall R, Baillie R (eds) Social determinants of Indigenous health. Allen & Unwin, Sydney

Skinner T, Ellis I 2009 Tale of two courthouses: a critique of the underlying assumptions in chronic disease self-management for Aboriginal people. Australasian Medical Journal 1(14):216–210

Thomson N, MacRae A, Burns J et al 2010 Overview of Australian Indigenous health status. Australian Indigenous HealthInfoNet, Perth

Turrell G, Mathers C 2000 Socioeconomic status and health in Australia. Medical Journal of Australia 172:434–438

Walter M, Saggers S 2007 Poverty and social class. In: Carson B, Dunbar T, Chenhall R, Baillie R (eds) Social determinants of Indigenous health. Allen & Unwin, Sydney, pp 87–94

Zubrick S R, Lawrence D M, Silburn S R et al 2004 The Western Australian Aboriginal child health survey: the health of Aboriginal children and young people. Telethon Institute for Child Health Research, Perth

CHAPTER 22

Connecting clinical and theoretical knowledge for practice

Jane Conway and Margaret McMillan

LEARNING OBJECTIVES

After reading this chapter you should be able to:

- appreciate the interaction between clinical practice and classroom-based learning activities
- identify strategies that maximise learning opportunities in a range of contexts
- explore strategies for acquiring knowledge-ABILITY
- view yourself as an autonomous, action-oriented learner
- appreciate the interaction between lifelong learning and professional development
- recognise the attributes you possess that will facilitate your practice as graduates.

KEY WORDS

Transition, graduate, accountability, lifelong learning, curriculum, clinical learning, clinical decision making

THE CLINICAL AREA: THE SITE OF NURSING PRACTICE

A confident, competent nursing workforce that has the capacity to provide comprehensive, person-centred care and is part of a cohesive, interprofessional healthcare team is dependent upon the effective transition from being a student to a recent graduate who makes connections between clinical and theoretical knowledge. The curriculum underpinning a nursing program focuses on educating students for clinical practice and uses educational strategies that support the integration of clinical and theoretical knowledge.

Nursing programs globally recognise that the clinical area is an important, if not the most important, area for practice professions such as nursing (Lambert & Glacken 2005, Sedgwick & Harris 2012). Definitions of clinical teaching and learning invariably include some notion that clinical practice is the place where students apply theory in practice, or where contradictions between theory and practice, and nursing and educational values, are highlighted (Brown et al 2011, Myrick & Yonge 2005, Nematollahi & Isaac 2012, Whitehead & Holmes 2011). The clinical environment is, in fact, where students begin to develop professional identities as nurses, but it is only the beginning of the pathway to personal confidence and competence. This pathway continues throughout the postgraduate transition year and beyond as both nursing and nurses engage in new roles within health service delivery (Institute of Medicine 2011, Newton & McKenna 2007).

Individuals, employers, supervisors, education bodies and regulatory authorities have a collective responsibility to ensure that the knowledge and skills base from which a nurse operates is not only extensive enough for the roles and functions of a given position, but is also up-to-date, within the law and directed towards client benefit. This provides a series of safeguards, enhances risk management and contributes to quality improvement through promoting application of the principles of ethics, which include doing good/not doing harm, justice and autonomy.

Clinical practice provides the stimulus for students and practitioners alike to use these skills in order to recognise best practice and, if necessary, enhance and modify existing practice. This chapter is designed to encourage students to view clinical and on-campus learning as one entity—a continuum of development and lifelong learning that has the unifying goal of achieving and maintaining competence within the complexities of contemporary practice.

Figure 22.1 depicts the interrelationship between clinical practice knowledge and the theoretical knowledge embedded in nursing-specific frameworks within nursing

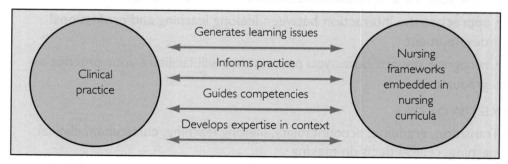

Figure 22.1
The interrelationship between practice and curriculum in nursing programs

curricula. This diagram indicates that clinical activity and on-campus learning are interdependent.

The curriculum provides formal structure to a student's learning. However, beyond graduation, nurses are able to create their own curriculum by framing work experiences as learning experiences and drawing upon their abilities as lifelong learners, reflective practitioners and information-literate graduates who appreciate the importance of continuing professional development for fulfilment of the competency standards for nursing practice.

The transition from student to graduate provides an opportunity to launch a career in nursing. This requires the development of the ability to critically examine one's own and others' practice and be accountable for individual action. These abilities underpin nursing competency and are often linked to the idea of being a lifelong, inquiring learner (Australian Nursing and Midwifery Council 2006, Australian Nursing and Midwifery Council 2009, Standing & Sama 2010), and are seen as increasingly important to professional nursing practice in the twenty-first century.

The changing nature of health service delivery continues to present challenges to both clinicians and students (Huntington et al 2011). In literature related to contemporary health service delivery, it is widely acknowledged that reduced average lengths of stay, an ageing clientele, increased throughput and acuity, developments in healthcare and educational technology and increasing numbers of learners requiring clinical experience impact on the clinical learning milieu and the extent to which it consistently fosters the cognitive skills required for professional practice (Jeffries 2008, Johnson 2009, Lunney 2008). Well-designed simulated learning experiences have the potential to address challenges in the quality and quantity of clinical placement (Rudd et al 2010) as well as promote sound judgement and enhance appreciation of professional accountability (Ertmer et al 2010). It is imperative that learners capitalise on events in both clinical and on-campus settings that foster their ability to critically analyse situations, identify underpinning knowledge and ideas and critically appraise their own professional development (Hartigan-Rogers et al 2007). Such critique needs to be managed carefully in order to maintain perspective and avoid overreaction.

Over decades, much has been written about the impact of a purported reality shock that students experience during clinical experience and/or upon entry into the workforce as a graduate. The transition period from graduate to practitioner has been seen as a time during which nurses are socialised into the workplace and its formal and informal rules, protocols, norms and expectations. It has been identified as an exciting, challenging and stressful period (Feng & Tsai 2012, Morrow 2009). A range of factors contribute to a sense of reality shock, including the need to adjust to the demands of shift work, time pressures associated with assuming a case load, coping with workplace staff shortages, experiencing potential intergenerational differences in work values and ethics, and the need to accept accountability for patient safety and to delegate to and supervise other staff (Duchscher 2009). Etheridge (2007) has reported that new graduates also experience a lack of confidence in their interpretation of assessment data and clinical decision making.

The transition from student to graduate has been likened to a grieving response (Halfer & Graf 2006) and is a period whereby the graduate initially focuses (we would say rightly) on themselves and their own development for the first six months in the workplace (Thrysoe et al 2011). The aspirations of the profession of nursing are for the transition period to be positive and supportive. However, despite these aspirations, new graduates continue to experience fragmentation and frustration as clinical demands conflict with access to support, mentorship and continuing development (Dyess & Sherman 2009, Fenwick et al 2012, Hatler et al 2011, Mooney 2007).

It is our contention that there is a need to focus on the positive rather than the negative aspects of transition and to acknowledge the extent to which graduates have a repertoire of portable knowledge and skills which provide a foundation for the development of social identity as a nurse rather than as a student nurse in order to further the development of individual agency as a practitioner. According to Ras (2012:199) social identity has 'both emotional- and values-based significance. Identifying with a group offers the individual positive self-esteem and empowered distinctiveness as a member of we'. Self-agency has been defined as the understanding of the self that enables shaping of motives, actions and possibilities (Ras 2012). Individual agency is the mechanism that enables knowledge-ABILITY through continuing development of self-insight, a sense of self-efficacy and recognition of the need for self-determination. It is associated with moving beyond the initial and natural sense of alienation experienced in an unfamiliar context to a sense of self-confidence, composure and resilience. Development of self-agency is an iterative rather than lineal process that requires that nurses take responsibility for themselves and their learning. This self-agency requires an ability to create meaning in a given context and to embrace a view of learning as 'volitional, curiosity-based, discovery-driven and mentor-assisted' (Janik 2005:144) and results in the continuing creation and transformation of perspective, through cognitive and affective engagement in reflective practice (Dirkx 2006).

The capacity to respond appropriately and effectively in nursing practice is dependent upon the extent to which we connect clinical and theoretical knowledge in order to make sense of the situations that students engage with during clinical learning experiences and that graduates encounter during their transition. Such sense making requires what we have termed knowledge-ABILITY. The concept of knowledge-ABILITY requires that learners are able to transfer concepts between the learning cultures typical of on-campus and clinical environments. Without clinical learning experiences which provide the opportunity to integrate classroom theory in 'real-life' practice situations, nursing students may have had little opportunity to develop the lifelong learning skills of critical thinking and reflective practice considered important to professional practice (Caputi 2010, Tanner 2010).

In her often cited, classical work about the development of registered nurses, Benner (1984) has identified that the ability to integrate theory and practice to the point of being able to generalise is essential to development from novice (newly qualified nurse) to more advanced levels of nurse. However, it is widely acknowledged that there are particular challenges in being able to transfer concepts across clinical contexts. Effective clinicians are aware that context is the crucial moderator in nursing practice, and have developed mechanisms for managing situations contextually, rather than seeking to manage all situations in the same way.

Such ability to transfer core concepts across situations and modify actions according to context is an indication of 'expert' nursing practice (Benner 1984, Conway & McMillan 2012). Expanding upon this, we believe there is a need for learners to be able to transfer concepts between the learning cultures typical of on-campus and clinical environments. In the remainder of this chapter, we seek to reinforce to readers that throughout their learning as students, they will acquire a set of knowledge and skills in both nursing and learning that are transferable to a range of contexts and which are foundational for professional practice as a nurse.

CONNECTING CLINICAL AND THEORETICAL LEARNING TO BECOME KNOWLEDGE-ABLE

We recognise that, for many student nurses, clinical practice is the goal of nursing education. Clinical educators, lecturers and clinicians often declare that they have a shared goal of ensuring quality education for nursing students. However, each of these sectors of the nursing community has what, at times, may seem to be very different definitions of nursing and, within that, different expectations of students and graduates. This results in what students may perceive as a lack of alignment between the values of, and experiences in, the education and health service sectors.

While much of this perceived lack of alignment has been attributed to what has been described as the theory–practice gap (Newton et al 2009, Sellman 2010), it is our view that nursing education has a single unifying focus—to assist people to be nurses. Being a nurse requires the ability to actively respond with nursing interventions, to think about the clinical judgements made and the consequences of action taken and to develop a capacity to articulate that thinking to others.

Contemporary nursing curricula include discipline-specific knowledge and integration of knowledge from other disciplines to inform the practice of nursing. This differs from previous practices of modifying knowledge from other disciplines to suit nursing situations. Thus, nursing education serves both an epistemological and a political purpose, and students should be able to articulate and conceptualise the nature of their discipline and apply their thinking to actual practice.

The overarching structure of all nursing courses is the nursing curriculum, which determines both the outcomes that should be achieved and the processes by which these will be achieved. Nursing education programs include both on-campus and clinical learning experiences, which provide students with opportunities to practise the skills of nursing, to develop and demonstrate their knowledge base about nursing and to acquire academic skills that support communication of their thinking about nursing. Increasingly, nursing curricula use problem-based teaching strategies to encourage development of the knowledge, skills and behaviours of effective clinicians. This type of learning fosters exploration of 'real-life' situations to enhance critical thinking and clinical decision making (Conway & Little 2003, Stubbings et al 2012).

Figure 22.2 demonstrates the continual process of conceptualisation and re-conceptualisation of nursing, which occurs through situation deconstruction, analysis and reconstruction. These enquiry and process skills are essential to professional practice and the development of knowledge.

The curriculum should cause students to think about what they do as nurses, why they do what they do and how they might do it differently. It is these enquiry skills that will cause the student to generate knowledge about nursing. For this reason, it is important that the nursing curriculum raises questions such as: 'What is nursing?', 'What does it mean to nurse?', 'Whom do nurses nurse?', 'Where do nurses nurse?', 'Is nursing the same as caring?' and so on, as well as helping students to learn the task-oriented content of how to nurse.

Conceptualising or thinking about nursing needs to both direct and emerge from practice. It is a process of enquiry in which students work with concepts and form networks of concepts that frame and impact on their practice. It is not our intention to

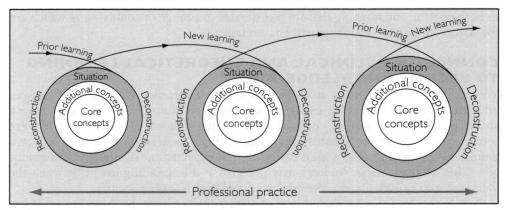

Figure 22.2
Relationship between situation analysis, learning and professional practice

give the impression that qualified nurses should only think about nursing. The goal of nursing programs is to develop a graduate who can apply concepts to practice, manage complex nursing situations and accept accountability for practice. Of course, this also demands skills in doing nursing activities.

However, we believe that students should be aware that nursing is about the ability to analyse situations and respond appropriately. How we interpret and analyse situations depends upon how we think about them. As our thinking about nursing develops, the meaning we give to situations changes and learning occurs. We then take this learning with us to the next situation and create new meanings and experiential knowledge.

Experiential knowledge is not merely being exposed to an experience. It is that which emerges when the experience is structured to achieve learning as an outcome of the experience. Therefore, students should use the theoretical base developed from on-campus, university-based activities to frame the clinical experience so that learning, rather than merely experiencing, occurs. Students should ask themselves: 'What is it that I want to achieve from this learning experience and how does this relate to my ability to practise nursing?'

Clinical learning experiences provide nursing students with the opportunity to begin to develop the skills of identifying general principles of practice, transferring these across contexts and modifying actions based on principles of management. While clinical experience is clearly a powerful motivator for students to learn how to nurse, the literature suggests that clinical experiences are an important part of the transfer of learning from the classroom to the practice setting.

How we think about nursing practice shapes what we learn from or about practice and how we direct the transition from student to recent graduate and subsequent movement along a career pathway. However, as noted by Heartfield (2006), there are differing representations or constructions of nursing practice dependent on individual, professional, industrial, regulatory and organisational perspectives. Irrespective of perspective and context, 'being a nurse' requires the ability to integrate the knowledge, skills and attitudes of nursing into who we are and how we practise.

Now, more than ever before, contemporary health service delivery demands that nurses demonstrate the full suite of skills representative of the knowledge-ABLE worker.

The knowledge-ABLE worker aspires to enhance patient and staff safety, minimise adverse circumstances, promote partnership initiatives, focus on 'fitness-to-function' and acknowledge that health service delivery is dependent upon multiprofessional team effort. Thus, the student nurse as a knowledge-ABLE learner sees connections between clinical and theoretical knowledge of nursing within a broader framework of learning that integrates his or her experience and the outcomes of education for a knowledge-ABLE worker.

Table 22.1 presents the elements of contemporary health service challenges and desired knowledge-ABLE worker responses. The table indicates that although the factors that impact on health service delivery and healthcare work can be viewed in isolation, nurses, as knowledge-ABLE workers, require a multifaceted education to respond meaningfully to the challenges in contemporary health service provision.

Table 22.1
Worker responses to a changing health service

Health service challenges	Knowledge-ABLE worker response
Technology: clinical and information systems interface.	Procedurally competent, information-fluent personnel.
Fragmented patient experience.	Contributors to systems review.
Changing health patterns: chronicity and consumerism.	Effective managers of consumer expectations, competing value systems and tensions in resource allocation.
Changing workforce: unaligned skill mix and case mix.	
Inappropriate structures and processes.	Coordinators of throughput and care processes.
Changing professional roles and functions.	Participants in networked organisation and healthcare teams.
Rigidity in professional frameworks and knowledge bases.	Personnel who focus on consumer needs and outcomes rather than profession-specific outcomes.

HOW TO BEST DEVELOP KNOWLEDGE-ABILITY

Classroom-based learning activity provides us with a relatively safe environment to explore what we know, what we do and who we are as nurses, so that we are more prepared for professional practice situations. Clinical learning activity provides us with the opportunity both to test out what we have learnt in practice and to confront new situations from which we can further our learning. However, we can only learn if we are prepared to do so. It is important that we value learning as much as we value what we have learnt. It is our ability to question ourselves and our practice that enhances our professional development.

In order to learn we need to develop the process skills for lifelong learning. These process skills are the basis of learning and are transferable across disciplines and facilitate the progression from what Benner (1984) has described as novice to expert nurse. In the case of nursing, nursing knowledge provides specific content which, when processed, results in nursing action. That is to say, when we become nurses we have developed general learning skills and we demonstrate our use of these through being able to 'think and act like a nurse'. In order to be lifelong learners in relation to nursing practice, we need to become what has been termed reflective practitioners. We need to reflect about what we do as nurses, how we respond as nurses and individuals and what we would do again in a similar situation. We then need to act when a similar situation occurs. The skills of reflective practice unite theoretical and clinical concepts; are both thought-oriented and action-oriented; allow for consideration of the affective aspects of nursing experience; and provide opportunity to explore how the learner as a reflective practitioner felt about the experience. Such an approach is particularly useful in nursing, as it acknowledges human and emotional, as well as intellectual, domains of decision making and encourages self-regulation and autonomy in learning. There are a number of useful frameworks for situation analysis that are oriented towards integrating thinking and action which are inclusive of consideration of the affective aspects of nursing experience. Gibbs (1988) developed a reflective cycle which encourages systematic thinking about situations as learning events. Gibbs' processes include description of the situation, determining thoughts and feelings about the situation, identifying what was good or bad about the experience and analysing the situation in order to draw conclusions and identify responses should a similar situation occur.

Little (1996) elaborated upon the elements of Gibbs' framework to develop a framework of questions which facilitate reflection about particular aspects of learning and is applicable in both classroom and clinical learning situations that can be used to facilitate reflection. These questions provide a useful guide to developing lifelong learning skills, yet are equally important questions for clinical decision making. The framework recognises that learning is inherently a personal experience and places emphasis on the subjective nature of learning. In order to be accountable for their practice, nurses need to become subjectively engaged in that practice and examine their perceptions and assumptions. Additionally, the framework integrates the abilities related to information literacy, application and transfer of knowledge and skills to novel situations and learning within a group. This framework of questions is useful because it encourages us to look at situations in context and to focus on learning. It enables us to appreciate that, as learners and professionals who make sound clinical judgements, we are required to interact effectively with others, provide reasoning and support for our actions and decisions and be aware that we are accountable for our own learning and practice actions. Little's approach is presented in the boxes below.

Situation/analysis or decision making

- What information do I have?
- What further information do I need?
- What options/alternatives do I have?
- What should I prioritise?
- What action/s should I take?
- Why?
- Can I justify this action (lawfully, ethically, effectively, theoretically)?

The learning process

- What do I already know?
- How do I know it?
- What do I need to know?
- Where will I find it?
- What resources can I use?
- How will I know I know?
- Why should I learn it?

Perceptions

- What are my feelings?
- What are my beliefs about the situation?
- What are my assumptions?
- How have I derived these beliefs/assumptions?
- How do my feelings/beliefs
  - affect my interpretation?
  - affect my response?
  - relate to espoused professional values?
- Why do I hold this belief/assumption?
- What are alternative beliefs/assumptions?

Learning processes

- What is the validity of my source?
  - Legislation
  - Data based on research
  - Opinion
  - Practice
  - Expertise
  - Experience
- What is the currency of the knowledge, skills, behaviour?
- What is the support for this view?
  - Political/ideological
  - Cultural
- What other ideas/concepts/skills does it relate to?
- How does it relate to my view of the world (current understanding)?

The situation revisited

- How does my learning relate to/apply in this situation?
- How does my learning relate to/affect my original ideas?
- What gaps/misconceptions did my learning identify?
- What ideas/skills did my learning confirm?
- What response would I give now in the situation?

Reflection on:

Situation analysis
- How well did I use the data?
- How well did I define the situation in need of a response?
- How comprehensive were my alternatives?
- How well can I justify my response?

The learning process
- How valid/relevant were my sources?
- How comprehensive were my sources?
- How effective was my learning?

The group process
- How well did I contribute?
- What was my role in the group?
- How effective was each member's contribution?
- Did the group remain on task?
- Did the group attend to process (i.e. how people were feeling/responding/ behaving)?

KNOWLEDGE-ABILITY AS ACTIVE LEARNING

While frameworks for reflection are relevant to a number of practice disciplines, including nursing, there is potential for nurses to utilise the 'learning' components of models such as these selectively and to overlook the critical elements related to action. In responding to the needs of individuals and communities, nursing is both reactive and proactive. As both the guardians of and visionaries for nursing's future, it is important that students take the opportunity to develop the skills to critically evaluate the nursing practice they observe and to create and consider alternatives to this practice. The imagination of possibilities can only occur when nurses think about nursing. In other words, each of us has a professional responsibility to conceptualise in context. We need to think about what needs to be done for the client and how this impacts on the care situation. There needs to be a relationship established between theory, judgement and action taking.

Ultimately, professional accountability is related to actions, not a capacity to generate ideas. Although theory is important, because it provides a framework for the work nurses do, it is of little consequence unless it results in effective nursing actions. Conversely, practice can become meaningless unless we seek to understand it through conceptualising the practice of nursing. Such integration of theory and practice leads to our moving beyond becoming nurses to being nurses who integrate our knowing, doing and being to produce what is meaningful, client-focused management of situations. Many educational theorists have consistently highlighted the importance of being reflective practitioners in order to be, both personally and professionally, constantly transformed and emancipated from our previous ways of thinking and acting (Brookfield 1993, Cranton 1994, Friere 1972, Mezirow 1985, Taylor 2008).

Figure 22.3 represents what we perceive to be the relationships between context and lifelong learning processes and curriculum and improved practice. Achieving improved practice requires the process skills of lifelong learning and reflective practice.

The knowledge-ABLE nurse develops awareness that the range of factors that impact upon nursing extend beyond the immediate client care situation (Meyer & O'Brien-Pallas 2010). Organisational theorists have developed PETS—a schema for examining these political, economic, sociocultural and technological factors. When nurses seek to enhance their knowledge-ABILITY, they should reflect upon the extent to which these factors shape what constitutes nursing service delivery. Figure 22.4 provides an example of the application of PETS to delivery of nursing services.

It has been reported that when nursing students, qualified nurses and their employers are asked to evaluate nursing education, they feel that the time in clinical placements was inadequate and this has led to suggestions that there needs to be an increase in clinical experience as part of undergraduate learning. However, it may well be that an increase in quality of the clinical experience is preferable to an increase in quantity of clinical placements (Henderson et al 2010, Mannix et al 2006). We believe that while clinical educators, lecturers and unit staff share in structuring the clinical experience, students are also accountable for ensuring that they gain a quality clinical experience. This accountability for self-learning links closely with the principles of adult learning and ongoing professional development (O'Shea 2003).

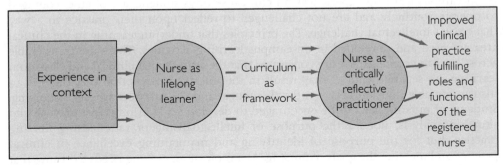

Figure 22.3
An educational equation for improved nursing practice

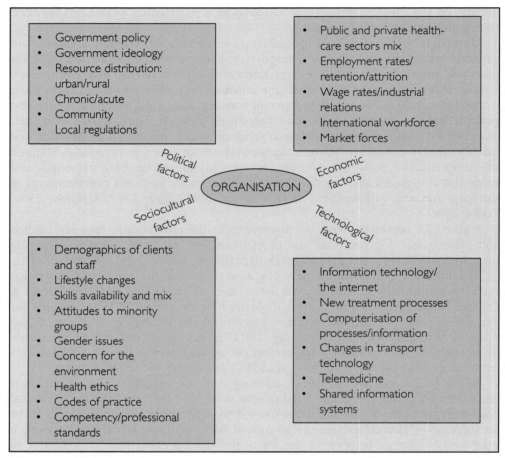

Figure 22.4
Application of the PETS framework to explore professional change in nursing

Despite the emphasis on critical thinking, problem solving and reflective practice as 'signature pedagogies' (Long et al 2012) to enhance nursing students' competence in on-campus learning experiences, in clinical settings students are often encouraged to operate routinely and are not challenged to reflect upon their practice in a way that creates intellectual challenge. The principles that underpin learning in the clinical area are used and developed in on-campus learning activities. These are transferable across learning contexts. We are concerned that the attitude that clinical and classroom learning are separate entities may result in the mistaken perception that there is an insurmountable division between the theoretical and the practical aspects of nursing. Students of nursing need to be encouraged to develop skills in reflective practice and situation analysis, not for the purpose of intellectualising or rationalising nursing practice, but for the purpose of identifying and maintaining excellence in clinical practice and meeting the goals of nursing. As a profession, nursing needs to ensure that the culture of healthcare supports and encourages positive, passionate and committed students and graduates who are able to embrace change and shape the profession of nursing for both the current and the future contexts in which it will flourish. This means the profession needs to acknowledge that when people are presented with novel experiences they may lack confidence, require instruction and demonstration and continuous feedback, require supportive cues and take some time to become proficient (Benner 1984) and set reasonable expectations of students and graduates.

Each student has a responsibility to integrate theory and practice experiences. With their colleagues in practice and education, students should seek intellectual challenge. A useful framework for this can be reflective practice models, which facilitate full participation in learning experiences. Underpinning reflective practice is a capacity to intellectualise and appraise one's performance in context.

APPRAISAL AS A STRATEGY FOR KNOWLEDGE-ABILITY

The ability to critically examine our own performance and be accountable for our own actions is essential to professional career development. It has been observed that transition requires the ability to conduct a realistic self-appraisal (Conway & McMillan 2012). Appraisal is a process by which people can:

- confirm outcomes of previous experience
- identify areas of strength
- identify areas for development
- remotivate and energise
- help predict and identify personal potential, and
- acknowledge performance against existing standards.

Appraisal is an ongoing process that can be informed by, but is not limited to, the formalised feedback sessions that occur among learners and educators. Appraisal consists of assessing accomplishments and performance to make an informed judgement about strengths and limitations in order to identify areas for improvement. It is a mechanism through which nurses can begin to self-manage their performance development (Conway & McMillan 2005).

Feedback is considered an essential part of the appraisal process. You should seek feedback that is constructive and includes comments about both things you have done well and areas (and suggested strategies) for improvement where necessary. All too often, feedback can be perceived as reactive and punitive, rather than as a vehicle for development through identifying one's own and others' strengths, availing yourself and others of opportunity and operating within and accepting processes (Hattie & Timperley 2007). Appraisal involves both openness and vulnerability. It should be authentic, active, meaningful and constructive for nurses as well as those they work with as clients and peers.

GAINING THE MOST FROM EXPERIENCE

In order to optimise learning, it is important that each experience be approached as a way of linking theory and practice, and as an opportunity for further learning and generation of new perspectives. Increasingly, nurses are required to engage in roles beyond that of direct patient caregiver and engage in 'systems level intervention', such as contributor in multidisciplinary teams, researcher and manager, through which they facilitate quality patient care. At the very least, students need to think about how the roles and functions that registered nurses perform have shaped, and have been shaped, by the practice situation.

Nursing students should explore roles other than direct caregiver. In most nursing programs the primary emphasis is placed on providing clinical experience in a range of settings (e.g. mental health, acute care and the community). However, it is unclear whether students are encouraged to explore a range of nursing roles and functions while in those settings. In order to prepare for the diversity of practice, students themselves should analyse each situation and try to determine what nursing roles and competencies are applicable. For example, students should ask themselves:

- What is the role of the registered nurse here? Is the registered nurse in this context a 'direct caregiver' or a 'care facilitator'?

- Does the role require skills as a clinician, supervisor, researcher, educator, manager or communicator, or a combination of these?

- If I were to be asked to manage this person's situation, what would I do and why?

- What nursing activities are most important and why?

- What knowledge base is required for sound clinical decision making?

- Where does this knowledge come from?

- How do I know what I know?

- What more could I know?

- How could I find out about this?

- How has my response to this situation been shaped by my beliefs about what practice is?

- What strengths do I have to respond to this situation?

- What are my learning needs in response to this situation?

Asking questions such as these encourages us to explore the diverse roles and functions of nurses and to differentiate between the roles of registered nurses and other levels of nurses. It also acknowledges that, in order to maintain effectiveness as clinicians, nurses need to learn continually from a range of situations. In order to achieve this, it is essential that someone (including the learner) facilitate their learning towards nursing outcomes. Learners often seek, indeed need, external support, guidance and assessment. Thus the clinical educator, the university lecturing staff and other personnel such as clinical educators and preceptors in practice settings can provide feedback and support to students.

The current trend in education to view educators as 'facilitators', rather than 'givers', of learning has been well-recognised in the nursing education literature. It implies that nurses as educators are increasingly adopting a more student-centred, collaborative model of education (Del Prato et al 2011). Moreover, the nurse as educator needs to model the way students or peers are expected to approach learning, as well as modelling exemplary nursing practice.

Clinical experiences provide the opportunity for students to observe and participate in nursing practice. Inherent in the notion of effective practice is the ability to make sound clinical judgements based on assessments and reassessments, to collaborate with others, to provide meaningful feedback to colleagues about performances and to establish and maintain professional relationships. Clinical experiences acclimatise students to the real world of practice and its culture, providing preparation for the reality of practice, which is dynamic and replete with novel situations.

Specifically, we have observed that students and clinicians in the clinical setting are often confused about when students should be observing another's practice and when they should be actively participating in the provision of client care. Understandably, students and clinicians alike want to be opportunistic and seize what they perceive to be limited practice learning opportunities and may, with the very best of intentions, place themselves and the client at risk because they are dealing with situations that are new to them. Our advice would be for the student to always consider the need for optimal client outcomes, to be sure of the core objectives and concepts of the clinical placement and determine the relationship between these goals and the activity to be performed. If the learning experience is highly desirable, students need to seek advice from the clinical educator about the scope of the student's practice and the need for close supervision.

When students are invited to perform care with which they do not feel comfortable, they might tell the qualified nurse that they are too busy or have other things to do. Sometimes the nurse, who has made an effort to give the student a meaningful learning experience, may interpret this response as disinterest in nursing. In situations such as these, we would suggest that students recognise the nurse's offer as a way to enhance their learning. The student should explain their situation to the senior nurse on duty, confirm that the qualified nurse is ultimately responsible for the client's care and engage in the activity as far as possible.

THE IMPORTANCE OF OTHER RESOURCES IN LEARNING

We have already made substantial reference to the reciprocity between theoretical and practical frameworks for learning, and identified the importance of focused experiences related to nursing in either classroom or clinical settings. Classroom learning provides opportunities to explore options and alternatives, to justify thinking and to learn from examples drawn from practice. It also gives students opportunities to develop the scholarly approaches necessary for contemporary nursing practice. An amplified enquiry approach is needed. Skills in clinical judgement are encouraged through the student developing nursing intervention strategies built upon explicit relationships between thought, judgement and action. Knowing about the person for whom students are caring requires a focus on our ability to acquire, recall and process information from a range of sources, including, but not confined to, the immediate care situation.

While this is important learning, in our experience, it is also essential that student nurses are able to access, retrieve and use information from reputable sources, to draw conclusions about implications of ideas for nursing practice and to communicate these in writing. Increasingly, nursing programs are integrating these skills into the core nursing program and instructing students in information literacy and writing skills (Ku et al 2007). Information literacy and fluency is required in both learning and practice settings.

Additional support in informative literacy and academic writing skills is available to students. Generic assistance to students ranges from short courses to individual consultations to assist in essay writing, including analysing and interpreting questions, planning, structuring and writing essays, referencing and assistance with mathematics for drug calculations. Students also benefit from spending time with the librarian, learning how to use the library effectively, to conduct literature searches and to use databases to access resources (Honey et al 2006, McNeil et al 2003).

While we encourage the use of these support services, we would caution students that they do not provide discipline-specific information, nor do they necessarily develop the skills for health information literacy, including the ability to effectively use health informatics. That is to say, staff of these units can assist you in structuring your writing, ensure your grammar and punctuation are correct and inform you about referencing, but they cannot provide the ideas for your work because they do not 'think and act like nurses'. It is important that students seek assistance from lecturing and library staff who are aware of current issues and debates in nursing, to clarify questions and check their understanding of aspects of nursing. The internet has made it possible to access a number of resources, including other students via the worldwide web. Of course, users should be cautious about disclosing personal information and should check the validity of any information obtained via 'the net'.

Furthermore, it is important that, in addition to using technology to support their own learning and development, nurses are able to use information systems within health services to better meet consumer expectations and needs and be informed by and contribute to service management and clinical research (Australian Nursing and Midwifery Council 2009, Hovenga et al 2010).

CONCLUDING THOUGHTS

While there is increasing emphasis on the development of cognitive abilities in nursing, this should not lead to what has been labelled as a dichotomy between clinical skills and theoretical knowledge. Despite claims made by some authors that emphasis on theoretical knowledge in nursing results in a devaluing of clinical skills and, consequently, a devaluation of clinical practice, practical and theoretical nursing knowledge are inevitably and infinitely intertwined. Nursing practice and nursing education have increasingly recognised the need to integrate thinking and doing to create informed action. Discussion of the separation of thinking and doing does little to promote integration of on-campus and clinical learning activity. Students should view their learning to be nurses as occurring in two distinct yet interdependent contexts: the classroom and the clinical setting. Furthermore, they should use their experiences as students to develop foundational knowledge and skills for effective, confident and competent transition to employment.

The past few decades have provided evidence that there is a paradigm shift in education, which now views learning as the construction of meaning in context rather than what to learn and how to do things. Nurse education is about the ability—indeed flexibility—to examine situations, deconstruct them from a number of perspectives and reconstruct them around core concepts essential to nursing practice. When students engage in reflective practice in a manner that enacts individual agency, they are able to reinforce self-worth, retain confidence and self-esteem and expand knowledge and skills.

Contemporary nursing practice demands that nurses question and justify decisions in context, and emphasises the ability to think about nursing, as well as the ability to perform nursing actions to best manage nursing situations. The challenge for students is to develop an integrated approach to practice, which values thoughtful, highly skilled and efficient action, and to continue with lifelong learning and professional development—that is, to be knowledge-ABLE rather than simply knowledgeable.

REFLECTIVE QUESTIONS

1. What principles can you identify that underpin your learning in on-campus and clinical settings and how do these assist you to transfer your learning across and between these contexts?

2. How can you become more responsible and accountable for your own learning, including planning and evaluating your learning?

3. Who can assist you with meeting these needs?

4. What are the strengths you take as a learner and a student of nursing to your future practice?

5. What strategies will you use to develop resilience, confidence and competence as a beginning professional?

RECOMMENDED READINGS

Benner P, Tanner C, Chesla C 2009 Expertise in nursing practice: caring, clinical judgment, and ethics. Springer Publishing Company, New York, New York

Duke M, Forbes H 2012 Dealing with the theory–practice gap in clinical practice. In: Chang E, Daly J (eds) Transitions in nursing: preparing for professional practice, 3rd edn. Churchill Livingstone, Sydney

Hatlevik I K 2012 The theory–practice relationship: reflective skills and theoretical knowledge as key factors in bridging the gap between theory and practice in initial nursing education. Journal of Advanced Nursing 68(4):868–877

Musker K 2011 Nursing theory-based independent nursing practice: a personal experience of closing the theory–practice gap. Advances in Nursing Science 34(1):67–77

Wolff A C, Regan S, Pesut B, Black J 2011 Ready for what? An exploration of the meaning of new graduate nurses' readiness for practice. International Journal of Nursing Education Scholarship 7(1):Article7. Epub 19 Feb 2010

REFERENCES

Australian Nursing and Midwifery Council 2006 National competency standards for the registered nurse, 4th edn. Australian Nursing and Midwifery Council, Canberra

Australian Nursing and Midwifery Council 2009 The standards and criteria for the accreditation of nursing and midwifery courses leading to registration, enrolment, endorsement and authorisation in Australia. Australian Nursing and Midwifery Council, Canberra

Benner P 1984 From novice to expert: excellence and power in clinical nursing practice. Addison Wesley, Menlo Park, California

Brookfield S 1993 On impostorship, cultural suicide and other dangers: how nurses learn critical thinking. Journal of Continuing Education in Nursing 24(5):197–205

Brown T, Williams B, McKenna L et al 2011 Practice education learning environments: the mismatch between perceived and preferred expectations of undergraduate health science students. Nurse Education Today 31(8):e22–e28

Caputi L (ed) 2010 Teaching nursing: the art and science, 2nd ed. College of DuPage Press, Glen Ellyn, IL

Conway J, Little P 2003 Adopting PBL as an institutional approach: considerations and challenges. Journal of Excellence in College Teaching 11(2–3):11–26

Conway J, McMillan M 2005 Making the transition to professional nursing: becoming a lifelong learner. In: Daly J, Speedy S, Jackson D et al Professional nursing: concepts, issues, and challenges. Springer, New York

Conway J, McMillan M 2012 Professional career development: development of the CAPABLE nursing professional. In Chang E, Daly J (eds) Transitions in nursing: preparing for professional practice, 3rd edn. Churchill Livingstone, Sydney

Cranton P 1994 Understanding and promoting transformative learning: a guide for educators of adults. Jossey-Bass, San Francisco

Del Prato D, Bankert E, Grust P, Joseph J 2011 Transforming nursing education: a review of stressors and strategies that support students' professional socialization. Advances in Medical Practice 2:109–116

Dirkx J M 2006 Engaging emotions in adult learning: a Jungian perspective on emotion and transformative learning. New Directions for Adult and Continuing Education 109:15–26

Duchscher J E 2009 Transition shock: the initial stage of role adaptation for newly graduated Registered Nurses. Journal of Advanced Nursing 65(5):1103–1113

Dyess S, Sherman R 2009 The first year of practice: new graduate nurses' transition and learning needs. Journal of Continuing Education In Nursing 40(9):403–410

Ertmer P, Strobel J, Cheng X et al 2010 Expressions of critical thinking in role-playing simulations: comparisons across roles. Journal of Computing in Higher Education 22(2):73–94

Etheridge S 2007 Learning to think like a nurse: stories from new nurse graduates. Journal of Continuing Education in Nursing 38(1):24–30

Feng R F, Tsai Y F 2012 Socialisation of new graduate nurses to practising nurses. Journal of Clinical Nursing 21:2064–2071

Fenwick J, Hammond A, Raymond J et al 2012 Surviving, not thriving: a qualitative study of newly qualified midwives' experience of their transition to practice. Journal of Clinical Nursing 21(13/14):2054–2063

Friere P 1972 The pedagogy of oppression. Penguin, Harmondsworth

Gibbs G 1988 Learning by doing: a guide to teaching and learning methods. Further Education Unit, Oxford Polytechnic, Oxford

Halfer D, Graf E 2006 Graduate nurse perceptions of the work experience. Nursing Economic$ 24(3):150–155

Hartigan-Rogers J A, Cobbett S L, Amirault M A, Muise-Davis M E 2007 Nursing graduates' perceptions of their undergraduate clinical placement. International Journal of Nursing Education Scholarship 4:1–12

Hattie J, Timperley H 2007 The power of feedback. Review of Educational Research 32:601–611

Hatler C, Stoffers P, Kelly L et al 2011 Work unit transformation to welcome new graduate nurses: using nurses' wisdom. Nursing Economic$ 29(2):88–93

Heartfield M 2006 Specialisation and advanced practice discussion paper. Online. Available: www.nnnet.gov.au/downloads/recsp_paper.pdf

Henderson A, Twentyman M, Eaton E et al 2010 Creating supportive clinical learning environments: an intervention study. Journal of Clinical Nursing 19(1–2):177–182

Honey M, North N, Gunn C 2006 Improving library services for graduate nurse students in New Zealand. Health Information and Libraries Journal 23(2):102–109

Hovenga E J S, Kidd M R, Garde S, Cossio C 2010 Health informatics: an overview. IOS press, Washington DC

Huntington A, Gilmour J, Tuckett A et al 2011 Is anybody listening? A qualitative study of nurses' reflections on practice. Journal of Clinical Nursing 20(9/10):1413–1422

Institute of Medicine 2011 The future of nursing: leading change, advancing health. The National Academies Press, Washington, DC

Janik D S 2005 Unlock the genius within neurobiological trauma, teaching, and transformative learning. Rowman and Littlefield Education, Lanham, Maryland

Jeffries P R 2008 Getting in STEP with simulations: simulations take educator preparation. Nursing Education Perspectives 29:70–73

Johnson S L 2009 International perspectives on workplace bullying among nurses: a review. International Nursing Review 56:34–40

Ku Y, Sheu S, Kuo S 2007 Efficacy of integrating information literacy education into a women's health course on information literacy for RN-BSN. Students Journal of Nursing Research 15(1):67–76

Lambert V, Glacken M 2005 Clinical education facilitators: a literature review. Journal of Clinical Nursing 14:664–673

Little P 1996 Questions for learning. Unpublished workshop material. PROBLARC University of Newcastle, Newcastle

Long T L, Telford J, Breitkreuz K et al 2012 Competence and care: signature pedagogies in nursing education. In: Chick N L, Haynie A, Gurung R (eds) Exploring more signature pedagogies: approaches to teaching disciplinary habits of mind. Stylus Publishing, Sterling, VA

Lunney M 2008 Current knowledge related to intelligence and thinking with implications for the development and use of case studies. International Journal of Nursing Terminologies and Classifications 19(4):158–162

Mannix J, Faga P, Beale B, Jackson D 2006 Towards sustainable models for clinical education in nursing: an on-going conversation. Nurse Education in Practice 6:3–11

Meyer R M, O'Brien-Pallas L L 2010 Nursing services delivery theory: an open systems approach. Journal of Advanced Nursing 66(12):2828–2838

McNeil B J, Elfrink V L, Bickford C J, Pierce S T 2003 Nursing information technology knowledge, skills and preparation of student nurses, nursing faculty and clinicians: a US survey. Journal of Nursing Education 42(8):341–349

Morrow S 2009 New graduate transitions: leaving the nest, joining the flight. Journal of Nursing Management 17:278–287

Mezirow J 1985 A critical theory of self directed learning. New Directions for Continuing Education 25:17–30

Mooney M 2009 Facing registration: the expectations and the unexpected. Nurse Education Today 27:840–847

Myrick F, Yonge O 2005 Nursing preceptorship: connecting practice and education. Lippincott Williams and Wilkins, Philadelphia, Pennsylvania

Nematollahi R, Isaac J 2012 Bridging the theory practice gap: a review of graduate nurse program in Dubai, United Arab Emirates. International Nursing Review 59(2):194–199

Newton J M, Billett S, Jolly B, Ockerby C M 2009 Lost in translation: barriers to learning in health professional clinical education. Learning In Health & Social Care 8(4):315–327

Newton J, McKenna L 2007 The transitional journey through the graduate year: a focus group study. International Journal of Nursing Studies 44(7):1231–1237

O'Shea E 2003 Self-directed learning in nurse education: a review of literature. Journal of Advanced Nursing 43(1):62–70

Ras N L 2012 What we do here is who we are. Advances in Educational Administration 13:197–222

Rudd C, Freeman K, Swift A, Smith P 2010 Use of simulated learning environments in nursing curricula. Online. Available: https://www.hwa.gov.au/sites/uploads/sles-in-nursing-curricula-201108.pdf

Sedgwick M, Harris S 2012 A critique of the undergraduate nursing preceptorship model. Nursing Research and Practice. Online. Available: http://www.hindawi.com/journals/nrp/2012/248356/

Sellman D 2010 Mind the gap: philosophy, theory, and practice. Nursing Philosophy 11(2):85–87

Standing M, Sama A 2010 Lifelong learning in judgement and decision-making. In: Standing M (ed) Clinical judgement and decision-making in nursing and interprofessional healthcare. Open University Press, Maidenhead, pp 80–99

Stubbings L, Chaboyer W, McMurray A 2012 Nurses' use of situation awareness in decision-making: an integrative review. Journal of Advanced Nursing 68(7):1443–1453

Tanner C 2010 From mother duck to mother lode: clinical education for deep learning. Journal of Nursing Education 49(1):3–4

Taylor E 2008 Transformative learning theory. New Directions for Adult and Continuing Education 119:5–15

Thrysoe L, Hounsgaard L, Dohn N, Wagner L 2011 Expectations of becoming a nurse and experiences on being a nurse. Nordic Journal Of Nursing Research & Clinical Studies / Vård I Norden 31(3):15–19

Whitehead B, Holmes D 2011 Are newly qualified nurses prepared for practice? Nursing Times 17–30(107):19–20,20–23

GLOSSARY

Aboriginal and Torres Strait Islander Health Services; Aboriginal Medical Services: Services that may be established and governed (controlled) by Aboriginal and Torres Strait Islander peoples in their communities or in partnership with Aboriginal and Torres Strait Islander peoples specifically to improve access to health services for Aboriginal and Torres Strait Islanders.

acceptability: The test applied to a premise or reason. In order to have a sound argument, a premise must be acceptable to the person evaluating the argument.

aesthetic: An abstract notion used in discussing the artistic aspect of nursing (and its creative expression). In this context, it relates broadly to theoretical and practical aspects of nursing art.

affective: Pertains to moods, feelings and attitudes.

altruism: Regard for others as a principle for action; unselfishness.

argument: A conclusion that is supported by a set of reasons intended to provide grounds for the acceptability of the conclusion.

autonomy: Personal or political independence, self-determination, self-sufficiency.

binary: Composed of two parts. *See also* dichotomy.

bioethics: An interdisciplinary field of inquiry characterised by a systematic and critical examination of the moral dimensions of healthcare and other associated fields (e.g. the life sciences) from the standpoint of various ethical perspectives.

biologism: A particular form of essentialism (see below) in which women's (or men's) essence is defined in terms of their biological capacities.

caring: Compassionate or showing concern for others. Can refer to behaviour used by those who belong to a profession such as nursing that involves looking after people's physical, medical and general welfare.

'close the gap': A campaign to reduce the gap in life expectancy, employment and educational opportunities between Aboriginal and Torres Strait Islander peoples and other Australians.

community assessment: A structured study of a specified community or targeted area that uses objective data to assess the current conditions and identify areas of strength and weakness.

congruency: Agreement or consistency in two or more views or positions. For example, in examining two or more theoretical views, one may find that there are areas of agreement across the same ground; hence, there is evidence of congruency.

construct: 'A type of highly abstract and complex concept whose reality base can only be inferred. Constructs are formed from multiple less abstract or more empirical concepts' (Chinn & Jacobs 1983:200).

critical friend: A trusted colleague who provides feedback on your work.

critical incident analysis: The use of clinical or personal incidents as a reflective tool.

critical thinking: The development of a questioning attitude to that which is normally taken for granted.

cultural competence: 'A set of behaviours, attitudes and policies that come together in a system, agency or among professionals to enable that system, agency or group of professionals to work effectively in cross cultural situations' (National Health and Medical Research Council 2005).

cultural safety: A philosophy of healthcare specific to working in a cross-cultural situation with Indigenous peoples. It is achieved by personal reflection and understanding of your own culture before you can meaningfully interact with Indigenous people (Ramsden 2002).

deductive reasoning: The process of inferring particulars from general laws or principles.

dialectic: Defined in the Australian Concise Oxford Dictionary (1987) as the 'art of investigating the truth of opinions, testing of truth by discussion [or] logical disputation or criticism dealing with metaphysical contradictions and their solutions; existence or action of opposing forces'.

dialectical: A process or perspective involving a dialectic. For example, in theory development using a dialectical approach to generation of knowledge, the process could involve debate with presentation of an argument (thesis), which is considered critically and challenged by a counterargument (antithesis), which is considered critically in relation to the thesis and other knowledge, possibly leading to new areas of agreement and understanding (synthesis).

dichotomy: A term that can be used to indicate a divide between two theoretical positions, which are polarised or incompatible.

discourse: An abstract notion used to label a collection of ideas or theoretical perspectives within an academic discipline. This may be composed of theses or arguments representing knowledge in the discipline, including areas of agreement and disagreement, fundamental assumptions, values and beliefs, expressed in disciplinary language and symbols. The notion reflects the idea of a conversation using language within these boundaries.

dissemination: The act of distributing or spreading something, especially information for it to become widespread.

diversity: A variety of something, such as opinion, colour or style; can refer to ethnic variety, as well as socioeconomic and gender variety, in a group, society or organisation.

early intervention: The initiation of supportive therapeutic strategies as soon as a problem or challenge is identified. Is often associated with disability, and involves longer-term engagement.

empiricist/logical positivist model: An approach grounded in the belief that the world can be viewed as a machine and that the task of science is to discover the laws by which the machine operated; emphasis on predictability, measurement and the quantification of observable data.

epistemology: The theory of knowledge; the origins, nature, methods and limits of human knowledge.

essentialism: The attribution of a fixed essence to women; that there are given, universal characteristics of women, including biological, psychological and social characteristics, which are not readily amenable to change.

ethical principalism: The view that moral decisions are best guided by appealing to sound universal moral principles, such as the principles of autonomy, beneficence, nonmaleficence and justice; ethical principalism is one of the most popular approaches used to examine ethical issues in healthcare.

ethical universalism: The view that there exists one set of universal values/standards that is applicable to all people throughout space and time, regardless of their histories and/or cultural backgrounds (contexts).

ethics: A branch of philosophic inquiry concerned with understanding and examining the moral life. It seeks rational clarification and justification of basic assumptions and beliefs that people hold about what constitutes right or wrong/ good or bad conduct. Can also be defined as a system of action guiding rules and principles that function by specifying that certain types of conduct are required, prohibited or permitted. The term 'ethics/ethical' may be used interchangeably with the term 'morality/moral'.

etiquette: A set of behavioural action guides concerned with the maintenance of style and decorum in social settings; often, although mistakenly, confused with ethics/morality.

evidence: Something that gives a sign or proof of the existence or truth of something, or that helps us to come to a particular conclusion.

feminisms: This term captures the variety of theoretical approaches to the support of equal rights for women, in all spheres of life, along with a commitment to improve the position of women in society; includes liberal feminism, socialist feminism, radical feminism, postmodern feminism and so on.

gender: A social construction that expresses the many areas of social life, as distinguished from biological sex; the socially learned behaviours and expectations that are associated with the two sexes.

generic: A characteristic that is 'general, not specific or special' (Australian Concise Oxford Dictionary 1987).

grounded theory: A research process designed to lead to generation of theory through study of a particular human situation or context.

grounds: The degree to which a set of reasons supports a conclusion.

health policies: 'The strategies and courses of action adopted as being advantageous and expedient to provide within the resources available from a health system that at least maintains, and preferably improves, health' (Hennessy & Spurgeon 2000:6).

health promotion: 'Health promotion is a broad field of activity ranging from actions that are essentially medically focused and individual (such as individual risk-factor assessment and counselling) to actions aimed at helping people to change their behaviour, and further along to actions that seek to create supportive environments and settings that address a broad range of social and environmental determinants of health' (Marshall 2004:185).

hermeneutics: A process of interpretive analysis, which is concerned with uncovering meaning and a technique for interrogating text. Van Manen states that 'hermeneutics is the theory and practice of interpretation. The word derives from the Greek god Hermes whose task it was to communicate messages from Zeus and other gods to the ordinary mortals' (van Manen 1990:179). Hermeneutics was originally a technique used to interpret religious text, which has made a transition into research activity in the social sciences and humanities. Hermeneutical refers to a process or perspective involving hermeneutics.

holism: A perspective in which people are seen as made up of biological, psychological, social and spiritual components, which are indivisible.

hypotheses: Tentative statements of relationships between two or more variables, which have little empirical support. The repeated confirmation of hypotheses changes their status to empirical generalisations (statements with moderate empirical support) and thence to law (statements with overwhelming empirical support).

iconography: 'Illustration of subject by drawings or figures; book whose essence is pictures; treatise on pictures or statuary; study of portraits especially of an individual' (Australian Concise Oxford Dictionary 1987).

inductive reasoning: The process of inference of a general law or principle from the observation of particular occurrences.

journalling: The technique of recording thoughts and feelings after reflecting on an event.

magnet hospitals: Hospitals that have particular quantifiable features, each of which is based on recognition of the contribution of nurses to patient care and the overall environment. These features include: 'effective and supportive leadership; nursing staff decision making; commitment to professional clinical nurse qualities; participatory management; autonomy and accountability, and a supportive environment' (Buchan 1999).

managed care: A health management system that controls the resources and delivery of services to people who are enrolled in a specific type of healthcare plan.

masculinist: Pertaining to the masculine; the male gender characteristics derived from social construction and expectation.

meta: A prefix commonly encountered in theoretical literature. In this context it means 'beyond or higher order' (Australian Concise Oxford Dictionary 1987). A meta-paradigm of any discipline is a statement or group of statements identifying the relevant phenomena to the discipline (Fawcett 1984).

model: A schematic representation of some aspect of reality, which may be empirical or theoretical. Empirical models are replicas of observed realities (e.g. a plastic model of the ear). Theoretical models represent the world in language or mathematical symbols (e.g. nursing's 'grand theories').

moral/morality: See ethics above.

moral duty: An act that a person is bound to carry out for moral reasons.

moral obligation: As above, an act that a person is obligated to perform for moral reasons; is generally regarded as being weaker than a moral duty and may be overridden by stronger moral duties.

moral principles: General standards of conduct that make up an ethical system of action guides and which carry particular imperatives (e.g. 'Do no harm').

moral right: A special interest that a person has and which ought to be protected for moral reasons (e.g. the right to life) (contrast with legal right; e.g. a special interest that a person has and which ought to be protected for legal reasons); moral rights generally entail correlative rights.

moral rules: Derived from principles and prescribed particular standards of conduct (e.g. 'Always tell the truth'). Rules have less scope than principles; they also do not have the same force and can be overridden by principles.

naturalism: A form of essentialism in which a fixed nature is assumed for women, not readily amenable to change.

nursing ethics: The consideration of various ethical and bioethical issues from the standpoint of nursing theory and practice.

Occam's razor: The principle that the simplest explanation is most likely to be the right one.

paradigm: A paradigm is a term used to describe accepted practices and techniques through which a discipline accumulates and refines its knowledge base.

patriarchy: The social system in which the masculine dominates, oppresses and exploits the feminine, within the spheres of reproduction, sexuality, work, culture and the state.

phenomenology: A philosophy and descriptive research method designed to uncover the essence and meaning of lived experiences—for example, suffering or grieving (Parse 2001). In a phenomenological research study, the focus is on the meaning of the phenomenon under investigation for the research participants who participate in the study.

philanthropic: 'Loving one's fellow men, benevolent, humane' (Australian Concise Oxford Dictionary 1987).

philosophy (alternative view): 'A way of reflecting not so much on what is true and false but on our relationship to the truth' (Foucault, cited in Lotringer 1989).

philosophy/philosophic inquiry (conventional view): An argumentative intellectual discipline concerned with the discovery of 'truth' and meaning. Unlike science, which seeks answers to questions that can only be answered by empirical evidence, philosophy seeks answers to questions that cannot be answered by empirical evidence.

postmodernism: Relates to the critique of modern, capitalist, industrialised society; new political and social strategies, which embrace pluralism and diversity of cultures and values.

poststructuralism: Refers to a range of theoretical positions in which the mode of knowledge production uses particular theories of language, subjectivity, social processes and institutions to understand existing power relations and to identify areas and strategies for change.

praxis: Praxis can be seen as the link between reflection and action. Freire (1972) defines praxis as 'reflection and action upon the world in order to transform it' (Cox et al 1991:385).

premise: A reason offered in support of a conclusion.

pre-reflection: Preparatory reflection that occurs before the experience.

preventive ethics: The study and practice of ethics (including ethics education) aimed at preventing (as opposed to remedying) moral problems.

professional development: Refers to skills and knowledge attained for both personal development and career advancement.

public health: 'The science and art of promoting health, preventing disease, and prolonging life through the organised efforts of society' (World Health Organization 1998:3).

qualitative research: Research that focuses on human experiences, including accounts of subjective realities, and conducted in naturalistic settings, involving close, often sustained contact between the researcher and research participants (Denzin & Lincoln 2005, Sarantakos 2005).

quantitative research: Refers to research that seeks to measure some concept of phenomenon of interest (e.g. blood pressure, pain or student attitudes to learning about research). It is also called positivist, reductionist or empirical. Quantitative research is termed deductive, which means the thinking leads from a known principle to an unknown, and is used to test a particular research hypothesis.

racism: A 'form of oppression/privilege which exists in a dialectical relationship with antiracism ... societal system in which people are divided into races with power unevenly distributed, or produced based on their racial classification' (Paradies 2006:68).

rationalism: A philosophical position that argues that the only way to truth is through the deliberations of the rational human mind.

realism: An applied appreciation and acceptance of the authentic nature of the world, rather than an idealised view of it.

reflection (also reflection-on-action): Reflection that occurs after the experience.

reflective practice: The incorporation of reflection into practice.

regulatory authorities: Those organisations responsible for the registration of nurses (e.g. the Queensland Nursing Council or the Nurses and Midwives Board of New South Wales).

relevance: A test applied to a premise or reason. If a premise or reason is relevant, it helps to support the conclusion of the argument.

shared governance: A concept based on the principles of partnership, equity, accountability and ownership (Porter-O'Grady 1991). It requires health professionals to be self-directive, effective decision makers, strongly involved in the activities of the organisation at every level of participation, and providing clinical leadership (Porter-O'Grady 1991).

social capital: 'Social capital represents the degree of social cohesion which exists in communities. It refers to the processes between people which establish networks, norms, and social trust, and facilitate co-ordination and co-operation for mutual benefit' (World Health Organization 1998:19).

social class: A broad concept encapsulating objective material, position and subjective understandings, and incorporating differing access to power (Walter & Saggers 2007:88).

social support: 'That assistance available to individuals and groups from within communities which can provide a buffer against adverse life events and living conditions, and can provide a positive resource for enhancing the quality of life' (World Health Organization 1998:20).

sound: An argument is sound when the premises are acceptable and provide adequate grounds for accepting the conclusion.

stereotype: A predetermined idea that ascribes particular characteristics to all members of a social group.

theory: A logically consistent set of propositions, which presents a systematic view of some aspect of reality.

universalism: Refers to the attributions of functions, social categories and activities to which women of all cultures are assigned; asserts what is shared in common by all women.

validity: An argument is valid when the premises that are offered provide adequate grounds for acceptance of the conclusion.

REFERENCES

Buchan J 1999 Still attractive after all these years? Magnet hospitals in a changing health care environment. Journal of Advanced Nursing 30(1):100–108

Chinn P, Jacobs M K 1983 Theory and nursing: a systematic approach. Mosby, St Louis

Cox H, Hickson P, Taylor B 1991 Exploring reflection: knowing and constructing practice. In: Gray G, Pratt R (eds) Towards a discipline of nursing. Churchill Livingstone, Melbourne, pp 373–389

Denzin N K, Lincoln Y S 2005 (eds) Handbook of qualitative research, 3rd edn. Sage, Thousand Oaks, California

Fawcett J 1984 The meta-paradigm of nursing: present status and future refinements. Image: Journal of Nursing Scholarship 16(3):84–86

Freire P 1972 The pedagogy of oppression. Penguin, Harmondsworth

Hennessy D, Spurgeon P 2000 Health policy and nursing. Macmillan Press, London

Lotringer S 1989 Foucault live (interviews, 1966–84). Semiotext(e), New York

Marshall B 2004 Health promotion in action: case studies from Australia. In: Keleher H, Murphy B (eds) Understanding health: a determinants approach. Oxford University Press, Melbourne

National Health and Medical Research Council (NHMRC) 2005 Cultural competency in health: a guide for policy, partnership and participation. NHMRC, Canberra

Paradies Y 2006 A systematic review of empirical research on self reported racism. International Journal of Epidemiology 35(4):888–901

Parse R R 2001 Qualitative inquiry: the path of sciencing. Jones and Bartlett, Boston

Porter-O'Grady T 1991 Shared governance for nursing. Association of Operating Room Nurses Journal Feb–Mar, 53(3):691–703

Ramsden I 2002 Cultural safety and nursing education in Aotearoa and Te Waipounamu, Thesis, Victoria University, Wellington

Sarantakos S 2005 Social research, 3rd edn. Palgrave Macmillan, London

van Manen M 1990 Researching lived experience. State University of New York Press, New York

Walter M, Saggers S 2007 Poverty and social class. In: Carson B, Dunbar T, Chenhall R, Baillie R (eds) Social determinants of Indigenous health. Allen & Unwin, Sydney

World Health Organization (WHO) 1998 Health promotion glossary. Online. Available: www.wpro.who.int.hpr/docs/glossary.pdf

INDEX